THE
DRUG
BOOK

Books by Michael C. Gerald

The Complete Idiot's Guide to Prescription Drugs
The Nurse's Guide to Drug Therapy
Nursing Pharmacology and Therapeutics
Pharmacology: An Introduction to Drugs
The Poisonous Pen of Agatha Christie

THE DRUG BOOK

FROM ARSENIC TO XANAX
250 MILESTONES IN THE HISTORY OF DRUGS

Michael C. Gerald

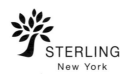

STERLING
New York

STERLING
New York

An Imprint of Sterling Publishing
387 Park Avenue South
New York, NY 10016

ISBN 978-1-4027-8264-0

Library of Congress Cataloging-in-Publication Data
Gerald, Michael C.
  The drug book : from arsenic to Xanax, 250 milestones in the history of drugs / Michael C. Gerald.
     p. ; cm.
  From arsenic to Xanax, 250 milestones in the history of drugs
  ISBN 978-1-4027-8264-0
  I. Title. II. Title: From arsenic to Xanax, 250 milestones in the history of drugs.
  [DNLM: 1. Pharmaceutical Preparations–history. 2. Drug Therapy–history. 3. Pharmacology–history. QV 11.1]

615.109–dc23
                              2012050737

Distributed in Canada by Sterling Publishing
c/o Canadian Manda Group, 165 Dufferin Street
Toronto, Ontario, Canada M6K 3H6
Distributed in the United Kingdom by GMC Distribution Services
Castle Place, 166 High Street, Lewes, East Sussex, England BN7 1XU
Distributed in Australia by Capricorn Link (Australia) Pty. Ltd.
P.O. Box 704, Windsor, NSW 2756, Australia

For information about custom editions, special sales, and premium and corporate purchases, please contact Sterling Special Sales at 800-805-5489 or specialsales@sterlingpublishing.com.

Manufactured in China

2 4 6 8 10 9 7 5 3 1

www.sterlingpublishing.com

This book is dedicated to my granddaughters Aila Tovia Jones and Io Esther Gerald, who will be the beneficiaries of future advances in drug development.

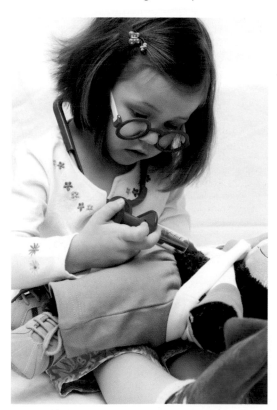

Contents

Introduction

Linking Past and Present

> *Because the newer methods of treatment are good, it does not follow that the old ones were bad; for if our honorable and worshipful ancestors had not recovered from their ailments, you and I would not be here today.*
>
> —Confucius (551–478 BCE)

The search for drugs that free humankind from suffering is a pursuit that crosses time and time zones. Humans have long relied upon natural substances to attain relief from ailments afflicting the mind and body. While most of these herbs satisfied an immediate need to fill an empty stomach, a select few altered physical or mental states. Depending upon the substance ingested and its quantity, the effects ranged from lifesaving to disastrous. Early local healers separated those herbs that were harmful or ineffective from those that provided benefits, and the latter emerged as the medicines of that era. A few survived the test of time, enhancing well-being even today.

Are herbal drugs only of historical interest? Not by a long shot. According to the World Health Organization, in some Asian and African countries about 80 percent of their population rely on traditional medicines to deal with their primary healthcare needs, with herbs the most popular component of these practices. And the use of herbal medicines is not restricted to developing countries. Herbal medicines are major ingredients in dietary supplements, which for many of us serve to complement, or even replace, modern medicines.

As you might guess, new drugs are now arising from dissimilar sources and by a different kind of researcher. No longer is the discovery of new medicines left to happenstance or accident, as was the case when our ancient ancestors fortuitously found an herb that corrected their digestive system problems or that soothed their irritated skin. Until the nineteenth century, most Western drugs were concoctions of herbs. During the early 1800s, major advances in extraction procedures led to the isolation of pure chemical constituents from herbs. These constituents include: morphine, responsible for the pain-relieving effects of opium; quinine, which accounts for the antimalarial properties of cinchona; and colchicine, underlying the anti-gout effects of meadow saffron. As we will see in this book, many contemporary drugs are chemicals or chemical modifications of herbs that bear considerable, little, or no resemblance to those in nature. In the late nineteenth century and well into the twentieth, scientists turned to animals for hormones used as medicines, and later to microbes as a valuable source of vaccines and antibiotics.

Drug discovery over the past century has capitalized on an increasing knowledge of the molecular biology and physiology of the healthy and disease-ridden body. This has led to the rational design and an outpouring of new chemical drugs that have successfully treated diseases that had previously evaded the best efforts of science. Now, during the most recent decade, and to an ever-increasing extent, there has been an explosion in the number of biologic drugs that specifically target disease mechanisms at the molecular level where they originate. These highly complex protein molecules are naturally produced in the body in minute quantities and, thanks to advances in molecular biology, can now be mass-produced. (Although readily available, biologic drugs are not necessarily readily affordable.)

As drugs have evolved, so have the laboratories in which they have been discovered. Medications are now rarely developed by lone scientists working in isolation in cold and damp basement laboratories, as did Marie and Pierre Curie when isolating radium from pitchblende. Their research was conducted at meager financial cost but at considerable cost to their health, and they did not even patent their discovery. Today, new discoveries are the creations of multidisciplinary teams of scientists and physicians bringing to bear their individual and collective expertise in state-of-the-art research facilities in universities or multinational companies, at costs of many hundreds of millions of dollars, with the anticipation of billion-dollar returns on the investment. Times have certainly changed!

What Do We Consider a Drug?

She had never forgotten that, if you drink too much from a bottle marked "poison," it is almost certain to disagree with you, sooner or later.

— Lewis Carroll (1832–1898)

You might surmise that I am using terms *drug* and *medicine* synonymously. Not so. I will consider *drug* to also encompass poisons, drugs of abuse, recreational substances, and those chemicals that are intended to improve the quality of our lives.

As you peruse *The Drug Book*, you will find scores of medicines that have prevented, managed, and even cured diseases that were once untreatable, incurable, and invariably fatal. We will look at the following: anti-HIV medicines that have reduced the AIDS death rate by 80 percent and, in three decades, have transformed this dreaded disease into a chronic disorder; oral contraceptives that have liberated women both sexually and economically, permitting them to decide if and when to have children; general anesthetics that have extended the range of the surgeon's scalpel from performing rapid, crude amputations to highly complex operations on vital organs; and drugs that have contributed to the significant reduction in the risk of heart attacks and strokes, the leading causes of death in the Western world.

Bearing in mind the five-century-old dictum by Paracelsus that "the dosage makes it either a poison or a remedy," we will also consider conventional poisons alongside medicines that function as poisons when used in excessive doses. For centuries, arsenic—the preferred poison of the infamous Renaissance Borgia family and their acolytes—was considered the "king of poisons and the prisoner of kings." Unwitting ingestion of tetrodotoxin in the innards of a puffer fish was a near epicurean disaster for Captain James Cook in 1774, and this potent nerve agent almost ended the world-saving career of 007, as recounted in Ian Fleming's *From Russia with Love*. In recent years, polypharmacy and abuse of prescription narcotics have been a frequent source of morbidity. Both the "King of Rock and Roll" and the "King of Pop" tragically died as a result of drugs injudiciously prescribed by their physicians.

Nonmedical purposes of some drugs have dwarfed their originally approved medical uses. Human growth hormone and anabolic steroids bring to mind bodybuilders or athletes seeking to improve their performance. These medicines were originally intended to treat growth disorders in children and increase muscle mass in such wasting diseases as cancer. Heroin was envisioned as an abuse-free substitute for morphine, but it is now a societal scourge.

Early medical interest in LSD was focused on its possible use in psychotherapy and for the treatment of alcoholism. However, over the decades, artists and intellectuals have used LSD in an attempt to enhance their creativity; it has also been used by scientists to probe the neurobiological basis for mental disease, and by the military and CIA to interrogate prisoners and other persons of interest. Alarmed by the recreational use of LSD, the government slashed funding for LSD research, and its medical potential remains nebulous to this day.

Must every drug cure or treat a life-threatening condition? I will visit a few drugs that simply make us feel better or improve the quality of our lives. Drugs such as Viagra augment sexual function in men, even when they are performing at a highly acceptable level. Other drugs have cosmetic effects, enhancing our appearance by reducing wrinkles or girth or by increasing the thickness or population of hair on our heads.

The Drug Book

My goal in writing *The Drug Book* is to inform and entertain general readers who are interested in drugs, the biomedical sciences, or scientific history, in addition to providing new and novel information on a wide range of drugs to scientists, doctors, and scholars. All of the essential background information and drug vocabulary is provided jargon-free, without subjecting the reader to highly technical explanations. In short, I will present a scientific perspective that is both accessible and engaging—and, in some cases, highly controversial.

Of the many thousands of drugs that have appeared over the ages, why have these 250 been chosen? While I may have omitted some drugs that you consider noteworthy, most of my selections have significantly improved our health and extended our lives. Many were groundbreaking in their day and used for decades or even hundreds of years until being replaced by "new and improved" generations of drugs. While the original medicines may have long fallen by the wayside or bedside, many of them have provided a foundation from which modifications, improvements, and spin-offs led to the creation of drugs considered essential today. (In passing, let me remind you that not all new drugs are necessarily safer or more effective than the older ones.) Moreover, the inclusion of some entries provides me the opportunity to share fascinating stories related to their development or developers. Just as the journey may prove more alluring than the destination, sometimes the backstory is more interesting than the drug.

Some of these drug discoveries, we shall see, were the products of brilliant conceptualization and deductive reasoning that could rival Sherlock Holmes in acuity. The German Nobel laureate Paul Ehrlich attributed his success in research to "four big G's": *Geduld* (patience), *Geschick* (ability), *Geld* (money), and *Glück* (luck), to which we might add a fifth G: *Geist* (intellect). Such drug discoveries were often methodically planned and executed in painstaking detail. However, other pathways can lead to success. Alexander Fleming attributed his discovery of penicillin—perhaps the most important of all drugs—to another factor: "[I]f I may offer advice to the young laboratory worker, it would be this—never to neglect an extraordinary appearance or happening."

Great discoveries are often made by great scientists, who often share the stage with their drugs: William Withering and foxglove (digitalis) for heart disease; Paul Ehrlich and

Salvarsan for syphilis; Frederick Banting/Charles Best and insulin for diabetes; Selman Waksman and streptomycin for tuberculosis. Other drugs have multiple lesser-known discoverers, such as ether, a general anesthetic that revolutionized the practice of surgery.

However, not all drug entries are stories of heroes, victories, cures, and accolades, and not all scientists are incarnates of German medical missionary and Nobel Peace Prize–winner Albert Schweitzer. Like the Greek gods, scientists suffer from human frailties, not the least of which is a strong, sometimes overwhelming, desire for recognition. For all the benefits it has bestowed on society, the pharmaceutical industry is composed of profit-making enterprises with stockholders to satisfy. In the interest of maintaining sales, some drug companies have delayed or even failed to disclose to the public and drug regulatory agencies the serious adverse effects their pharmaceuticals have caused. And you can draw your own conclusion as to whether the high cost of some newer medicines—in the order of many tens of thousands of dollars—is fair recompense for extending the life (but not necessarily the quality of life) of terminal cancer patients by a few months.

While arranged chronologically, each entry can be read in any order you choose. To permit you to easily trace the threads extending from one drug to another, cross-references are included in **boldface** in the entries, and a Notes and Further Reading section provides additional information and sources for curious readers. In keeping with tradition, the first letters of drug trade names are capitalized, while generic names are denoted in lower case. The dates assigned to the entries understandably vary in precision, and experts are not always of a single mind regarding a drug's date of discovery. Then, what constitutes "discovery"? In some instances, the year that scientists produced the drug in the laboratory may be of secondary importance when compared with the year the medicine appeared on the market and was available to thankful patients or the year that the concept was generally embraced by the biomedical world or the year that the drug first appeared in a manuscript or when it captured the public's attention and gained front-page prominence.

Now, more than ever before, drugs permeate our lives. Some drugs have literally saved countless souls. Far from rescuing us from the jaws of death, other drugs have greatly improved our health and happiness. Still others have destroyed lives. In magnificent color and historical breadth, *The Drug Book* will provide the inside scoop on an array of mind- and body-altering substances that have had the most notable impacts on the course of human history, shining a light on the scientists, doctors, and healers who have brought them to us.

Acknowledgments

The support of the editorial staff at Sterling Publishing is greatly appreciated—in particular Melanie Madden, my editor for this book. My warmest thanks to my son, Marc, for introducing me to Sterling and providing encouragement and support throughout the course of this project.

Greatest thanks of all and love to my wife, Gloria, who has been my unnamed collaborator on all phases of this project, primarily serving as my first and most critical reviewer of all drug entries and creatively identifying the most suitable images to accompany these entries.

Herbs

Galen (129–c. 199)

Humans and animals have always needed food in order to survive. Their challenge was locating and differentiating those herbs that could serve as sources of nutrition from those that were hazardous to their health. Our ancestors likely observed and emulated the choices made by their animal neighbors. The lucky ones learned, through trial and error, that when lesser amounts of some hazardous plants were taken, they produced changes in bodily function, mood, or behavior. Perhaps, the herb relieved an illness or injury they were experiencing.

Initially, this "drug-related" information was shared orally and, later, more permanently, on papyri, clay tablets, parchments, and paper. Among the herbs known to be used as medicines in prehistoric times is black cohosh, employed by Native Americans to treat gynecological and kidney disorders, depression, sore throats, and rheumatism. White willow bark has long been cultivated in Europe and China for pain relief, and yarrow—used throughout history as an astringent to reduce bleeding and as a diaphoretic to promote sweating—was excavated at Shanidar IV, a Neanderthal flower burial in northern Iraq dated to around 60,000 BCE. Birch polypore, an edible mushroom used as a laxative, was carried by Ötzi the Iceman, a 5,000-year-old mummy found in western Austria. Various human societies in antiquity have consumed mallow to cleanse the colon.

Experience revealed that not all parts of the plant were equivalent in producing their health-promoting effects. The most powerful responses might occur after eating the leaves, roots, bark, fruits, seeds, or juices. After fragmenting that plant part and mixing it with a liquid, such as **alcohol**, a more concentrated mixture of active constituents could be extracted in either the liquid solvent or the solid residue. Such liquid and solid plant extracts—collectively referred to as galenicals, after the Greek physician Galen—continued to be used as medicines into the twentieth century. In fact, many contemporary dietary supplements consist of herbal mixtures.

SEE ALSO Opium (c. 2500 BCE), Colchicine (c. 70), Smith and Ebers Papyri (c. 1550 BCE), Morphine (1806), Alkaloids (1806), Dietary Supplements (1994).

While searching for food, our gatherer ancestors uncovered herbs that did not satisfy nutritional needs but rather, to their surprise, ameliorated some of their common health problems.

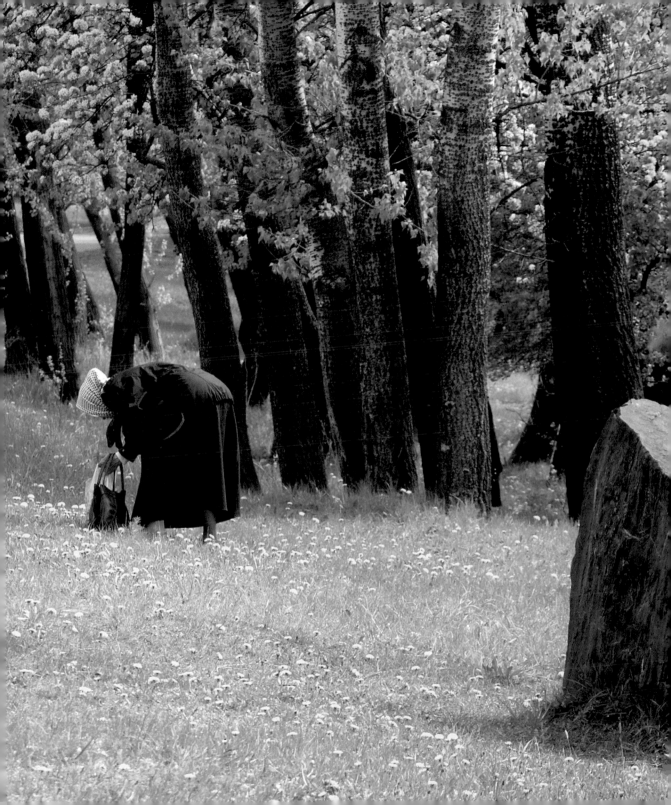

Alcohol

Alcohol is the oldest and most widely used drug in the world. Whereas its accidental discovery was undoubtedly made tens of thousands of years ago, proof of the intentional manufacture of beer dates back some 12,000 years. Numerous references to wine appear in the Bible, including Noah's planting of some of the earliest vineyards on Mt. Ararat in eastern Turkey.

Crushed grapes, other wild fruits, and honey contain glucose (sugar). When glucose is exposed to water and yeast (a fungus present on plants), the process of fermentation begins. When the alcohol content reaches 15 percent, the yeast dies and fermentation stops. To produce beverages with much higher alcohol content, distillation is required. Distillation was developed during the eighth and ninth centuries by medieval Arabic alchemists and utilized by Europeans in the twelfth century for the manufacture of high-alcohol beverages. Using the indigenous raw plant materials available to them, our forebears prepared brandy, whisky, rum, gin, and vodka, which have alcoholic contents ranging from 40 to 55 percent.

Societal uses of alcohol are many and varied. Its past uses included serving as a painkiller (analgesic) before operations, as an antiseptic on the skin, as an aid to digestion, and as a "pick-me-up" tonic or stimulant after fainting episodes. Although its importance in medicine faded decades ago, alcohol is still used in religious ceremonies and as a source of nutrition and calories. Contrary to popular belief—and despite the animated behavior of imbibers in social settings—alcohol acts as a depressant on the nervous system.

Examples of the intemperate use of alcohol can be found in the Bible and in ancient Greek and Roman writings and, in this respect, remind us that we are closely linked to the past. As the Italian general Giuseppe Garibaldi noted, "Bacchus has drowned more men than Neptune." Worldwide, alcoholism is a major public health problem: Alcohol is the most commonly abused substance and is the third leading cause of preventable death in the United States.

SEE ALSO Alchemy (c. 5000 BCE), Absinthe (1797), Ether (1846), Phenol (1867).

The Gospel Temperance Railroad Map *(1880) takes riders to very different terminals. Starting from Decisionville on the left, one can take either the Great Celestial Railroad, which leads to the Celestial City, or the Great Destruction Railroad, whose terminus is the City of Destruction.*

GOSPEL TEMPERANCE RAILROAD MAP

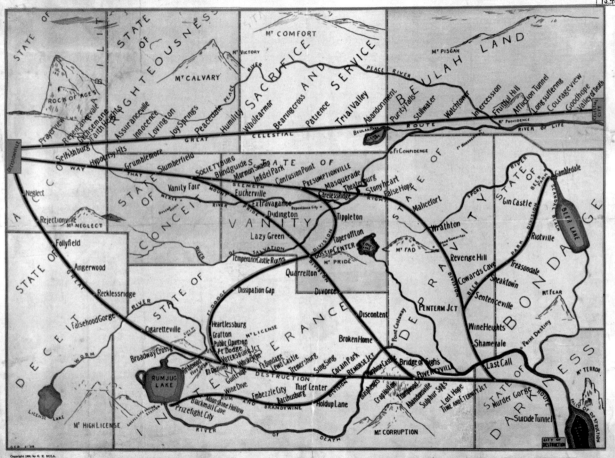

Copyright 1908, by G. E. BULA

166D

Alchemy

Jābir ibn Hayyān (721–815), **Nicholas Flamel** (1330–1418), **Paracelsus** (1493–1541)

CREATING GOLD AND IMMORTALITY. Alchemists have been with us for thousands of years, continuing into the nineteenth century, and its practitioners have included such scientific giants as Francis Bacon, Paracelsus, and Isaac Newton. They combined primitive science with a magical-mystical-religious view of the world, focusing on the discovery of a "philosopher's stone" to transmute base metals into gold or into drugs that permit attainment of immortality or extension of life.

The origins of alchemy may extend back some 7,000 years to a time when ancient Egyptian artisans worked with alloys of gold and silver to fabricate jewelry. With Alexander's conquest (322 BCE) of Egypt, the art moved from Alexandria to ancient Greece, where the objective was conversion of imperfect base metals such as lead into silver and gold, the most perfect of all metals. By contrast, the alchemical focus in the Eastern world was medical. Some 2,500 years ago in China, an elixir of life was sought, enabling the user to enjoy perpetual existence. In India, the aim was more modest: a product that could cure all diseases.

In the seventh century, the epicenter of science moved to Arabic countries, where their greatest alchemist was the Persian Jābir ibn Hayyān (Latinized as *Geber*), who is credited with transforming alchemy into chemistry. His written works on alchemy, which merged the quests for the philosopher's stone and the elixir of life, were translated into Latin and became standard references for later European alchemists. The German-Swiss physician-alchemist Paracelsus pursued the elixir of life further: "Many have said of Alchemy, that it is for the making of gold and silver. For me such is not the aim, but to consider only what virtue and power may lie in medicines." Paracelsus was a major influence in exhorting alchemists to replace herbal mixtures with chemical medicines of known identity.

In J. K. Rowling's *Harry Potter and the Philosopher's Stone* (1997), Harry seeks information about Nicholas Flamel, a French alchemist who claimed to have discovered both the philosopher's stone and an elixir of life for his and his wife's use.

SEE ALSO Alcohol (c. 10,000 BCE), Antiaging Drugs (2020).

The Alchemist's Laboratory is an engraving featured in a book by Heinrich Khunrath in 1595. Signs inscribed with Latin aphorisms surround the laboratory and serve as a source of inspiration for the alchemist.

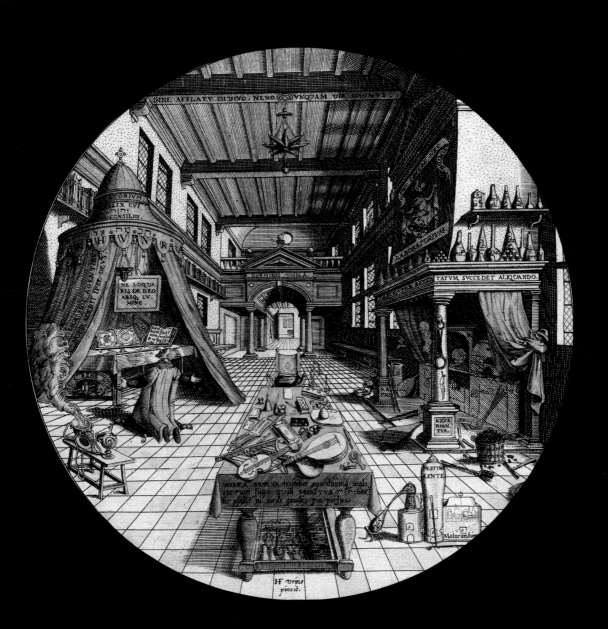

Cannabis

Cannabis sativa, the hemp plant, is indigenous to central and western Asia, where its use can be traced back thousands of years. In earlier times, as today, the benefits and hazards of cannabis have been the focus of controversy. It has been alternately described as a "delight giver" and a "liberator of sin."

The magnitude of the effects of cannabis (also called marijuana) is attributed to the different concentrations of delta-9-tetrahydrocannabinol (THC) in its plant parts and whether it is smoked and inhaled or taken orally. The physiological effects are generally modest and include an increase in pulse rate and a reddening of the conjunctiva of the eye. Low "social" doses of marijuana cause early stimulation, followed by sedation. During the initial period, the user experiences a "high" and enhanced perception of the senses. During the longer-lasting sedative period, the user passes in and out of a dreamlike state and has a shortened attention span, along with an impairment of short-term memory.

The literature describing the dangers associated with the long-term use of cannabis on lung function, reproduction, the immune system, mental health, motivation, and progression to "harder" drugs (the gateway theory) is contradictory and often infused with personal bias. One fact is clear: Not even very high doses cause a fatal outcome. High doses can, however, cause a panic reaction with disorganized thinking, fear of loss of control, and hallucinations.

The World Health Organization estimates that 147 million people, or 2.5 percent of the world's population, now consume cannabis annually. Nevertheless, the cultivation, distribution, or possession of cannabis is illegal in most countries, with some exceptions for medical uses. The enforcement of these laws and the penalties imposed for violations can vary considerably, even within a given country. Penalties for possession of small amounts range from modest fines to long jail sentences. Possession of larger amounts, likely for purposes of trafficking, can result in death penalties in a number of Southeast Asian countries, most notably Singapore. It is highly likely that reasonable people will be debating the wisdom of decriminalizing cannabis for the foreseeable future.

SEE ALSO Medical Marijuana (1839).

Cannabis is a weed that grows freely in most parts of the world. In addition to its recreational applications, stalks of this plant have been used for thousands of years to produce hemp for highly durable clothing and industrial-strength rope.

قنَّاوِي

قنب بستانى

Tea

Lao Tzu (600–517 BCE)

Many myths surround the discovery of tea as a beverage. In the earliest myth (c. 2737 BCE), several leaves of *Camellia sinensis* fell into Shen Nung's pot of boiling water. This mythical emperor of China was impressed by the taste and stimulating properties of his newly discovered beverage, which his attributed writings claim were beneficial for the treatment of tumors, bladder problems, abscesses, and lethargy. The founder of Taoism, Lao Tzu, viewed tea an essential ingredient in the elixir of life. The Chinese custom of offering tea to guests was predicated on the belief that it improved health and extended life.

Over the centuries, the pleasures of tea drinking spread throughout the East and reached Europe in 1610, when green tea leaves were brought to Amsterdam. The seventeenth century saw the taste for tea spread throughout Europe, including England in 1660, where it became the national drink by 1750.

There are three primary varieties of tea—green, black, and oolong—which differ based on how the leaves are processed. Tea leaves contain some 700 chemicals, the most important of which are polyphenols, caffeine, and theophylline. Greatest attention has been focused the polyphenols—in particular, catechins, which are antioxidants. Antioxidants can reduce free radicals that may play a role in heart disease and cancer. Green tea has the highest concentrations of catechins.

The results of studies on the health benefits of green tea are not clear, consistent, or convincing. The risk of colorectal cancer and cancers of the breast, stomach, and prostate are reduced in many tea studies but not in all. Green tea may prevent stroke, but it is far more inconsistent in its ability to reduce cholesterol levels and blood pressure or decrease the risk of diabetes or Alzheimer's disease.

Why the contradictory results? Many studies testing green tea were conducted in the East, where lifestyles and diets differ significantly from the West. In addition, an excessive number of cups of tea must be consumed to obtain the reported results.

SEE ALSO Alchemy (c. 5000 BCE), Coffee (c. 800), Caffeine (1819), Theophylline (1888).

There are some 3,000 varieties of tea worldwide, in six general categories: white, green, oolong, black, pu-erh, and flavored. The taste of tea depends on where it is grown and how it is harvested, dried, and processed.

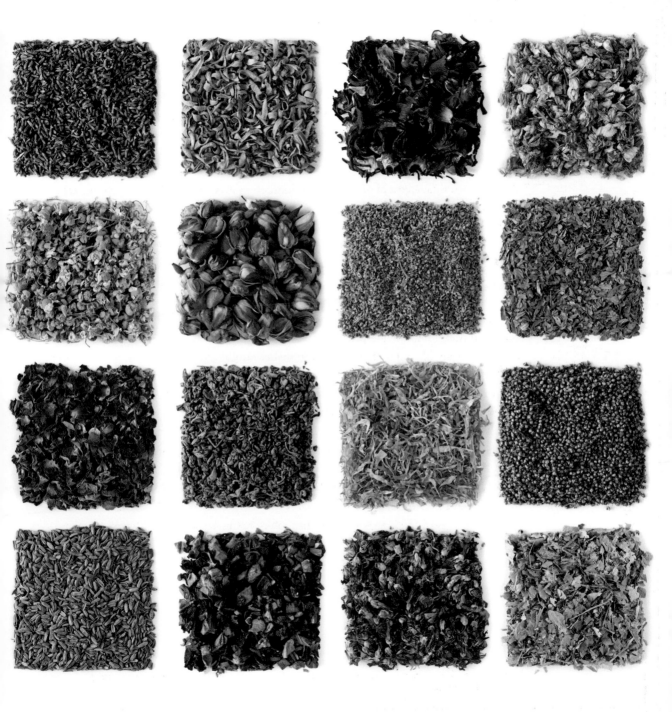

Opium

"Thou hast the keys of Paradise, oh just, subtle, and mighty opium!"
—Thomas de Quincey, *Confessions of an English Opium Eater* (1821)

Opium has held a preeminent role in the treatment of disease since the earliest days of recorded history. The medical writings of the ancient Assyrians, Greeks, and Romans extolled its wondrous properties for the relief of pain and inducement of sleep. Islamic traders introduced opium to China in the ninth century, and it was used for the next 800 years for the treatment of diarrhea resulting from dysentery. Even until the turn of the twentieth century, it was one of the few truly effective and reliable drugs available. Harvard Medical School professor and writer Oliver Wendell Holmes (1809–1894) noted that, with the exception of opium and anesthesia, "I firmly believe that if the whole **materia medica** [medical drugs], as now used, could be sunk to the bottom of the sea, it would be all the better for mankind—and all the worse for the fishes."

Opium is obtained from the poppy, *Papaver somniferum*, a plant historically cultivated in southeastern Asia, Iran, Turkey, and now primarily (more than 90 percent) in Afghanistan. Atop the plant's main stalk are five to eight egg-shaped capsules. Ten days after the poppy blooms, incisions are made into the capsule permitting a milky fluid to ooze out. This gummy mass is scraped off the capsule and pressed into cakes of raw opium, from which some twenty **alkaloids** are obtained. The two most important of these are **morphine** and **codeine**, which are responsible for opium's effects. **Heroin** is readily synthesized from morphine.

Long before heroin was abused, English traders began shipping opium into China from India. In an attempt to curb the widespread opium-smoking habits of its nationals, the Manchu government seized the opium cargo of a British ship. Two Opium Wars (1839–1842, 1856–1860) ensued, with disastrous defeats of the Chinese that led to, among other onerous concessions, legalization of opium importation, loss of the island of Hong Kong to Great Britain from 1842 to 1997, and the opening of China to Western trade and influences.

SEE ALSO Laudanum (1676), Morphine (1806), Alkaloids (1806), Codeine (1832), Heroin (1898), Opioids (1973).

These seemingly harmless balloon-like opium poppies have had a profound effect on society for good and evil. Opium was among the earliest medicines that physicians relied on. It is the source of morphine and a starting material for heroin synthesis, sparking the Opium Wars and China's subsequent interaction with the West. More recently, opium has functioned as a cash crop, supporting the wars in Afghanistan.

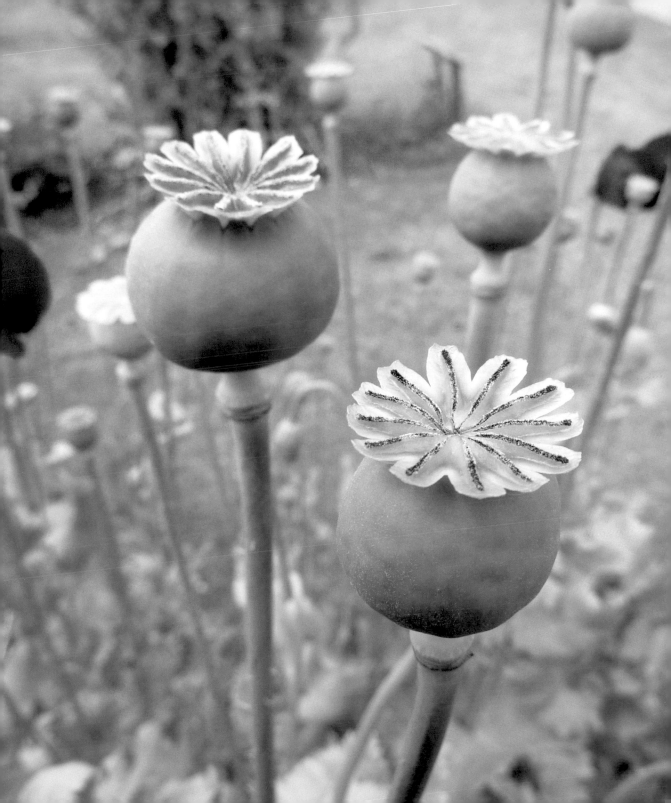

Smith and Ebers Papyri

Edwin Smith (1822–1906), **Georg Ebers** (1837–1889)

JEWELS OF THE NILE. Edwin Smith, an American collector of antiquities residing in Egypt during the second half of the nineteenth century, was responsible for bringing to the modern world the two most important ancient Egyptian medical manuscripts: the Ebers Papyrus and the eponymous Edwin Smith Papyrus.

The practice of medicine was highly advanced in ancient Egypt, thanks to physician, engineer, and architect Imhotep (2650–2600 BCE). A small fragment of Imhotep's writings survives in the 17-page, 377-line Edwin Smith Papyrus (c. 1600 BCE), a manuscript rich in anatomical figures and treatments of battlefield injuries. A far more comprehensive and significant medical record is contained in the Ebers Papyrus (c. 1550 BCE). This 110-page medical jewel consists of 877 section entries (rubrics) and some 700 prescriptions and remedies, as well as magic spells to combat demons and descriptions of such medical problems as diabetes, intestinal disorders, depression, asthma, arthritis, and crocodile bites. Among the many medicinal plants described are myrrh, frankincense, cardamom, dill, fennel, and thyme.

Smith purchased both papyri in Egypt in 1862. The Edwin Smith Papyrus remained in his hands until his death in 1906 and is now housed at the New York Academy of Medicine. The Ebers Papyrus was supposedly found wrapped in mummy cloth, in an excellent state of preservation between a mummy's legs in the Theban necropolis. Smith sold the manuscript in 1869, and in 1872 it was purchased by Georg Ebers, a German Professor of Egyptology at the University of Leipzig, where the manuscript now resides. Written in hieratic script, a cursive hieroglyphics, the manuscript was translated into German in 1890 and into English in the 1900s.

Ebers was a man of letters. In addition to his scholarly works, he authored several Egyptian guidebooks and historical romantic novels (e.g., *The Bride of the Nile: A Romance*, 1887), the most successful of which popularized Egyptian customs.

SEE ALSO Colchicine (c. 70).

The world's oldest surviving surgical document describes in extensive detail the examination, diagnosis, treatment, and prognosis of forty-eight medical conditions. Among the entries is the curing of infection with moldy bread, pre-dating Fleming's discovery of penicillin by some 3,500 years.

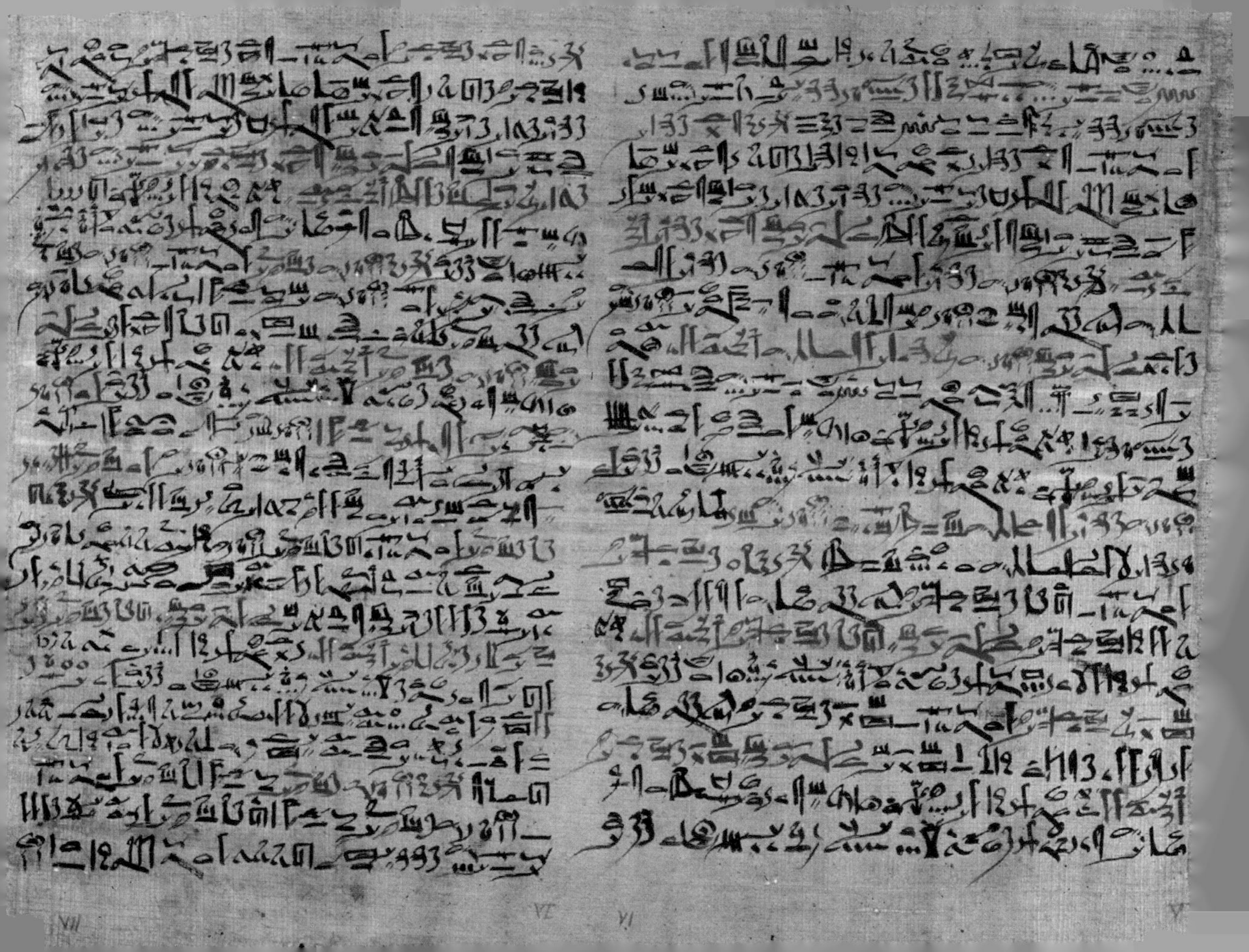

Rauwolfia

Garcia de Orta (1501–1568), **Leonhard Rauwolf** (1535–1596), **Ram Nath Chopra** (1882–2002), **Rustom Jal Vakil** (1911–1974)

The Indian snakeroot plant, *Rauwolfia serpentina*, has an ancient history in traditional Ayurvedic medicine. Hindu texts dating from approximately 500 BCE indicated rauwolfia (termed *Sarpaghanda* in Sanskrit) for the treatment of a host of disparate medical conditions, including epilepsy, insomnia, mental disorders, hypertension (high blood pressure), dysentery, and worm infestation. It is also used as an antidote for snake and insect bites, to reduce fever, and to stimulate contractions of the uterus. Mahatma Gandhi was said to have used it to achieve a state of calm contemplation. Some of these conditions benefited from rauwolfia treatment; others did not; and a few (epilepsy, diarrhea) actually worsened.

Garcia de Orta, a Portuguese physician who moved to India in 1534 to escape the Inquisition, first introduced rauwolfia to Western physicians. He was the earliest European to describe, in a 1563 book, tropical diseases (most notably cholera), as well as Indian spices and herbal remedies. Rauwolfia (also spelled "rauvolfia") was named in honor of Leonhard Rauwolf, a physician and botanist who, after a three-year trip to the Near East and Asia, returned to his native Germany with samples and extensive descriptions of plants used for medicinal purposes.

The earliest scholarly reports of powdered rauwolfia root for mental illness and hypertension appeared in Indian journals during the 1930s but attracted little outside attention. Thereafter, rauwolfia was intensively researched by two of India's most distinguished medical scientists—Ram Nath Chopra and Rustom Jal Vakil, the fathers of Indian pharmacology and clinical pharmacology, respectively.

Chopra was the first to study, over many years, the effects of the crude extract in animals. He described its calming effects on blood pressure, but not until a 1949 paper by Rustom Jal Vakil in the *British Heart Journal* described its antihypertensive effects did Western medicine take note. Rauwolfia's active component, **reserpine**, was isolated in 1952. Reserpine was also found to possess antischizophrenic properties, but the far more effective **chlorpromazine,** made available at the same time, upstaged it.

SEE ALSO Chlorpromazine (1952), Reserpine (1952).

Lord Dhanvantari, a Hindu avatar (deity incarnation) of healthcare and the founder of Ayurveda, developed medical treatments utilizing herbs, including snakeroot (rauwolfia). He is typically depicted with four hands, holding medicinal herbs in one hand and a pot containing the nectar of immortality in another.

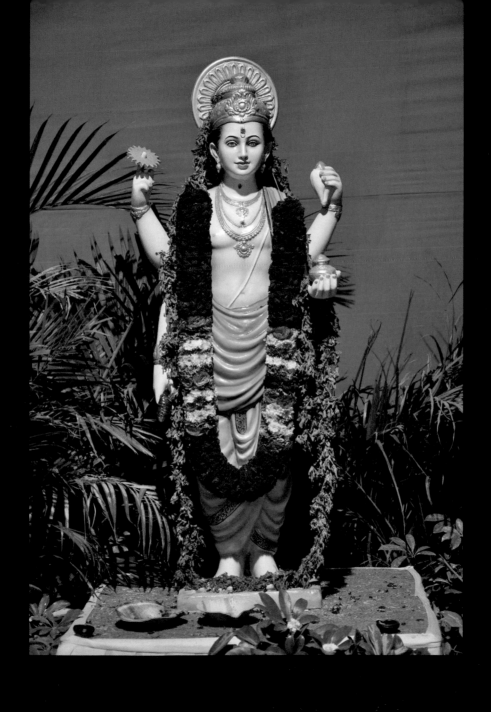

Hemlock

Plato (c. 428–c. 348 BCE), **Socrates** (469–399 BCE), **Derek Humphrey** (b. 1930)

The ancients knew hemlock as a drug, but its everlasting fame rests on its use as a state poison that ended the life of a key founder of Western philosophy. The plant, also called conium and poison hemlock, is native to Europe and grows alongside roads and ditches. It was used medically into the nineteenth century as a sedative and to relieve spasms in whooping cough and asthma. In higher doses, the active **alkaloid**, coniine, is a nerve poison.

FINAL DRINK FOR THE WISEST MAN. In 399 BCE, charged and convicted of impiety against the Greek gods and for corrupting the youth of Athens, Socrates was given a choice: exile or death by drinking from a cup containing hemlock. He selected the latter. In the *Phaedo* dialogue, his student Plato describes the progressive and marked paralysis and coldness of Socrates' body from the feet upward (death results from paralysis of the muscles of respiration). The peaceful ending described by Plato suggests that herbs, such as opium poppy juice, may have been added to produce a painless and more rapid death. The final scene is visually depicted in Jacques-Louis David's 1787 painting *The Death of Socrates*.

When old men ceased to be of service to the state in ancient Greece and were burdened by daily existence, they assembled at a banquet of death and voluntarily ended their lives by drinking hemlock. In 1980, Derek Humphrey founded the Hemlock Society USA in California with the dual aim of providing information to terminally ill persons and of promoting the legalization of physician-assisted suicide. After a number of name changes and mergers, the organization is now called Compassion & Choices and claims to have 40,000 supporters. On a far lighter note, the heavy metal band Hemlock has been in existence since 1993.

SEE ALSO Alkaloids (1806).

Hemlock, long forgotten as a medicine, has been immortalized as the poison given to Socrates. In David's painting, The Death of Socrates, *Plato, a disciple, is red-robed and sitting to the right of his master.*

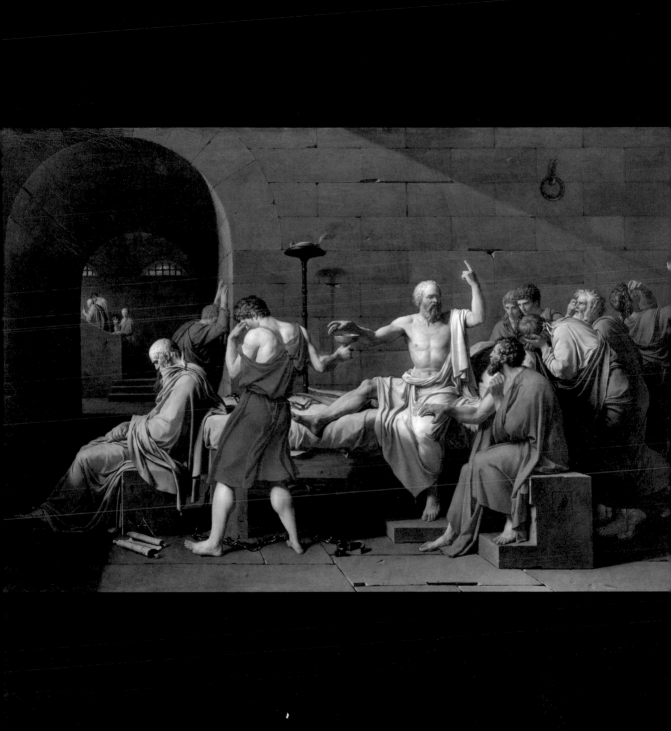

Mandrake

Titus Flavius Josephus (37–c. 100)

A BIBLICAL LOVE DRUG. References to mandrake, a plant indigenous to the Middle East as well as central and southern Europe, appear in the Bible, the writings of Shakespeare, and the tales of witchcraft and magic. The roots of mandrake (*Mandragora officinarum*) are spindle-shaped and often branched in a way that suggests a human figure, which led the ancients to believe that it possessed fertility-promoting and libidinous properties.

In the book of Genesis, the infertile Rachel offers her fecund sister Leah their mutual husband Jacob's sexual favors in exchange for Leah's mandrake. Years later, without the benefit of mandrake, Rachel becomes pregnant for the first time, giving birth to Joseph. In the biblical "Song of Songs," reference is made to its love-promoting fragrance.

In addition to its aphrodisiac properties, mandrake was said to be a charm against evil spirits and a universal cure. However, legend has it that, when wrenched from the earth, the plant would shriek and cause all who heard it to go mad and die. The first-century Jewish-Roman historian Josephus warned of its hazards and described a method for collecting the plant using a dog—at the expense of the dog's life.

Ancient Roman physicians were said to have administered a wine prepared from the root to dull pain and to induce a deep and prolonged sleep before operations. In a similar vein, this "morion" or "death-wine" was given to persons subjected to ancient Roman torture or painful deaths, such as crucifixion. Using mandrake's alternate name, *mandragora* Shakespeare refers to its effects in *Antony and Cleopatra*: "Give me to drink mandragora / That I might sleep out this great gap of time. / My Antony is away."

Over the centuries, mandrake was used to treat a variety of ailments but, because of its toxicity, was relegated to mere historical interest before the twentieth century. Some of the biological effects of this **belladonna**-related plant are attributed to a variety of active **alkaloids**, including **atropine** and **scopolamine**.

SEE ALSO Belladonna (1542), Alkaloids (1806), Atropine (1831), Scopolamine (1881), Viagra (1998), Female Viagra (2015).

Mandrake, from the manuscript Tacuinum sanitatis in medicina *(1390), a handbook on health and well-being written in Latin.*

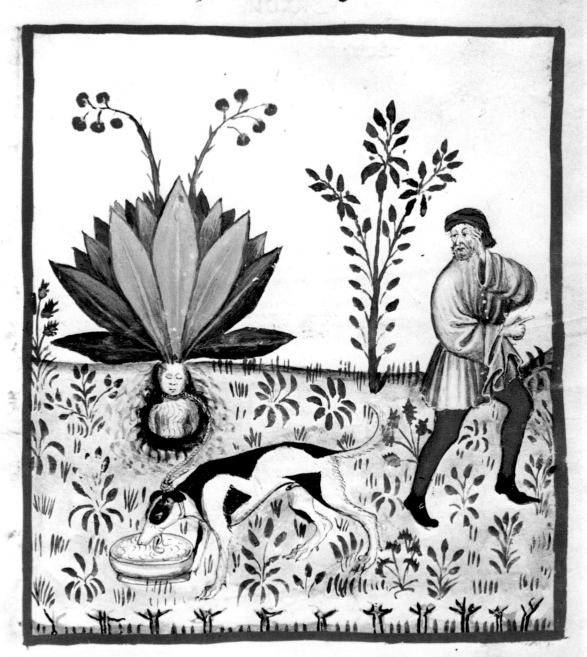

fructus mandragore. ợfio. fri. iij. sic. i ꝫ. Electo magni odonferr. uinam. odorado ꝫ tra foli.
calam. ꞇ uigilias. emplando elefantie ꞇ ifectoib; nigris cutis. nocini. ebetat sensus Re
noti. cu fructu edere. Quid qⁱt ꝴ ẽ comestibile ọuenit ca……ib; estate ꞇ miꝺianis.

Theriac of Mithridates

King Mithridates VI (132–63 BCE)

THE UNIVERSAL ANTIDOTE. To protect himself against all poisons and reptilian venoms—and he had reason to be concerned—King Mithridates concocted a single all-purpose universal antidote that he drank daily in increasing doses. This mithridatium or mithridate, variously described as consisting of some 36 to 65 ingredients, survived into the twentieth century (albeit with modifications), becoming the oldest prescription in history.

King Mithridates VI was ruler of the Kingdom of Pontus (northeastern Turkey) from 120 until 63 BCE. During the early decades of his rule, Mithridates significantly and ruthlessly expanded the size of his state into Asia Minor and Greece at the expense of the Roman Empire. During one such campaign in 88 BCE, his armies killed 80,000 Roman citizens and up to 150,000 of their allies. After his defeat at the hands of Pompey the Great in 63 BCE, Mithridates attempted to poison himself, his wife, and children. As the story goes, his antidote protected him alone from the effects of the poison but not against the sword, his backup choice of suicide.

We have not abandoned the notion of a universal antidote. For many years, families were instructed to keep a mixture of activated charcoal, magnesium oxide, and tannic acid at the ready in their first aid kits in the event of accidental poisoning. It is now known that both this recent antidote and Mithridates' theriac are ineffective, and the search for an effective universal antidote continues.

The English poet A. E. Houseman makes reference to the Theriac of Mithridates in his collection *A Shropshire Lad* (1896): "They put arsenic in his meat / And stared aghast to watch him eat; / They poured **strychnine** in his cup / And shook to see him drink it up."

SEE ALSO Ipecac (1682).

Theriac was an ancient multi-ingredient preparation intended as a cure against the bites of venomous serpents and wild animals—and later under Mithridates VI's direction, an all-purpose poison antidote. By the Middle Ages, theriac was considered a panacea. A sample of the preparation is contained in this eighteenth-century French pharmacist's urn.

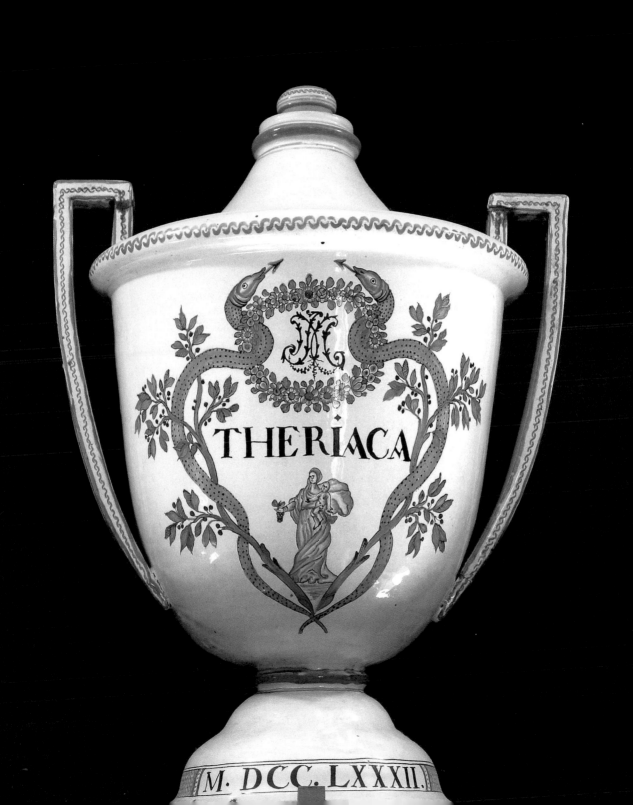

THERIACA

M. DCC. LXXXII.

Materia Medica

Pedanius Dioscorides (c. 40–90), Samuel Hahnemann (1755–1843)

For almost two millennia and through the nineteenth century, if you sought information about drugs, you consulted a **materia medica** source. What might be included in such a reference? Simply stated, "medical materials" encompassed everything relating to drugs, including the study of plants, with their identification and chemistry; the preparation of drugs from plant sources and (later) chemicals; a description of how drugs produce their beneficial and adverse effects in the body; and the use of drugs for the treatment of disease.

In the first century, the famous Greek physician Dioscorides compiled the first such work, which he entitled *De Materia Medica*. This classic collection—used continuously for about 1,500 years—consisted of descriptions of some 500 plants, contained in five volumes. Based on scientific experimentation and clinical experience over the centuries, subsequent works supplemented the descriptions with more objective information on the plants' effects in humans.

The use of materia medica remains alive and well among devotes of **homeopathic medicine**. The origins of homeopathic medicine date back to the 1780s, when Samuel Hahnemann translated a conventional materia medica text into his native German. Finding it lacking, he devised one of the fundamental principles of homeopathy: "like cures like." Contemporary homeopathic books, following Hahnemann's example, are a compilation of remedies and "provings" of their effectiveness. They are typically arranged alphabetically by their Latin names and accompanied by dosage information and symptoms they are intended to treat.

As knowledge accumulated, it became unreasonable to assume that "everything relating to drugs" could be contained in one materia medica source, and during the early twentieth century, each of its components became a specialized course of study. Increasing emphasis was placed on how drugs worked (pharmacology), their medicinal or natural product chemistry, and the rational basis for their use to treat medical disorders (therapeutics), while botanical descriptions (pharmacognosy) were scaled back.

SEE ALSO Herbs (c. 60,000 BCE), Homeopathic Medicine (1796), Dietary Supplements (1994).

For the thousand years between the fall of the Roman Empire and the Renaissance, scholars in the Arab world preserved the scientific knowledge of the ancient Greeks, which was later translated into Latin. This 1224 leaf depicting a mad dog biting a man is an Arabic translation of the De Materia Medica *by Dioscorides.*

وَيَعْرُقُونَ وَمِنْهُمْ مَنْ يَهْرُبُ مِنَ النُّورِ وَمِنْهُمْ مَنْ يَسْتَلِذُّهُ
وَمِنْهُمْ مَنْ يَنْبَحُ مِثْلَ الْكِلَابِ وَبَعْضٌ مَنْ اوْتُرِبَ مِنْهُ قَصَبُهُ
تِلْكَ أَيْضًا وَقَدْ ذَكَرْنَا أَنَّهُمْ رَأَوْا إِنْسَانًا وَإِنْسَانَيْنِ عَضًّا فَإِنْ فَعَلْنَا

صُورَةُ طَبِيبٍ حَلَبَ
وَيَرْعَضُ إِنْسَانًا.

وَإِنْ أَوْرَدَ مُوسَى إِلَى بِهَذِهِ الْآفَةِ وَمَسُّونَ وَإِنْ أَحَدَهُمَا عَضَّ وَإِنْ تُلِيَ
بِهَذِهِ الْبَلِيَّةِ وَخَلَصَ عَ عَ عَ عَ عَ عَ عَ
وَأَمَّا الْأَخَرُ وَكَانَ الْسَّامِعُ صَدِيقُهُ لَخَافَ الْمَاءَ فَلَا دَوَاءَ إِنْ

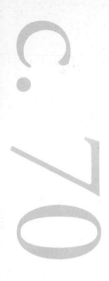

Colchicine

Pedanius Dioscorides (c. 40–90), **Benjamin Franklin** (1706–1790), **Pierre-Joseph Pelletier** (1788–1842), **Joseph Bienaimé Caventou** (1795–1877)

Descriptions of gout date back almost 5,000 years to ancient Egypt and are included in the **Smith and Ebers Papyri**. The most prominent symptoms of gout—a type of arthritis—are swelling, redness, and intense joint pain that most commonly affects the big toe and that may persist for days to weeks. In this condition, crystals of uric acid—the normal end-product of purine metabolism—deposit in the joints.

In his classic work *De Materia Medica* (*Regarding Medical Matters*), written in approximately the year 70, Dioscorides describes the use of *Colchicum* (meadow saffron) seeds to treat gout. Extracts of the seeds were used well into the nineteenth century. Colchicine, an **alkaloid** and the active constituent in *Colchicum*, was extracted and isolated from the seeds in 1820 by the French chemists Pierre-Joseph Pelletier and Joseph Bienaimé Caventou.

Colchicine is very selective and effective in its ability to relieve the pain and swelling seen with acute attacks of gout but not with other types of arthritis. It is also used to prevent attacks in individuals afflicted with frequent and recurrent episodes of gout. Colchicine use has declined and has been replaced by less toxic drugs, such as **Benemid**, which increases the elimination of uric acid in the urine, and **Zyloprim**, which reduces uric acid synthesis in the body.

COMBATING THE "DISEASE OF KINGS." Gout has long been considered a "disease of kings," or at least of the very wealthy, because of their overindulgence in rich foods and alcohol. (It has now been downgraded to a middle-class disease.) Among the many famous gout sufferers were King Henry VIII, Thomas Jefferson, Martin Luther, Charles Darwin, and Benjamin Franklin. Franklin used *Colchicum* extract while serving as the Ambassador to France (1776–1785) and introduced the drug to his fellow Americans. He also offered the following sage advice: "Be temperate in wine, in eating, girls, and cloth, or the Gout will seize you and plague you both."

SEE ALSO Smith and Ebers Papyri (c. 1550 BCE), Alkaloids (1806), Benemid (1951), Zyloprim (1966).

Benjamin Franklin brought colchicine extract to his fellow gout sufferers in America. This 1799 print, titled The Gout, *is by James Gillray.*

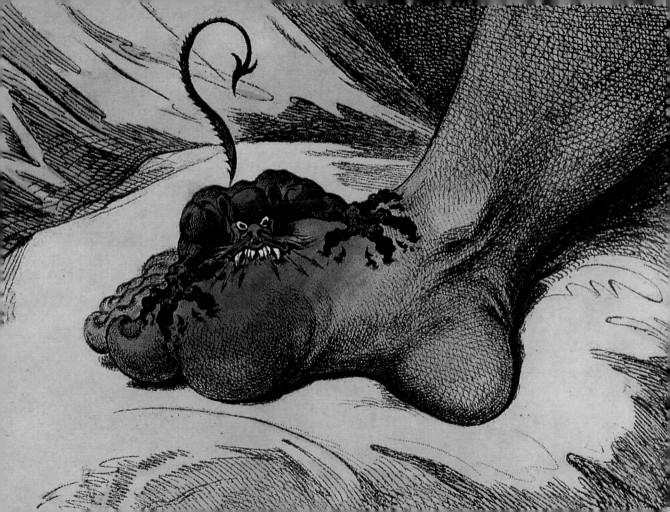

Coffee

Coffee is said by some to be the second most consumed beverage in the world—behind water. Every day, 52 percent of Americans older than eighteen (~100 million people) drink a cup of coffee, and another 30 percent consume coffee occasionally. Among coffee drinkers, one source reports that an average of 3.2 cups, each containing 9 oz. of coffee, are consumed daily.

What we know about the discovery of coffee is based upon legend. In one popular rendition, a ninth-century Arabian goatherd named Kaldi observed his goats merrily running instead of sleeping after feeding on coffee plant berries. By the fifteenth century, berries were brewed to prepare coffee. A century later, coffee was exported from the Ottoman Empire, and thousands of coffeehouses sprang up throughout Europe in the 1600s.

Early medical authorities were polarized in their assessment of coffee's benefits and hazards. Supporters claimed that it relieved kidney stones, gout, and migraine headaches, alleviated hangovers, promoted digestion, strengthened the heart and lungs, and was effective against the bubonic plague. Detractors emphasized that it caused loss of sexual desire, impotence, and weight loss leading to emaciation.

We have had almost 400 years of extensive experience sorting out and evaluating the health vs. hazard claims for coffee. What do we now believe? Coffee decreases the risk of type 2 diabetes, Parkinson's disease, breast and liver cancer, and cirrhosis of the liver. It increases mental alertness, improves reaction time, and elevates the mood. On the other hand, coffee increases the risk of osteoporosis and first trimester miscarriages. Moderate consumption is unrelated to the risk of heart disease, colon and rectal cancer, and overall mortality.

What caveats should you consider when evaluating these and other findings? Coffee contains caffeine and hundreds of other chemicals that might contribute to its effects (many of which are dose dependent), and not all coffees contain the same ingredients and proportions. Of critical importance to consider: How many cups of coffee were consumed daily? Were the findings obtained in human or animal subjects? If history is a guide, these findings will likely change with time.

SEE ALSO Tea (c. 2737 BCE), Caffeine (1819).

Coffee beans, which rank among the world's most widely traded commodities, are grown on small trees cultivated in more than seventy countries, primarily in Latin America, Southeast Asia, and South Asia. The red or purple fruits generally contain two seeds referred to as coffee beans.

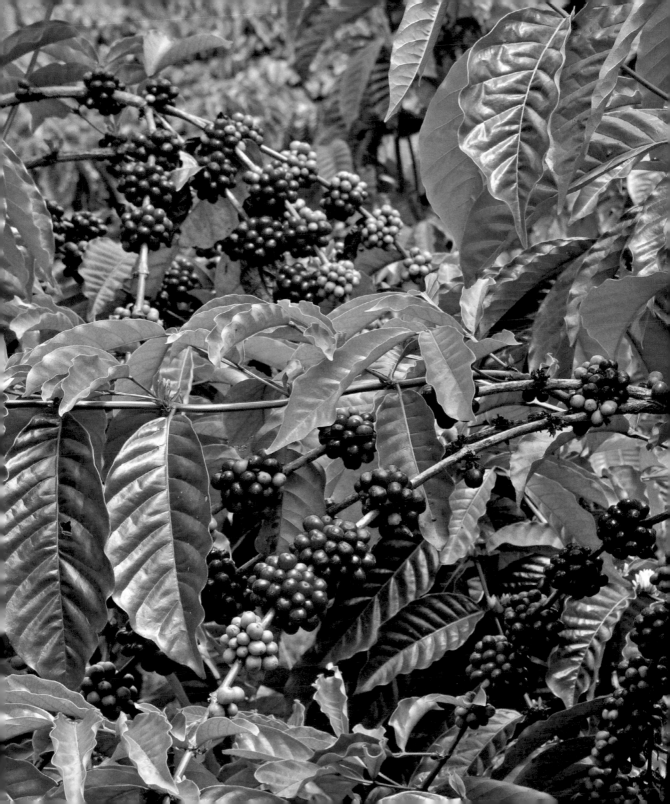

Arsenic

Agrippina the Younger (15–59), **Rodrigo Borgia** (1431–1503), **Cesare Borgia** (1476–1507), **Lucrezia Borgia** (1480–1519), **James Marsh** (1794–1846)

When arsenic comes to mind, few think of its medical uses, which date back to ancient Greece and China more than two millennia ago. More recently, potassium arsenite—now a reputable anticancer treatment—was sold as an early cure-all medication in 1786. Of far greater significance, arsphenamine (**Salvarsan**), an organic arsenic-containing drug, was the first authentic cure for syphilis, which plagued humankind beginning in the sixteenth century.

THE KING OF POISONS. Arsenic's role as a medicine, however, is dwarfed by its esteemed reputation as a poison between the times of ancient Rome and the nineteenth century. It was first isolated as an element in 1250. The poison of choice for nefarious professionals, arsenic trioxide (white arsenic) is colorless, nearly tasteless, and readily dissolvable in water and other drinking liquids. Thus, victims are oblivious to their impending doom. While the signs and symptoms of strychnine and cyanide poisoning are obvious, family members, physicians, and authorities might unwittingly attribute arsenic-induced vomiting, diarrhea, and muscle cramps to any number of ailments.

Among the most infamous and highly successful early poisoners was Agrippina the Younger. Sister of Caligula, she used arsenic to dispose of her husband, freeing her to marry the Roman emperor Claudius, her uncle. Many poisonings later, her sixteen-year-old son Nero became emperor. "La Cantarella" arsenic trioxide powder was a family trademark perfected by the Borgias of Renaissance Italy—particularly Rodrigo (Pope Alexander VI) and his children, Cesare and Lucrezia. La Cantarella was said to induce a deep, death-simulating sleep lasting for four hours, during which time the user had no detectable pulse. Juliet may have taken this potion while awaiting Romeo. Two centuries later, Tofana of Sicily's arsenic solution *Aqua Tofana* was reportedly responsible for the deaths of 500–600 persons.

The epoch of the "inheritance powder" declined significantly in 1836, when the British chemist James Marsh developed an irrefutable and highly sensitive chemical test for the presence of this poison in tissues.

SEE ALSO Atoxyl (1905), Salvarsan (1910).

The Borgias were patrons of the Renaissance arts and influential in Church and political affairs during the 1400s and 1500s. To advance their quest for power, they resorted to a variety of crimes, including murder, with arsenic as their favorite tool. A Glass of Wine with Caesar Borgia was painted by John Maler Collier in 1893.

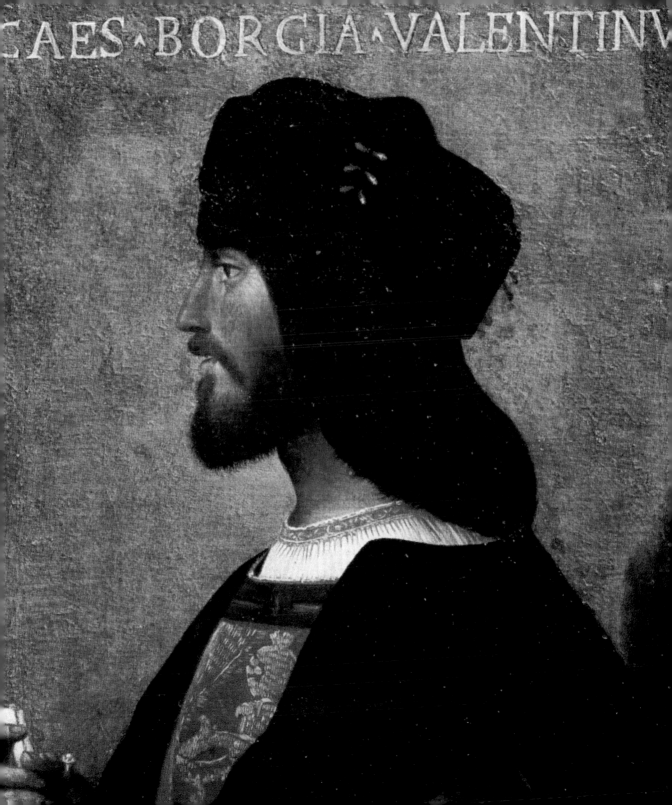
CAES · BORGIA · VALENTINV·

Witches' Flying Ointments

Johannes Hartlieb (1410–1468), **Alfred J. Clark** (1885–1941)

Accounts of the Sabbat or Black Mass, dating from the fifteenth to eighteenth centuries, related stories of nighttime meetings attended by witches, demons, and Satan, in which wild dancing and sexual orgies occurred. Why did the accused women confess that they were consorting with the devil when the penalty for witchcraft was death, either by hanging or burning at the stake? Torture, perfected by the Inquisitors, undoubtedly loosened many guiltless tongues. The use of "flying ointments," first described in 1456 by the Bavarian physician Johannes Hartlieb, may have also played a role in their heartfelt confessions.

Witches were said to fly to the Sabbat on brooms, cats, or other animals. They acquired this "power of flight" by applying a sooty green ointment containing plant extracts, which may have produced physiological changes that simulated the sensation of flight. A number of questions have been raised about the nature of these ointments, including their supposed ingredients and where they were applied.

If, as was generally accepted, they slathered their bodies with the ointment, the active chemicals would have had to cross the formidable barrier of the skin to enter the bloodstream. However, if the ointment were applied to the vaginal area, perhaps with a broomstick as some writers suggest, absorption would have been more certain and perhaps account for the sexual fantasies accompanying the Sabbat.

Flying ointments were many in number and varied in composition. Several such ointments were analyzed by the distinguished University College, London, pharmacologist A. J. Clark, who concluded that, among the multiple ingredients, **aconite** and **belladonna** were most worthy of consideration. Clark speculated that the sensation of flying might have arisen from a fluttering, irregular heartbeat caused by the aconite, as well as an excitement progressing to delirium caused by the belladona.

In 1692, nineteen women and men were convicted of witchcraft and executed in Salem, Massachusetts. Executions for witchcraft ended in Europe at the close of the eighteenth century.

SEE ALSO Belladonna (1542), Aconite (1762).

A 1508 woodcut by Hans Baldung depicts Hexen *(witches) preparing for the Sabbat.*

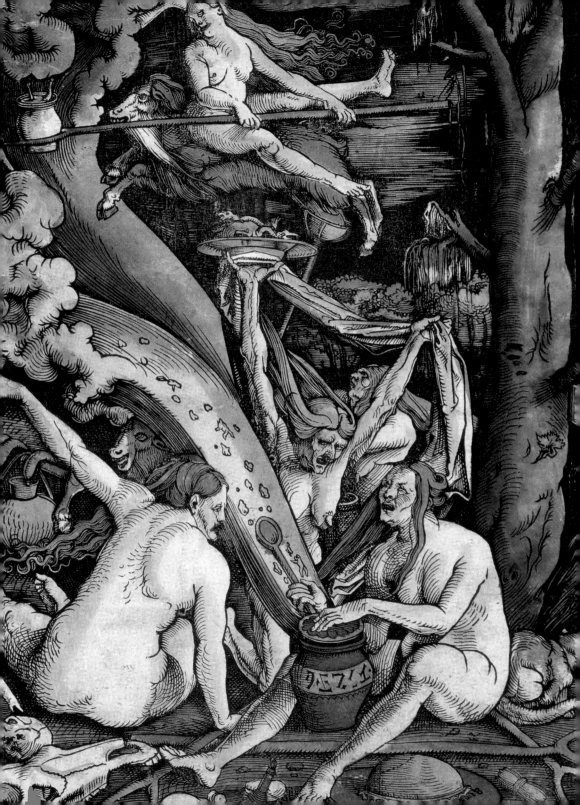

Coca

John Pemberton (1831–1888), Angelo Mariani (1838–1914)

In the late 1520s, when Francisco Pizarro and his conquistadores arrived in what is now Peru, the Incan Empire was the largest sovereignty in the Americas. Architecture was the most notable of the Incan arts, as exemplified by Machu Picchu, located 50 miles (80 km) from Cuzco, the empire's historic capital.

For hundreds of years before the Spanish appeared, the coca leaf was viewed as a divine gift, chewed only by the Incan nobility and select groups in religious ceremonies. After the conquest in 1532, coca was democratized, enabling Andeans laboring in the gold and silver mines to work harder and longer, enduring pain and hunger more successfully.

Coca leaves were brought to Spain toward the end of the sixteenth century, but almost three centuries passed before European interest was aroused. In 1863, the French chemist Angelo Mariani introduced Vin Mariani. This coca-containing tonic in Bordeaux wine, proudly bearing Pope Leo XIII's visage on advertising posters, was marketed for insomnia, nervousness, melancholy, impotence, and influenza.

The overwhelming financial success of Vin Mariani likely did not go unnoticed by John Pemberton, a Georgia druggist. In 1885, he originated Pemberton's French Wine Cola, which was modified the following year to the nonalcoholic Coca-Cola; the coca was retained. *Cola* referred to the inclusion of an extract of the African kola nut that contained 2 percent caffeine. After enactment of the Pure Food and Drug Act in 1906, Coca-Cola was reformulated to substitute "decocainized" coca leaves for the natural leaves.

The coca leaf (*Erythroxylon coca*) grows on small trees native to the lower slopes of the Andes. As in earlier times, the leaves are sold in local markets and widely used by the indigenous people of the central Andean highlands of Bolivia, Colombia, Ecuador, and Peru. Several leaves are chewed at once, producing a favorable numbing and tingling sensation and mild stimulation, while suppressing feelings of hunger and pain.

SEE ALSO Cocaine (1884), Novocain (1905), Pure Food and Drug Act (1906), Xylocaine (1948).

Growing on the lower slopes of the Andes, coca leaves continue to be chewed or imbibed as brewed teas by the indigenous people. Over the years, the leaves have been used not only as a stimulant but also for a variety of medical conditions and as a component of worship services.

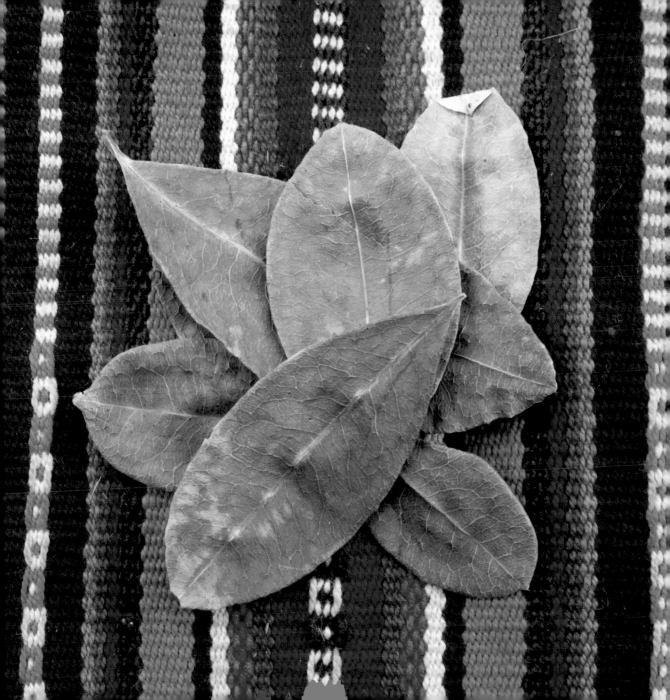

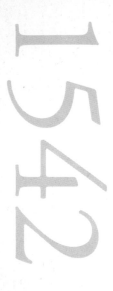

Belladonna

Leonhart Fuchs (1501–1566), **Carl Linnaeus** (1707–1778)

Belladonna, or "beautiful lady," was the objective of sixteenth-century Italian women, who squeezed the juice of the plant's berries into their eyes to achieve alluring widened pupils. Commonly called the deadly nightshade, the Swedish naturalist Linnaeus scientifically classified this plant *Atropa belladonna* in honor of the Greek goddess Atropos, the oldest of the three Fates, who cut the threads of life.

The belladonna plant was well known and respected by the ancient Hindus and Greeks, who employed it for medical purposes, some of which continued into the twentieth century. In addition, it enjoyed favor among ancient Roman and medieval poisoners and was a component of **witches' flying ointments**. In his classic book, *De Historia Stirpium* (1542), Leonhart Fuchs, German physician and a founding father of botany, included a description of belladonna, among hundreds of other medicinal plants.

Belladonna is a member of the *Solanaceae* or "potato" family, a highly varied group of plants that include ornamentals (petunia, matrimony vine), foods (potato, tomato, eggplant, peppers), and drugs such as **mandrake**. The belladonna plant contains generous quantities of the **alkaloids atropine**, **scopolamine** (hyoscine), and hyoscyamine, which serve as the basis for its medical and poisonous properties. The belladonna plant is indigenous to central and southern Europe and is cultivated in England, Germany, and the United States. All parts of the plant are potentially toxic because of the presence of the alkaloids. Its berries are sweet and colorfully attractive to children, often with fatal consequences.

Over the years, pharmaceutical preparations of this plant's leaf and root have been used to treat peptic ulcers and spastic disorders of the intestinal tract, including diarrhea. Isolation of the active alkaloids from their natural sources during the nineteenth century and, in some cases, improvement by chemists led to the availability of more specific drugs. Among the first of the homeopathic remedies in the 1790s, belladonna continues to be recommended for fever reduction and relief of headaches, labor pain, and pain in teething children.

SEE ALSO Mandrake (c. 200 BCE), Witches' Flying Ointments (1456), Homeopathic Medicine (1796), Alkaloids (1806), Atropine (1831), Scopolamine (1881).

These colorful, enticing berries contain high concentrations of the alkaloids atropine and scopolamine, which when ingested by children can cause severe toxicity and death.

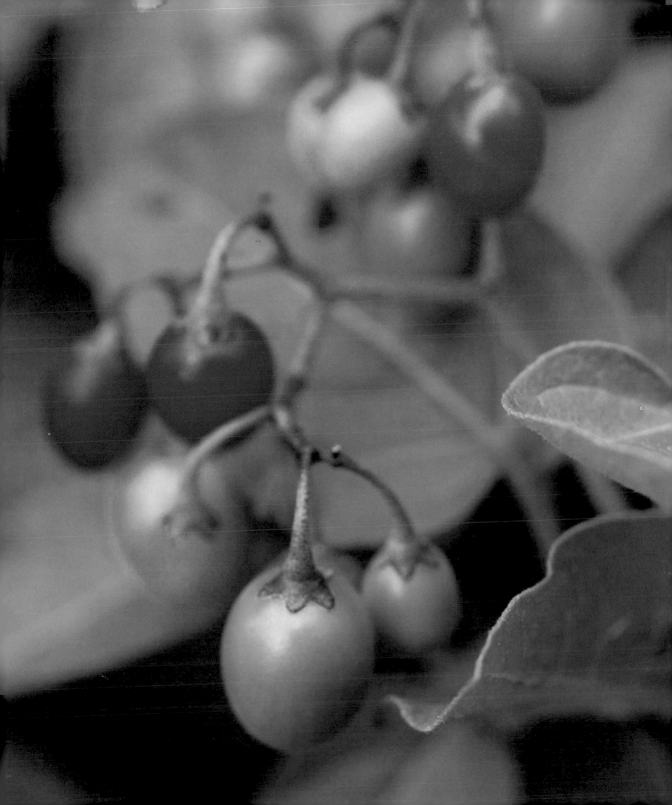

Antimonials

Johann Tholde (1565–1614)

Antimonials (antimony-containing compounds), now better known for their use in flame-proofing and microelectronics, have been employed as medicines since ancient times, emerging and then departing from the spotlight over the centuries. Writing under the pseudonym Basil Valentine, a purported Benedictine monk, the German alchemist Johann Tholde promoted their medical use. In his work *The Triumphal Chariot of Antimony* (c. 1602), he describes the properties of the element and its compounds and extols its virtues for syphilis, fevers, and the bubonic plague. Numerous deaths resulted from the use of antimony remedies, and it fell into disfavor—at least for a time.

Later in the seventeenth century, antimony potassium tartrate appeared and was used for reducing fevers until the late nineteenth century, when safer **aspirin**-like drugs became available. Its still-popular name, tartar emetic, refers to the extreme emesis (vomiting) it causes. Emetics were formerly recommended for the treatment of swallowed poisons; vomiting is now thought to do more harm than good.

The early twentieth century witnessed the introduction into medicine of organic compounds containing such metals as arsenic, gold, mercury, and antimony. Tartar emetic and other organic antimonials, when injected, were found effective against a number of parasitic diseases, including leishmaniasis.

Leishmaniasis is caused by a protozoan parasite transmitted via the bite of a sandfly. The World Health Organization estimates that 12 million people are currently infected, primarily in tropical and subtropical countries, with 1–2 million new cases appearing each year. There are two primary types of leishmaniasis: the common cutaneous form and the severe visceral form (kala-azar), which spreads in the bloodstream and causes swelling of the liver and spleen. If untreated, kala-azar fatality rates approach 100 percent within two years.

The organic antimonial Pentostam (sodium stibogluconate), introduced in the 1940s, is the most effective drug for all forms of leishmaniasis when injected for 20–28 days. Whereas it previously produced cure rates of 85–90 percent, with the development of protozoan resistance, treatment failure rates now approach 60 percent in some parts of India, where the disease is widespread. Antimonials may be once again descending from the summit.

SEE ALSO Aspirin (1899), Atoxyl (1905), Salvarsan (1910), Merbaphen (1920).

A sandfly feasting on a blood meal provided by a victim. In the process, the sandfly spreads the vector-borne protozoan parasite responsible for leishmaniasis.

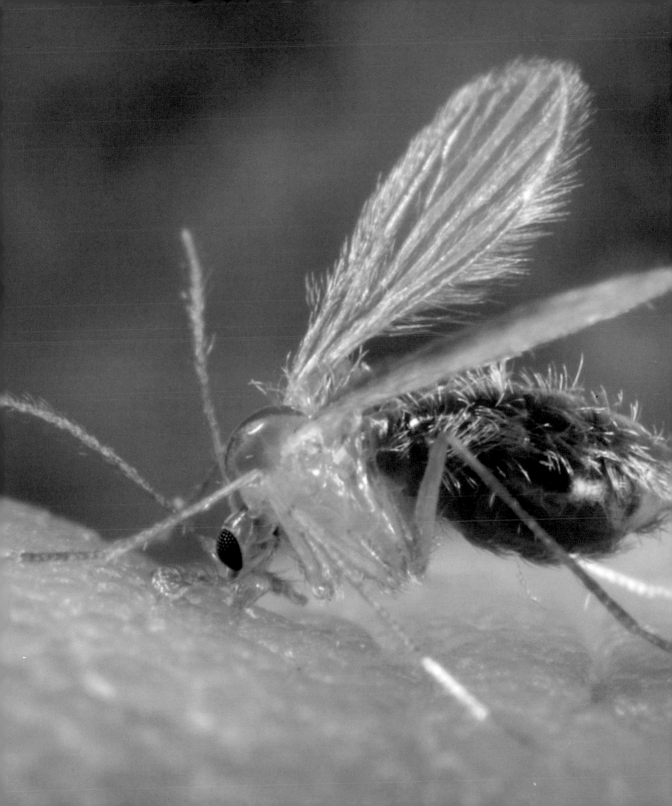

Patent Medicines

GOOD ADS TRUMP SOUND SCIENCE. Patent medicines are not patented medicines. Patents provide inventors exclusive rights to market their product for a limited time in exchange for a public disclosure of their invention. The designation *patent medicines* was based on the "letters patent," granted by the English Crown during the seventeenth century, which gave the maker exclusive rights to that formula and a royal endorsement in their advertising—a practice codified by the Statute of Monopolies (1623). However, although most of these medicines were trademarked, few were ever patented. To do so, the maker would have been obliged to disclose the secret ingredients, some of which were of dubious effectiveness or potentially harmful.

Capitalizing on the belief that American Indians were healthy and "at one with nature," many patent medicines bore American Indian names and contained supposed healing plant parts. Notwithstanding claims to the contrary, nineteenth-century patent medicines often contained addictive alcohol and narcotics.

The success of patent medicines in the nineteenth century was closely linked to the rise of the advertising industry. Products bearing inventive names were advertised in newspapers and mail-order catalogs and were purported to cure virtually all disorders afflicting humankind, without exception or qualification. Not burdened by legislation requiring makers to demonstrate the effectiveness of their products, advertisements relied upon endorsements by famous public figures and testimonials by supposed long-suffering (and now cured), grateful users. Medicine shows, traveling primarily to the midwestern and rural southern United States, presented entertainment acts and celebrity appearances, interspersed with promotions of "miracle cures."

During the early twentieth century, investigative journalists exposed the health hazards and addictive properties of many patent medicines. These articles led to the passage of the **Pure Food and Drug Act** in 1906. Over the years, while the familiar and lucrative trade names of patent medicines were retained, medical claims were restrained and formulas were modified to remove unsafe or ineffective ingredients.

SEE ALSO Pure Food and Drug Act (1906), Food and Drug Administration (1906), Placebos (1955), Dietary Supplements (1994).

"Snake oil" was a derogatory designation that referred to quack medicines widely promoted during the nineteenth century in the United States. Such products, containing undisclosed ingredients, were expansive on claims of effectiveness and silent on potential dangers.

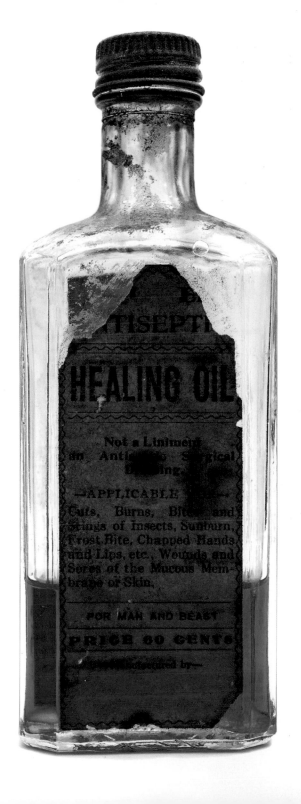

Cinchona Bark

Pierre-Joseph Pelletier (1788–1842), **Joseph Bienaimé Caventou** (1795–1877)

Conflicting tales have circulated regarding the history of cinchona, but there is little doubt that cinchona was effective for the treatment of fever and malaria, thanks to its active chemical, **quinine**. Written records of the medical use of cinchona date back to 1633, when a Jesuit publication described how indigenous Peruvians used the bark to successfully treat their "ague," a malarial type of fever. The most popular tale—albeit of very questionable historic accuracy—relates that, in 1639, the bark miraculously cured the Countess of Chinchón, wife of the Viceroy of Peru, of ague. Large quantities of the powdered bark were shipped to Spain in 1640, and European physicians very rapidly adopted it. The drug was variously called Peruvian bark; cinchona bark, an unintentional misspelling of the Countess of Chinchón's name; Jesuit's bark for its primary importers, distributors, and users; and Cardinal's bark, in honor of Cardinal de Lugo, its chief advocate in Rome.

Protestants, who discredited the drug, did not view endorsement by the Jesuits positively. However, its popularity grew immeasurably in the 1670s, when the English charlatan Robert Talbot successfully treated Charles II in England and Louis XIV's son in France of malaria with his cinchona-containing secret formula. When the secret ingredient was disclosed, cinchona's popularity soared. The cinchona bark contains two important alkaloids long used in medicine: the antimalarial drug quinine, isolated in 1820, and quinine's optical isomer **quinidine**, isolated in 1833 and used for abnormal heart rhythms.

In the mid-nineteenth century, the Dutch smuggled cinchona seeds from Bolivia and cultivated extensive plantations in Java; by 1918, the Dutch were the world's major supplier of quinine. Malaria was a major health threat facing the armed forces in Asia during World War II. After the 1942 Japanese occupation of Java, the Allies' supply of quinine evaporated. This fueled the effort to synthesize quinine in the laboratory—an effort that proved successful in 1944.

SEE ALSO Alkaloids (1806), Quinine (1820), Quinidine (1914), Chloroquine (1947).

In this seventeenth-century engraving, Peru offers a branch of cinchona to Science.

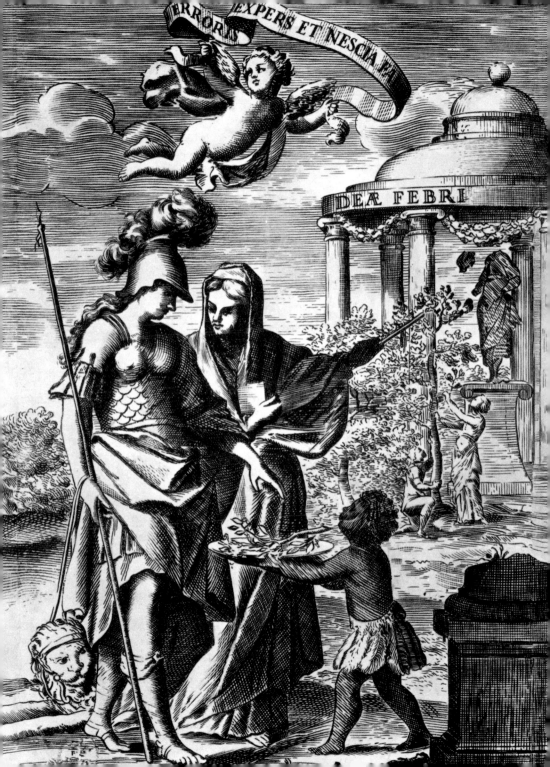

ERRORIS EXPERS ET NESCIA FALLI

DEÆ FEBRI

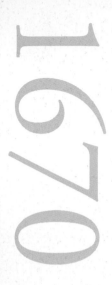

Ergot

Henry Hallett Dale (1875–1968)

FUNGAL TREASURE CHEST. During the Middle Ages, written reports from France described an unusual epidemic associated with extreme constriction of blood vessels, causing tissues to become cold, dry, and black. Victims experienced intense pain and gangrene in the extremities. In severe cases, limbs would drop off without the loss of blood. Some afflicted had convulsions, while pregnant women experienced severe uterine contractions that caused abortions. This condition, known commonly as holy fire or Saint Anthony's fire, after the order of monks who ministered to the suffering, was not limited to France or to the Middle Ages; epidemics sporadically occurred in Germany, Russia, and Ireland into the twentieth century.

A French physician named Thuillier proposed an association between this condition and the ingestion of rye in 1670. The cause of "ergotism," as it is now known, is ingestion of ergot **alkaloids** produced by the fungus *Claviceps purpurea*, which contaminates rye and other grains.

The medical use of ergot powder began with French midwives, who administered it to hasten labor. The word spread to medical practitioners in 1808, when a letter in the *Medical Repository of New York* described its use in the hastening and induction of labor. With its increased use came an increased number of stillbirths, and in 1824 a warning that ergot's use be restricted to controlling postpartum bleeding was issued.

Ergot, a "veritable treasure house of pharmacological constituents," was extensively researched during the early decades of the twentieth century. The eminent pharmacologist Henry Hallett Dale discovered the keys to this treasure house while working at the Wellcome Research Laboratory in London from 1904 until 1914. He found that extracts of ergot contained chemicals that blocked epinephrine and that contained histamine, acetylcholine, and a mixture of chemicals assigned the prefix *ergo-* and the accepted suffix for alkaloids, *-ine*. His findings were a starting point for the study of ergot alkaloids and the involvement of acetylcholine in the transmission of nerve impulses, the latter for which he received the 1936 Nobel Prize in Physiology or Medicine.

SEE ALSO Alkaloids (1806), Neurotransmitters (1920), Ergotamine and Ergonovine (1925), LSD (1943), Neo-Antergan (1944).

The most infamous of the colonial witch trials was conducted in Salem, Massachusetts, in 1692, resulting in the hanging of nineteen men and women and the death of five others. The accusers were two young girls who experienced hysterical fits—behavior attributed to their being bewitched. Some modern scholars have proposed that the accusers' affliction was caused by ergotism after ingesting ergot-contaminated rye bread.

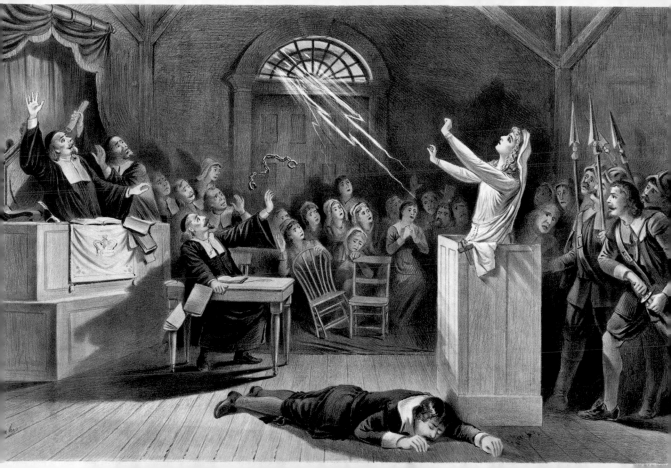

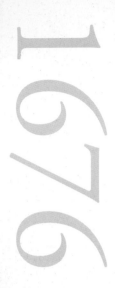

Laudanum

Galen (131–c. 199), **Paracelsus** (1493–1541), **Thomas Sydenham** (1624–1689), **Samuel Taylor Coleridge** (1772–1834), **Thomas de Quincey** (1785–1859), **Hector Berlioz** (1803–1869)

Illustrious figures from medicine, literature, and music have been linked to laudanum. For 1,500 years, the practice of medicine was dominated by the teachings of Galen, whose prescription "galenicals" contained dozens of plant and extraneous ingredients. These prescriptions remained unchallenged until the sixteenth century, when the Swiss-German scientist and physician Paracelsus vociferously advocated the use of simple, specific compounds for the treatment of disease. Paracelsus's "simple" laudanum (from Latin *laudare*, "to praise") contained **opium**, gold, and pearls in an alcohol base and was recommended for pain relief. Thomas Sydenham, the so-called English Hippocrates, further simplified this prescription in 1676 with his opium powder (10 percent) in alcohol. With Sydenham's imprimatur and further promotion by his medical successors, laudanum was prescribed for a range of maladies.

The wonders of opium and its proclivity to cause addiction were popularized by Thomas de Quincey, who first used laudanum in 1804 to treat trigeminal neuralgia (extreme facial nerve pain) and remained a life-long addict. In his autobiographical 1821 book, *Confessions of an English Opium-Eater*, he wrote, "Here was a panacea . . . for all human woes; here was the secret of happiness . . . at once discovered." Samuel Taylor Coleridge, another longtime addict, famously reconstructed a laudanum-induced dream about thirteenth-century Chinese emperor Kublai Khan as a poem but was interrupted after writing only 54 of 200–300 lines. The fourth movement of French composer Hector Berlioz's *Symphonie Fantastique* (1830)—said to be inspired by de Quincey's work— describes the protagonist attempting suicide with opium (perhaps laudanum) and instead experiencing a frightening dream in which he murders his beloved.

During the nineteenth century, laudanum was widely used by the general population—frequently as an undisclosed ingredient in **patent medicines** to treat "female disorders" and to quiet crying infants. Opium tincture (the contemporary designation of laudanum) and camphorated **opium** tincture (paregoric), which contains $\frac{1}{25}$ the opium content of laudanum, are still sometimes used to treat diarrhea.

SEE ALSO Opium (c. 2500 BCE), Patent Medicines (1623).

Samuel Taylor Coleridge at the age of forty-two still had not completed his planned poem from twenty years earlier—a poem that stemmed from his laudanum-induced sleep and ensuing dream of the Chinese emperor Kublai Khan.

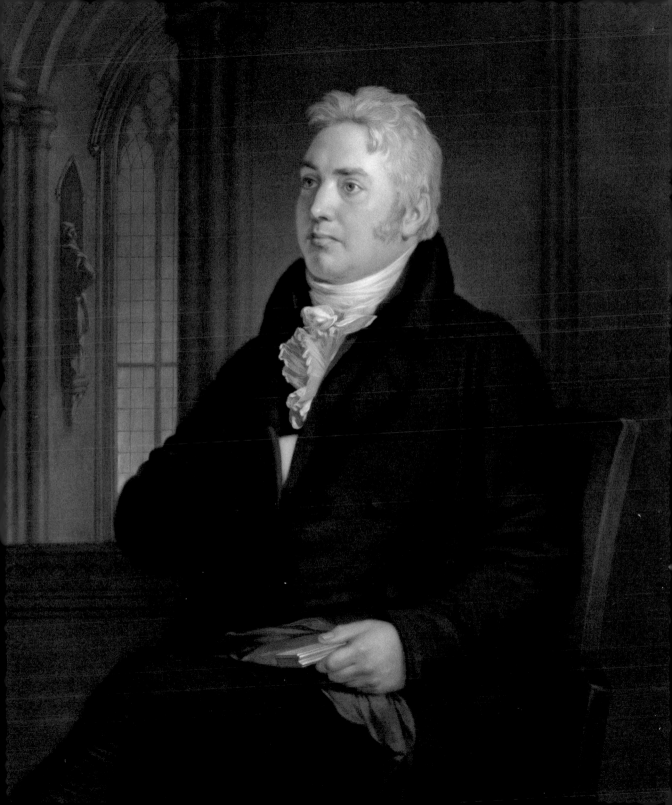

Ferrous Sulfate

Thomas Sydenham (1624–1689), Pierre Blaud (1774–1858)

Most of the body's nutritional requirements for iron are needed for the synthesis of hemoglobin, a protein in red blood cells (RBCs) that carries oxygen to the tissues. Anemia, a decrease in RBC number, size, or hemoglobin content, results in listlessness, fatigue, and skin pallor.

By far, iron deficiency is the most frequent cause of anemia worldwide, with more than one billion persons affected. In developing countries, the usual cause of iron-deficiency anemia is parasitic infection causing intestinal blood loss or destruction of RBCs. By contrast, in developed countries, volume expansion during pregnancy and blood loss during menses in premenopausal women are the principal causes. The body attempts to correct this iron loss by producing more RBCs, a process that further increases the body's need for iron.

Although the relationship between iron, hemoglobin, and RBCs was not known until the 1890s, ancient Greek physicians used iron to treat weakness, a major symptom of anemia. The rationale was to impart the patient with the strength of smelted iron. In 1681, Thomas Sydenham, often referred to as the English Hippocrates, used pills containing iron or steel filings, followed by wine, to treat chlorosis, a condition variously referred to as virgin's disease and green sickness because of the greenish tinge of the patient's skin. During the early decades of the eighteenth century, iron was found in blood, and it became apparent that iron-rich foods could raise the iron content of blood. In 1831, French physician Pierre Blaud introduced the first pills for the treatment of anemia, containing ferrous (iron) sulfate and potassium carbonate. His pharmacist nephew capitalized on this discovery and distributed the product worldwide as the "veritable pills of Doctor Blaud."

Blaud's pills, used until the middle of the twentieth century, have been replaced by a variety of other ferrous salts. Ferrous sulfate, the least expensive, is the first choice for the treatment and prevention of iron deficiency anemia in individuals whose daily requirements cannot be met by diet alone.

SEE ALSO Epoetin (1989).

During the seventeenth century, Thomas Sydenham—called by many the greatest English physician—used iron-containing pills to treat chlorosis (iron-deficiency anemia). Iron was extracted from the filings of rusted iron or steel objects.

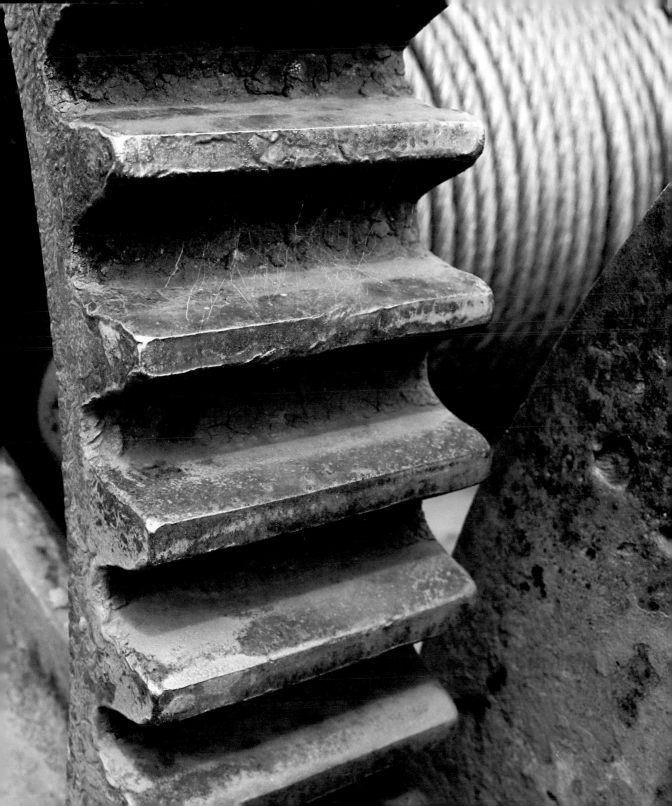

Ipecac

Jean Adrien Helvétius (1662–1727), **Pierre-Joseph Pelletier** (1788–1842)

Long before Portuguese explorers arrived in Brazil, the indigenous people used ipecac, a dried root, to treat diarrhea. Missionaries rapidly carried back news of this miraculous drug to Europe. In 1682, Jean Adrien Helvétius, a Parisian-based physician, administered his secret remedy to Louis XIV, whose son was suffering from a severe and prolonged case of dysentery. The concoction worked, and Helvétius was richly rewarded in exchange for divulging his secret ipecac-containing formula. In 1817, French chemist Pierre Joseph Pelletier extracted emetine, the most important of several **alkaloids**, from the root.

Although it had been used for centuries to treat dysentery, ipecac was judged by many authorities to be without value. As it turned out, ipecac is highly effective for treating dysentery caused by ameba (amebiasis) but not by bacteria. Its benefits were, unfortunately, accompanied by side effects including severe gastrointestinal upset, nausea, and vomiting.

Cough medicines are of two types: antitussives that suppress coughs and expectorants that liquefy and clear mucus from the airways. For many years, ipecac was used as an expectorant, but as with other expectorants, past and present, its effectiveness is unproven.

Starting in the 1960s, all parents were urged to keep a bottle of syrup of ipecac in their medicine chest to induce vomiting and empty their child's stomach of ingested poisonous substances. That all changed two decades later when parents were told to discard the drug. Why the revised thinking? It turns out that, while ipecac effectively provokes vomiting within 20–30 minutes, it does more harm than good when corrosive chemicals are ingested or when individuals are experiencing seizures or are not fully conscious. Its regular use by bulimics has led to potential heart problems and even death. Today, authorities recommend that the American Association of Poison Control Centers be immediately contacted at 1-800-222-1222 in the event of poisoning.

SEE ALSO Theriac of Mithridates (c. 65 BCE), Alkaloids (1806).

While serving the longest reign in European history (1643–1715), the "Sun King," Louis XIV, consolidated the absolute power of the king, advanced France as the leading European power, expanded its overseas empire, and was a patron of the arts. However, in the process, he impoverished France. Ipecac was used to successfully treat the king's son, who was stricken with a potentially fatal case of dysentery.

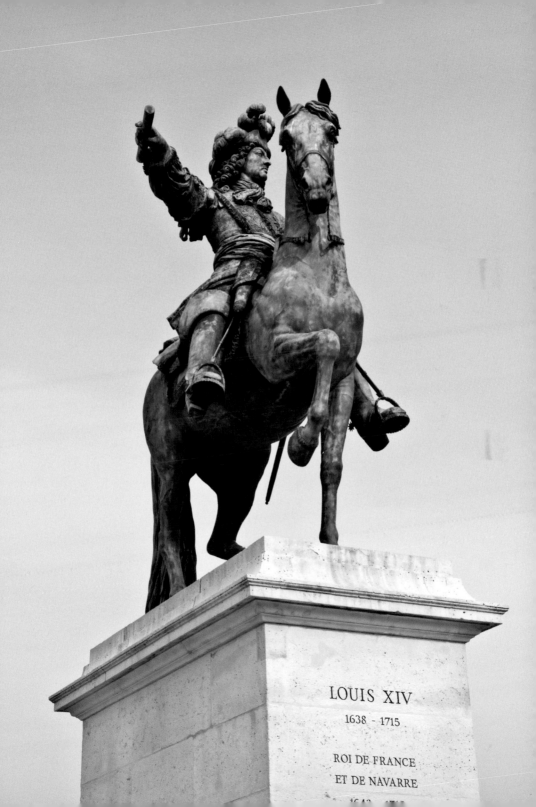

LOUIS XIV

1638 - 1715

ROI DE FRANCE
ET DE NAVARRE

Hydrogen Cyanide

When cyanides come to mind, we first think of poison, not medicine. This is not surprising, as the cyanides have very limited medical uses: Laetrile was widely promoted in the 1970s for the treatment of cancer, without established benefit, and sodium nitroprusside is currently used in emergency situations to reduce markedly elevated blood pressure.

The cyanides are extremely effective poisons used to kill humans, animal pests, and insects. Among the most rapid-acting poisons, hydrogen cyanide (prussic acid)—the most important cyanide—is a colorless gas with a characteristic bitter almond odor. Depending on the concentration inhaled, it can cause toxic effects and death from cardiac arrest within seconds to minutes. By inhibiting the tissue enzyme cytochrome oxidase, it prevents all body cells from using oxygen.

POISON OF CHOICE FOR SUICIDE. Berlin colormaker Heinrich Diesbach first synthesized hydrogen cyanide in 1704 from the dye Prussian blue. It has been most extensively used for executions and suicides. Although lethal injection is the most commonly used method of capital punishment in the United States, several states utilize gas chamber executions using cyanide gas. Hydrogen cyanide's most infamous use was for the mass extermination of inmates at Nazi concentration camps during the Holocaust. Because of its speed and dependability, such senior Third Reich members as Goebbels, Himmler, and Göring used liquid hydrogen cyanide for suicidal purposes in 1945–46. In 1978, more than 900 members of the Peoples Temple cult died in Jonestown, Guyana, after ingesting a flavored drink containing potassium cyanide.

Poisonings have resulted from exposure to cyanide in agricultural fumigants and chemical laboratory accidents. Combustion of certain plastics release hydrogen cyanide and are thought to have been responsible for airplane fires that killed 119 passengers in Paris (1973) and 303 pilgrims in Riyadh, Saudia Arabia (1980).

Hydrogen cyanide is rarely used in criminal poisonings because the rapid onset of death and the bitter almond odor provide a strong inference of foul play. In 1982, seven individuals in the Chicago area died after ingesting Tylenol (**acetaminophen/ paracetamol**) capsules to which potassium cyanide had been criminally added; the perpetrator was never apprehended. To prevent such scenarios, tamper-resistant drug containers are now routinely used.

SEE ALSO Acetaminophen/Paracetamol (1953).

In this Nazi gas chamber located at the Sztutowo concentration camp in Poland, more than 60,000 people are estimated to have perished from hydrogen cyanide gas between 1939 and 1945.

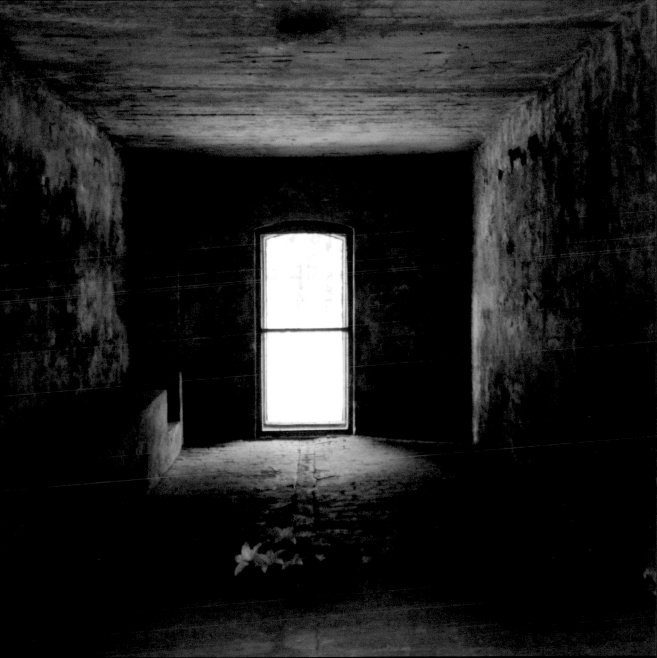

Clinical Testing of Drugs

James Lind (1716–1794)

In 1747, James Lind, a Scottish physician in the British Royal Navy, conducted the first controlled clinical drug trial on 12 sailors. Six year later, in 1753, he published the results in *A Treatise on the Scurvy*, in which he established that scurvy could be prevented and cured by the simple addition of citrus fruits to the diet. By contrast, it now takes approximately ten years, at a cost of some billion dollars, from the time a drug is merely a chemical of interest until it is approved for marketing by a drug regulatory agency, such as the **Food and Drug Administration** or the European Medicines Agency.

Animals or animal cells are the first test subjects. If the test drug looks sufficiently promising based on its effectiveness versus its toxicity, it is evaluated in humans, but only one in a thousand test drugs reach this stage. Human (clinical) trials are conducted in three phases, and a drug can be dropped at any step. Phase 1 trials primarily assess the drug's safety at different doses and are conducted in small groups of 20–100 healthy volunteers. During Phase 2, dozens to several hundred subjects are tested to determine whether the drug works in subjects with a specific medical condition.

Phase 3, the longest and most expensive stage, may involve hundreds to thousands of subjects with the medical disorder, at multiple institutions. Researchers rigorously compare the effectiveness of the test drug with a **placebo**, and to eliminate investigator bias, double-blind studies are conducted, in which neither the researcher nor the subject knows whether the drug or a placebo has been administered. Drug versus placebo effectiveness is compared by statistical analyses, and the results of animal and clinical trials—including toxicity data and adverse effects—are submitted to the drug regulatory agency for a benefits-to-risks analysis.

If the drug has been approved for marketing, Phase 4 (Post-Marketing Surveillance) studies may be conducted to determine whether rare or long-term adverse effects occur. These effects can only be detected when the drug is used under "real-life" conditions in large patient populations over an extended time. Not all marketed drugs survive Phase 4 evaluation. Some, such as **Vioxx** and **Avandia**, have been unceremoniously withdrawn from the market.

SEE ALSO Placebo (1955), Off-Label Drug Use (1962), Celebrex and Vioxx (1998), Avandia (2010), Weight-Loss Drugs (2010).

On board a ship like this one, Scottish physician James Lind conducted the first systemic clinical trial in 1747. His results, published in 1753, demonstrated that citrus fruits (containing vitamin C) cured scurvy.

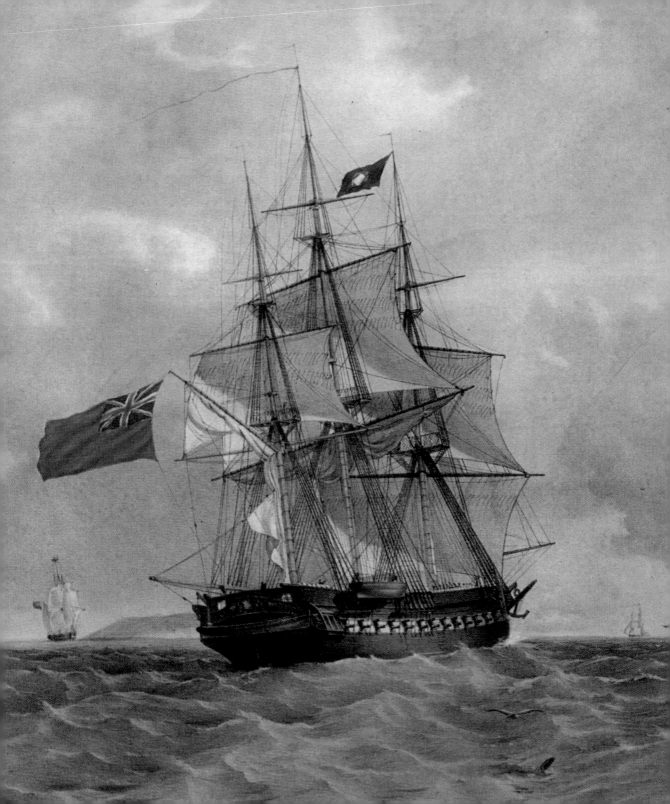

Aconite

Anton von Störck (1731–1803)

For more than two millennia, aconite has appeared in folklore, legend, and literature, playing many roles as a poison and as a medicine. Ancient Chinese and Gauls used it as an arrow poison in warfare. Old, infirm men on the island of Ceos in the Aegean Sea, who were no longer of benefit to the state, made a graceful exit with an aconite-containing poison.

WOLFMAN, FLYING WITCHES, FATAL ATTRACTION. Legends claim that aconite was used as a "love poison" in ancient Gaul, where men were allegedly poisoned via sexual contact with women who had taken aconite daily since infancy. During the Middle Ages, aconite (a.k.a. monkshood, wolfsbane) was used as a werewolf poison/repellent/cure and mixed with **belladonna** in **witches' flying ointments**.

During the 1760s and 1770s, Viennese physician Baron Anton von Störck undertook a detailed examination of eight poisonous plants known from ancient times, including **hemlock**, colchicum (**colchicine**), and aconite, with the intention of utilizing them as drugs. His test subjects were dogs and the good doctor himself. In 1762, Störck introduced aconite into medical practice for the treatment of gout, rheumatism, fevers, and glandular swellings. When applied to the skin, it was used as a liniment, and it was taken internally to reduce fevers. Aconitine was identified as the active principle in aconite in 1833. It continued to be used, with little medical justification of effectiveness, for decades into the twentieth century.

Aconite is the dried root of *Aconitum napellus*, a garden plant sometimes mistaken for horseradish with potentially lethal consequences from heart or respiratory failure. In 2004, Canadian television and film actor André Noble died from such a poisoning in Newfoundland. Far less accidental has been the use of aconite as an instrument of suicide and criminal poisoning.

References to aconite appear in the literary works of Shakespeare (*Henry IV, Part II*, c. 1597), John Keats (*Ode on Melancholy*, 1884), Agatha Christie (*What Mrs. McGillicuddy Saw!*, 1957), and J. K. Rowling (*Harry Potter and the Prisoner of Azkaban*, 1999).

SEE ALSO Hemlock (399 BCE), Colchicine (c. 70), Witches' Flying Ointments (1456), Belladonna (1542).

Aconite was used as a werewolf repellent in the Middle Ages. This gargoyle, said to be a werewolf, is located on the Cathedral of Moulins and was intended to frighten the faithful into attending church. The secular purpose of gargoyles is to serve as waterspouts conveying water from the roof and away from the building.

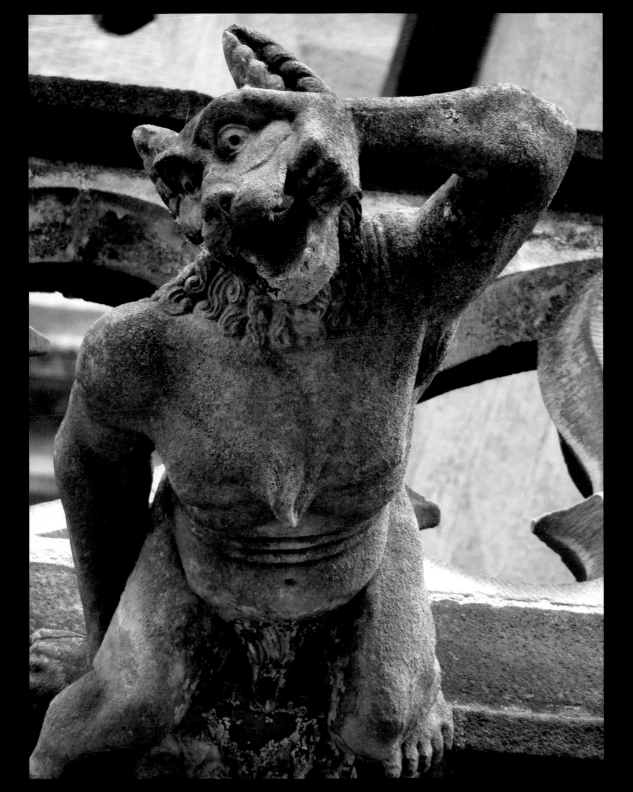

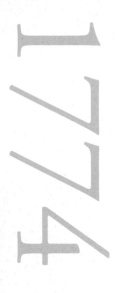

Tetrodotoxin

Captain James Cook (1728–1779)

Tetrodotoxin (TTX) was used in the 1930s in Japan to treat pain attributed to terminal cancer and migraine headaches. As a laboratory tool, it helped scientists to better understand how electrical impulses are carried down nerves. Far more interesting, however, is its toxic nature. Said to be 1,000 to 10,000 times more poisonous than cyanide, it is among the most poisonous substances and lacks a known antidote.

The ancient Japanese and Chinese recognized the dangers associated with eating selected parts of the puffer fish several thousand years ago. The first recorded case of poisoning appears in Captain James Cook's logbook entry of September 7, 1774, during the course of his second voyage around the world. Cook and the ship's naturalist ate the liver and roe of an unfamiliar fish in New Caledonia and hours later experienced numbness of sensation similar to "exposing one's hands and feet to fire after being pinched much by frost." By morning, they recovered. Not so fortunate were the ship's pigs, which died after eating the entrails.

In 1909, TTX was isolated from the puffer fish, an inhabitant of the Indian and Pacific oceans and named by the Japanese scientist Yoshizumi Tahara. TTX acts like **Novocain** and related local anesthetics. It blocks the movement of electrical impulses on sensory nerves, which results in a loss of sensation and paralysis of voluntary muscles—particularly the breathing muscle (diaphragm)—resulting in death by respiratory failure. Puffer fish (*fugu* in Japanese) is a delicacy in Japan, and only licensed chefs can prepare and cook it (without the TTX-rich liver, ovaries, and skin) after completing a two- to three-year apprenticeship.

Ian Fleming's fans recall that at the conclusion of his novel *From Russia with Love* (1957), SMERSH villain Rosa Klebb poisoned 007 with TTX, and he remained conscious but paralyzed, waiting to die from asphyxiation. In the 1980s, TTX was a purported ingredient in Haitian "Zombie powder," as the poison can render the victim near death but conscious for several days. However, the idea that such a powder accounted for descriptions of "voodoo zombies" was soon dismissed by scientists.

SEE ALSO Cocaine (1884), Novocain (1905), Xylocaine (1948).

The puffer fish is said to be the world's second most poisonous vertebrate, following only the golden poison frog of Colombia. Individuals who survive the profound respiratory-depressing effects of tetrodotoxin remain conscious for extended periods with their brain function intact.

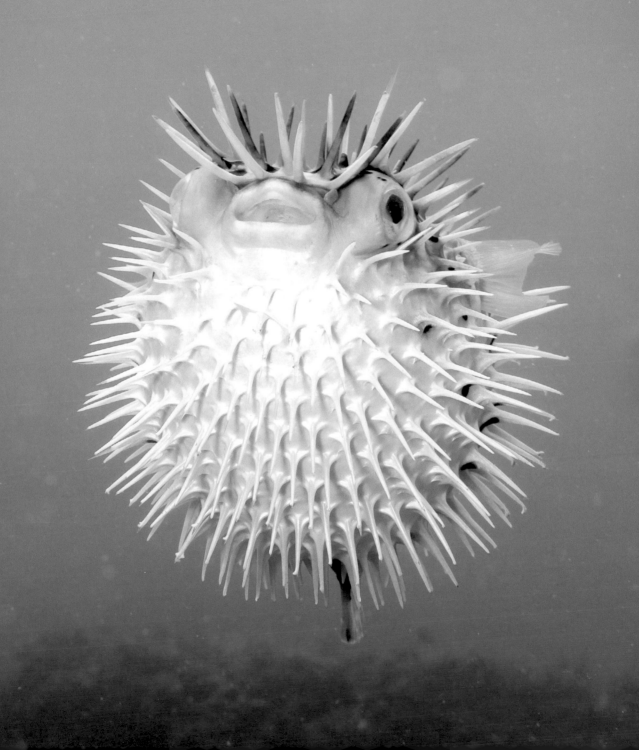

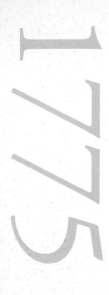

Digitalis

William Withering (1741–1799)

Medical reports of the foxglove first appeared in Wales in the thirteenth century, and its scientific name *Digitalis purpurea* (purple gloved finger) was given some 300 years later. English physician William Withering transformed this folk remedy into what many authorities believe is the most important herb-derived drug and one of the most important of all drugs.

Shortly after his arrival in Birmingham in 1775, Withering was asked to assess a secret family tea recipe of an "old woman in Shropshire" for the treatment of dropsy—excessive fluid accumulation resulting from congestive heart failure. The tea's recipe contained more than twenty herbal ingredients, but Withering, an active botanist, readily recognized the active herb to be foxglove.

Over the next decade, Withering administered foxglove to 163 patients with dropsy, meticulously studying the patients most likely to benefit from the drug, as well as noting early signs of its toxicity. In his 1785 medical classic, *An Account of the Foxglove and Some of Its Medical Uses*, Withering mistakenly attributed foxglove's lifesaving effects in heart failure to profuse diuresis (fluid loss). Notwithstanding the strong warnings Withering sounded about the appropriate medical uses of digitalis and the narrow margin of safety between effective and toxic doses, the drug was carelessly used during the nineteenth century and, because of deaths associated with its administration, fell into disfavor among the physicians of the day. Fortunately, early in the twentieth century, digitalis was rescued from oblivion, and guidelines were established for its use for heart failure and abnormal heart rhythms. The plant product has since been replaced by its purified active ingredients—**digitoxin** and digoxin—as well as other chemical drugs.

Withering was not only an active practicing physician and botanist, but also an accomplished mineralogist and chemist. As a member of Birmingham's prestigious Lunar Society, his fellow "Lunatics" included James Watt, steam engine inventor; Joseph Priestley, discover of oxygen; and Erasmus Darwin, physician, scientist, and grandfather of Charles Darwin.

SEE ALSO Herbs (c. 10,000 BCE), Digitoxin (1875), Propranolol (1964).

Portrait of Dr. Gauchet *was painted by Vincent van Gogh in 1890, several months before van Gogh's suicide. Gauchet is thought to have treated van Gogh for mania and/or epilepsy with digitalis (purple foxglove). Some writers attribute the yellow tone present in many of van Gogh's paintings to xanthopsia, a side effect of digitalis in which a person perceives a yellow tint in his surroundings.*

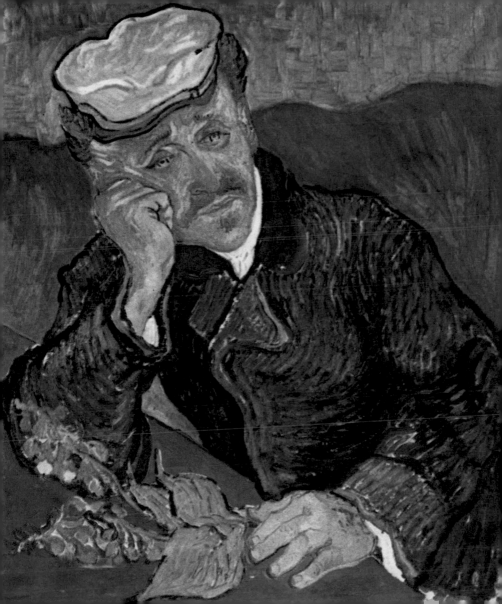

Calomel

Paracelsus (1493–1541), Benjamin Rush (1746–1813)

From about 1780 to the mid-nineteenth century, "heroic medicine" strongly influenced American medical practice. Intended to rid the body of disease-causing impurities from all possible egression sites, treatment approaches included methods to induce vomiting and profuse sweating, blistering to draw out infections, cleansing the bowel with calomel, and bloodletting with help of leeches. The treatment of George Washington's presumed infection of the epiglottis involved the removal of more than five pints of blood over a sixteen-hour period, which likely hastened his demise in 1799.

Benjamin Rush, the most illustrious physician of the period and among the most influential and aggressive practitioners of heroic medicine, used bloodletting and calomel (mild mercurous chloride) to treat a 1793 yellow fever epidemic in Philadelphia. He also used mercury salts to promote copious salivation when treating syphilis, typhus, and tuberculosis. Rush's influence far transcended his active medical practice. He was a professor of medicine at the University of Pennsylvania, author of the first American textbook of psychiatry, and signer of the Declaration of Independence.

The use of calomel did not originate with Rush; Paracelsus first proposed it for use as a diuretic, cathartic, and treatment of syphilis. Between the first documentation of syphilis in Europe before 1500 and the introduction of **Salvarsan** in 1910, mercury compounds were the primary drug treatments for the disease. Successful treatment required continuous and painful weekly injections of mercury over a two-year period and was invariably accompanied by hair loss, loosened and lost teeth, kidney damage, and other symptoms of mercury toxicity.

One response to the harsh—some would say, barbaric—treatment approaches of the "heroic period" was the introduction of **homeopathic medicine** at the end of the eighteenth century. Another far more powerful counterbalancing influence was the rise of scientific medicine.

SEE ALSO Homeopathic Medicine (1796), Salvarsan (1910), Merbaphen (1920), Penicillin (1928).

A "cure" with calomel was often worse than the disease, as was experienced by George Washington in his final hours in 1799. This portrait of Washington was painted by Augustus Weidenback in 1876.

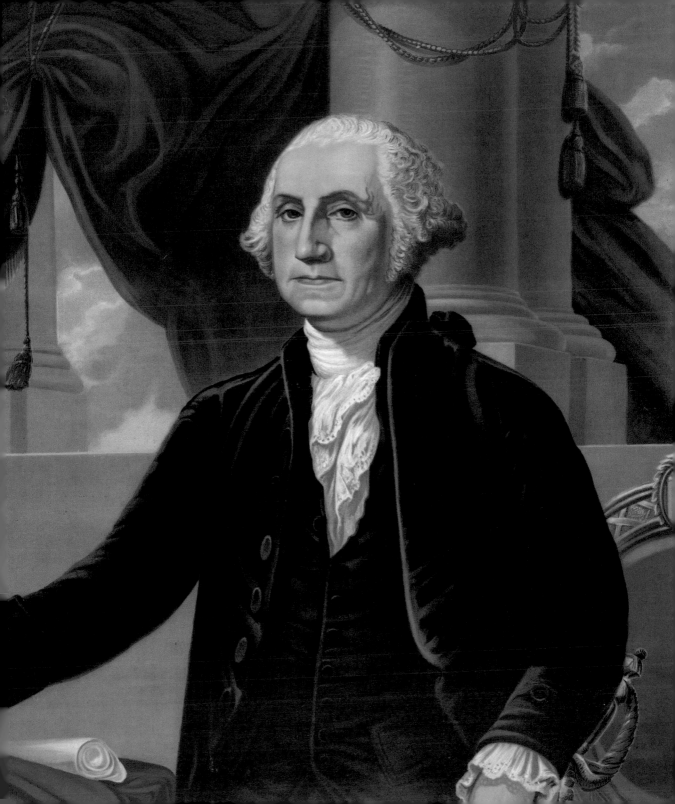

Smallpox Vaccine

Lady Mary Wortley Montagu (1689–1762), **Edward Jenner** (1749–1823)

Smallpox is the most devastating disease ever to afflict the human race. During the eighteenth century, it killed some 400,000 Europeans each year and caused one-third of all cases of blindness. As recently as the twentieth century, smallpox was reported to be responsible for 300–500 million deaths worldwide.

This highly contagious disease has infected humans for more than 10,000 years. As the result of aggressive vaccination programs during the nineteenth and twentieth centuries, smallpox became the first disease successfully exterminated through the efforts of science when it was certified by the World Health Organization to be eradicated in 1979. Quite clearly then, the smallpox vaccine ranks among the most significant of all drugs.

Writer and poet Lady Mary Wortley Montagu initially sparked European interest in a vaccine. Upon her return to England from Constantinople in the early 1720s, she aggressively promoted the local practice of *variolation*, or the inoculation against smallpox using materials obtained from a smallpox lesion—a practice that was rapidly and widely adopted in English-speaking countries and in the American colonies.

Folk experience in the English countryside suggested that dairymaids who had contracted the mild cowpox were spared from smallpox. Between the 1770s and 1790s, a number of individuals tested a cowpox vaccination, but English physician Edward Jenner validated the approach. In 1796, Jenner inoculated an eight-year-old boy with cowpox material, and the boy remained healthy after being exposed to smallpox. Jenner then replicated these results in twenty-three individuals and published his results. Although there was initial opposition, smallpox vaccinations soon became a routine practice in Europe and the United States. Closely related to the cowpox virus, Vaccinia virus has been used since the nineteenth century for smallpox vaccinations, which were so successful that, by 1986, routine vaccinations were no longer necessary in any country.

Smallpox was used as a biological weapon during the French and Indian War (1754–1763) when the British gave two blankets exposed to smallpox to Delaware tribe members. Contemporary interest has focused upon smallpox's potential use by rogue governments or terrorists in biological warfare.

SEE ALSO Polio Vaccine (1954), Cipro (1987), Gardasil (2006).

This poster, exhorting parents to get their children vaccinated against smallpox, was distributed between 1936 and 1941 by the Chicago Board of Health.

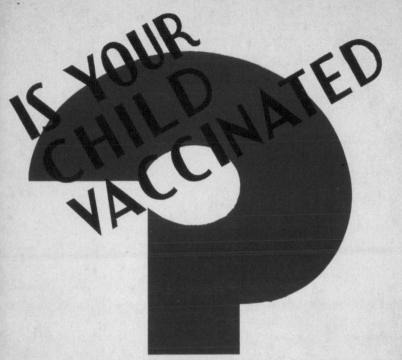

IS YOUR CHILD VACCINATED **?**

Vaccination
PREVENTS
SMALLPOX

CHICAGO DEPARTMENT OF HEALTH

MADE BY ILLINOIS WPA ART PROJECT CHICAGO

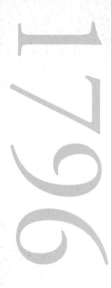

Homeopathic Medicine

Samuel Hahnemann (1755–1843)

As a general rule, the greater the dose, the greater the effect. This concept is well accepted by pharmacologists, who study how and why drugs act, as well as by physicians and other health professionals who prescribe drugs as medicines.

LESS IS MORE. By contrast, one of the basic tenets of homeopathic medicine states that the more a drug is diluted, the greater its effects. The active ingredient is subject to successive dilutions until literally none of the original drug molecules remain. Homeopathic advocates argue that, according to the "law of infinitesimals," with dilutions of the drug in water or **alcohol**, accomplished with forceful shaking, the diluent acquires a "memory" that enables the preparation to work.

Homeopathic physicians see diseases as being caused by "miasms," which create disturbances in vital (life) forces. Treatments are based on the law of similars (let like be cured by like)—that is, whatever causes a disease can cure it. Drugs must produce symptoms in healthy persons that are similar to the symptoms being treated in the patient. For example, exposure to an onion causes a running nose, sneezing, and coughing; thus, a homeopathic onion remedy can be used to treat a cold or allergic attack that produces similar symptoms. Homeopathic remedies are selected on the basis of symptoms and not, as in conventional medicine, on diseases.

German physician Samuel Hahnemann founded homeopathy, based on his opinion that medicine as practiced in the late eighteenth century was doing as much harm to patients as good. Whereas the effectiveness of homeopathic medicines may be questioned—many products have been demonstrated to be no more effective than **placebos** in controlled scientific studies—they are generally acknowledged to be safe.

SEE ALSO Materia Medica (c. 60), Calomel (1793), Placebos (1955), Dietary Supplements (1994), Direct-to-Consumer Ads (1997).

The eighteenth-century practice of "heroic medicine" employed highly aggressive approaches to rid the body of disease-causing impurities. In response, homeopathic medicine was introduced, based in part on the principle that less is more. Alexander Beydeman's painting depicts Homeopathy Watching the Horrors of Allopathy *(1857).*

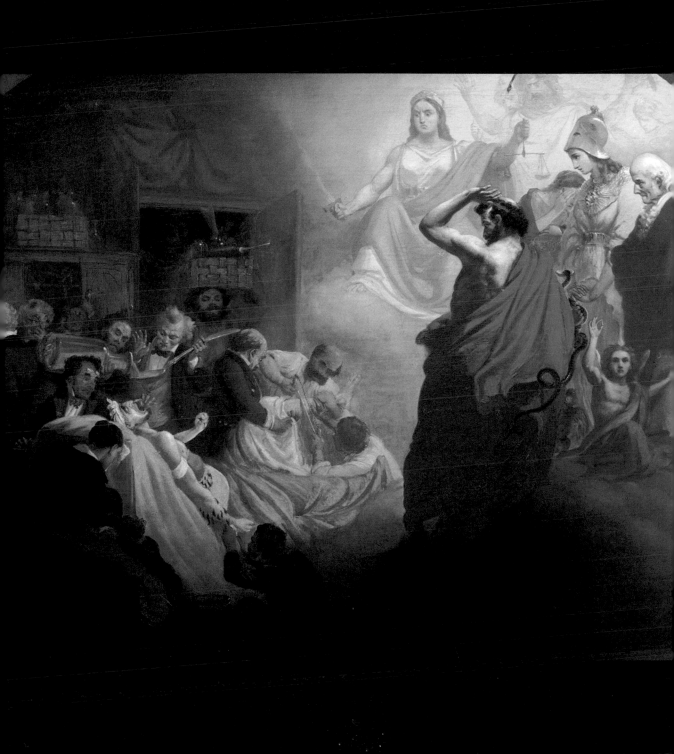

Absinthe

THE GREEN FAIRY OF ART AND LITERATURE. Switzerland has the dual distinction of being the first country to commercially manufacture absinthe in the 1790s and among the first in Europe and North America to ban it one century later. During the intervening period, the "green fairy" was mythicized in the works and by the drinking habits of artists and writers living in France, including van Gogh, Manet, Toulouse-Lautrec, Picasso, Baudelaire, Hemingway, Rimbaud, and Wilde.

During the early years of the twentieth century, absinthe drinking lost its mystique and was linked to violent crimes and social disorder. This led to bans on its manufacture in much of Europe (excluding the United Kingdom) and the United States. In the 1990s, the hazards of absinthe were reevaluated, and the potent liquor was returned to the shelves worldwide.

Absinthe is a spirit containing 50–75 percent **alcohol**, anise (imparting its flavor), fennel, and the leaves of wormwood (*Artemisia absinthum*). The wormwood leaves contain thujone, absinthe's chief behaviorally active constituent, and its characteristic green color is the result of chlorophyll in the herbs. The method used to prepare the drink generally involves pouring ice-cold water over a sugar cube into a glass that contains the spirit.

Purported effects of absinthe on behavior, including increased clarity of thinking and enhanced creativity or hallucinations and madness, have been the subject of continued controversy and debate. In a 2008 report, chemical analysis revealed that, contrary to expectations, the thujone content of early twentieth century "pre-ban" absinthe was about the same as absinthe produced after 1988, when the European Union lifted its ban. Absinthe's behavioral effects could also be attributed to its high alcohol content: Absinthe containing 70 percent alcohol is 140 proof, whereas most gins, vodkas, and whiskeys are only 80–100 proof. Because there are now no legal or industrial standards or definitions as to what constitutes "absinthe," its content varies widely worldwide.

SEE ALSO Alcohol (c. 10,000 BCE).

This 1896 lithograph advertising Absinthe Robette, drawn by the Belgian artist Henri Privat-Livemont (1861–1936), is considered among the most iconic Art Nouveau images.

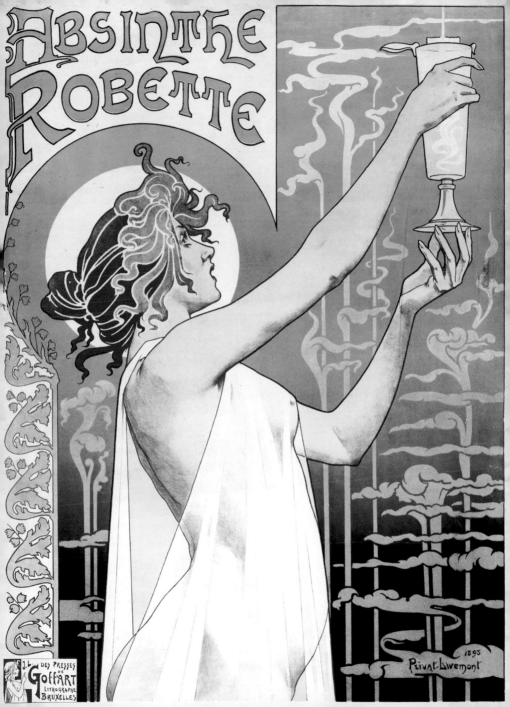

Alkaloids

Friedrich Wilhelm Sertürner (1783–1841), **Pierre-Joseph Pelletier** (1788–1842), **Joseph Bienaimé Caventou** (1795–1877)

Herbs, the primary source of drugs for thousands of years, are typically classified from a biomedical perspective on the basis of the chemistry of their active constituent. Of these constituents, the alkaloids are the largest in number and variety and are of greatest biological interest. Experts have found it difficult to precisely define *alkaloids*, but they are naturally occurring compounds, usually of plant origin, that typically contain a basic nitrogen within a ring molecular structure. Their chemistry, biological effects, and medical uses are far too varied to describe here even briefly, but they have one thing in common: chemists have agreed to end all alkaloid names with the suffix *-ine.*

Why do plants manufacture alkaloids? It seems reasonable to assume that it's not to provide humans with potential medicines. Rather, the bitter taste or toxicity conferred by the alkaloids may protect the plant against insects and herbivores. Alternatively, alkaloids may be synthesized as by-products of the normal chemical reactions that occur within plants.

Plants that are highly biologically active and even poisonous have attracted the keenest interest of scientists and physicians seeking potential drugs for the treatment of disease. In the early nineteenth century, laboratory procedures permitted the extraction and isolation of active chemicals, most notably alkaloids, from their natural sources. The first and arguably the most important of these was by the German apothecary apprentice Friedrich Sertürner, who, in 1806, isolated the alkaloid **morphine** from the opium poppy. In fewer than two decades, French chemists Pierre-Joseph Pelletier and Joseph Bienaimé Caventou proceeded to isolate **strychnine** (1818), **atropine** (1831), and **quinine** (1820), among other alkaloids. Throughout this book, several dozen other examples of alkaloids—including their modifications and improvements in the laboratory to increase effectiveness or reduce toxicity—are presented.

SEE ALSO Morphine (1806), Strychnine (1818), Quinine (1820), Codeine (1832), Atropine (1831), Physostigmine (1875), Scopolamine (1881), Cocaine (1884).

Chemical procedures developed during the early nineteenth century enabled scientists to isolate and extract active chemicals from their plant sources. Of greatest interest and medical promise were alkaloids, which are often responsible for the medicinal and toxicological effects of biologically active plants.

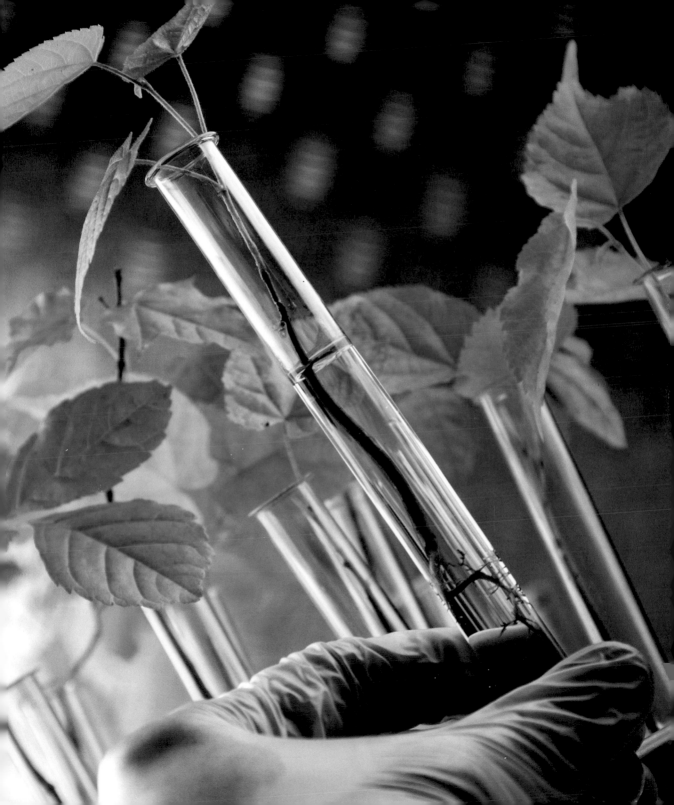

Morphine

Friedrich Wilhelm Sertürner (1783–1841), **Alexander Wood** (1817–1884)

IN THE ARMS OF MORPHEUS. The pain-relieving and sleep-inducing properties of **opium** were well known to ancient healers, but which chemical was responsible for its effects? In 1806, Friedrich Wilhelm Sertürner, then an obscure German apothecary apprentice working in Paderborn, reported that he had isolated a chemical from opium that was able to induce profound sleep in dogs. These findings and subsequent others attracted little attention until 1817, when Sertürner announced that he had isolated pure "morpheum," which he had taken himself and given to three boys under the age of seventeen. Although historically groundbreaking, the experiment was a near disaster, as all subjects almost died from drug overdoses. Morpheum, named after the Greek god of dreams and later renamed morphine, was the first of many **alkaloids** isolated from plants. In 1822, Sertürner purchased the major pharmacy in Hamelin, Germany (of "Pied Piper" fame), where he worked until his death in 1841.

Although effective when given by mouth, morphine's use as an analgesic (painkiller) exploded after the Scottish physician Alexander Wood perfected the hypodermic syringe in 1853. It was indiscriminately administered to wounded soldiers during the American Civil War (1861–1865), Prussian-Austrian War (1866), and Franco-Prussian War (1870), and as a result, the prevalence of postwar morphine addiction was so high that it was termed the *army disease* and the *soldier's disease*.

Newer drugs may cause less abuse and addiction than morphine and they may act longer or be more effective by mouth, but no drug has been discovered that is more effective than morphine for the relief of severe pain of all kinds. It acts by reducing the patient's subjective awareness of pain—i.e., the patient still feels the pain but is no longer bothered by it. In addition to being used to relieve pain, morphine-related drugs are used for the treatment of cough (**codeine, dextromethorphan**), diarrhea (Lomotil), **heroin** addiction, and poisoning by morphine-like drugs (naloxone). Morphine remains the gold standard against which all other analgesics are compared and is one of the most significant drugs ever discovered.

SEE ALSO Opium (c. 2500 BCE), Alkaloids (1806), Codeine (1832), Heroin (1898), Methadone (1947), Dextromethorphan (1958), Fentanyl (1968), Opioids (1973), OxyContin (1996).

Morpheus, the Greek god of dreams, is depicted with Iris, the personification of the rainbow and messenger of the gods, in this 1811 painting by Pierre-Narcisse Guérin.

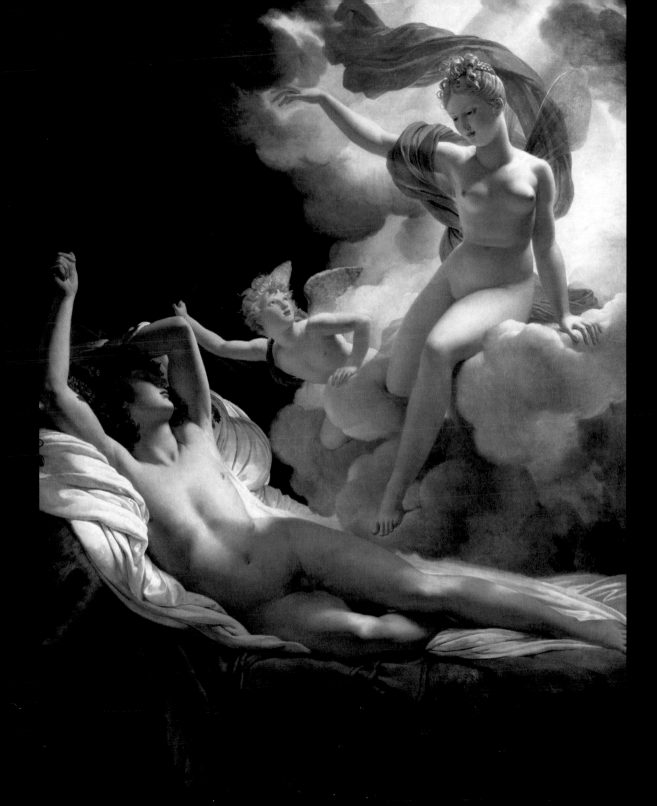

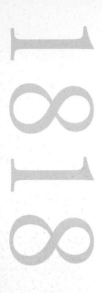

Strychnine

Pierre-Joseph Pelletier (1788–1842), Joseph Bienaimé Caventou (1795–1877)

Seeds of the small tree *Strychnos Nux-vomica* were brought to Europe from India during the fifteenth century to eliminate the growing rat population. Its purported beneficial effects and established toxic effects are primarily attributed to strychnine, isolated in 1818 by the French chemists Pierre-Joseph Pelletier and Joseph Bienaimé Caventou. Strychnine was among the first plant **alkaloids** identified.

One of the most bitter substances known, strychnine can be detected even after being diluted 1 in 700,000 parts of water! It was long used as a major ingredient in bitters (preparations used to stimulate the appetite) and in tonics intended to restore energy to a fatigued mind and body in the elderly and infirm. Strychnine was also an ingredient in a number of sugarcoated laxatives.

GRIN OF DEATH. Far more interesting are strychnine's characteristic toxic effects that affect the spinal cord and usually appear within 15–60 minutes after its ingestion or inhalation. Sudden contractions of all voluntary muscles are followed by their complete relaxation, and the body may arch backward so that both the crown of the head and the heels are simultaneously touching the ground. The jaw is clamped shut, and the muscles of the face are contracted, producing a hideous grin (*risus sardonicus*). During these convulsions, victims are both conscious and acutely aware of their impending fate. Death, which typically occurs after two to five convulsions, results from respiratory failure.

In Agatha Christie's first published novel, *The Mysterious Affairs at Styles* (1920), there was never doubt that Mrs. Inglethorp was poisoned with strychnine; how and when it was given to her was the key to the puzzle.

Strychnine is not selectively toxic, and many of its unintended victims have been small children and household pets rather than rodents and birds. Far safer is its laboratory use as a tool to study neurotransmission in the spinal cord.

SEE ALSO Alkaloids (1806), Neurotransmitters (1920).

For hundreds of years, strychnine enjoyed a reputation as the preferred rat poison. This 1919 poster, prepared by the U.S. Food and Drug Administration, urged, "Kill the Rat! The Most Destructive and Dangerous of Animal Pests."

KILL THE RAT!

By spreading fatal diseases the rat has killed more people than bullets have. He is just as filthy and dangerous as ever.

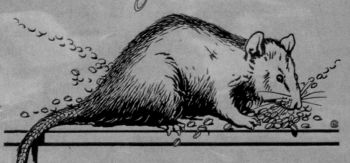

THE MOST DESTRUCTIVE AND DANGEROUS OF ANIMAL PESTS

While America is trying to feed the Allies, this pest annually destroys foodstuffs in the United States worth $200,000,000.

POISON RATS! TRAP RATS!
NEVER LET ONE GO!

MAKE HOUSES, STORES, GRANARIES, ELEVATORS RAT-PROOF

FOR PRACTICAL METHODS OF DESTROYING RATS, APPLY TO

U. S. DEPARTMENT OF AGRICULTURE

BUREAU OF BIOLOGICAL SURVEY, WASHINGTON, D. C.

Caffeine

Johann Wolfgang von Goethe (1749–1832), **Friedrich Ferdinand Runge** (1795–1867)

The worldwide popularity of **coffee**, **tea**, cocoa, mate, and cola-containing soft drinks can be traced to their stimulating properties—properties attributed to their caffeine content. Caffeine is the world's most commonly used stimulant, and indeed, the leading behaviorally active drug. As one Turkish proverb says, "Coffee should be black as Hell, strong as death, and sweet as love."

GOETHE'S GIFT TO SCIENCE. In 1819, an unknown twenty-five-year-old German chemist named Friedrich Ferdinand Runge met seventy-year-old Johann Wolfgang von Goethe, the most important writer in the German language. In addition to his diverse works of literature, Goethe authored a number of scientific treatises on plant morphology and color. During this meeting, Goethe presented Runge with a gift of Arabian mocha coffee beans, from which, months later, the young chemist extracted one of the first **alkaloids**: caffeine.

What effects are we likely to see after ½–2 cups of coffee (50–200 mg of caffeine), two cans of a cola beverage (12 oz. can /35–45 mg of caffeine), or one "stay-awake" pill (100–200 mg/pill)? Our mood brightens and mental alertness increases, while any feelings of drowsiness and fatigue dissipate. Our intelligence does not increase, but, as countless students can attest, our attention span lengthens. Physical endurance also increases. Doses much above 200 mg do not further improve mental or physical performance; rather, they have detrimental effects due to nervousness, tremors, and irregular or rapid heartbeats.

When multiple cups of coffee or energy drinks (12 oz./50–70 mg of caffeine) become a regular, daily ritual, tolerance develops and the stimulating effects of caffeine diminish. In addition, the body becomes physically dependent upon the presence of caffeine, as evidenced by withdrawal symptoms, which generally appear 12–24 hours after the last drink. These are relatively mild and may include irritability, nervousness, and a characteristic throbbing headache. With fresh caffeine input, the symptoms rapidly disappear. When used in moderation, however, caffeine is a very safe drug.

SEE ALSO Tea (2737 BCE), Coffee (c. 800), Alkaloids (1806).

Coffee's popularity is attributed not only to its appealing aroma and taste but also to the mental and physical uplift its caffeine provides.

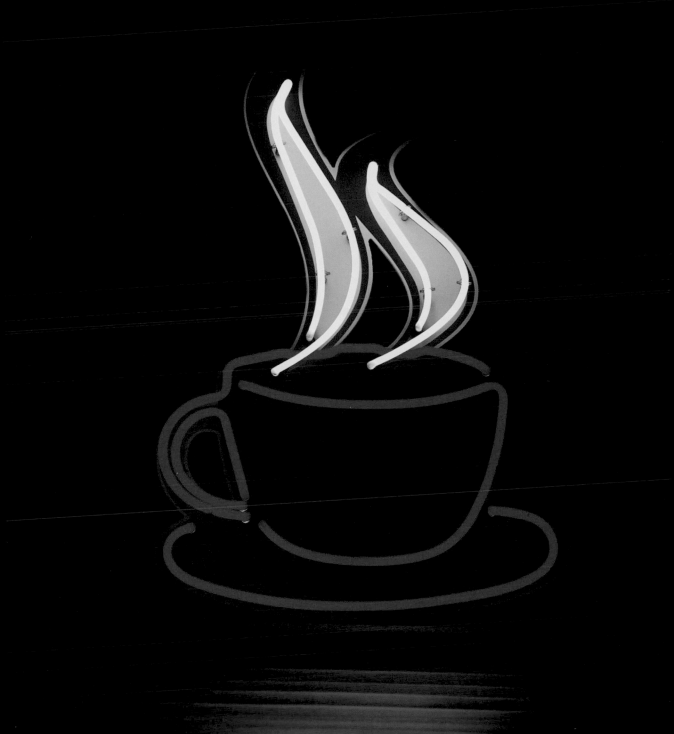

Quinine

Pierre-Joseph Pelletier (1788–1842), **Joseph Bienaimé Caventou** (1795–1877)

Malaria, a mosquito-transmitted disease caused by the *Plasmodium* parasite, may have afflicted humans 50,000 years ago. It appeared in Chinese medical records almost 5,000 years ago, may have contributed to the fall of the Roman Empire, and remains the most significant parasitic disease, affecting humans in 90 countries. Each year, there are 250–500 million new cases and 1 million deaths worldwide.

Cinchona bark, used by the indigenous people of Peru to treat malarial fevers, was brought to Europe in 1639, where it soon gained favor. In 1820, French chemists Pierre-Joseph Pelletier and Joseph Bienaimé Caventou isolated quinine—the active antimalarial **alkaloid** in cinchona—which is said to have played a major role in permitting Europeans to combat malaria and colonize Africa in the latter half of the nineteenth century. It remained the primary drug to treat acute attacks of malaria until the 1920s, when more effective and less toxic drugs, such as **chloroquine**, displaced it. However, with the worldwide emergence of chloroquine-resistant strains of *Plasmodium falciparum*—the most common cause of malaria, responsible for 90 percent of all deaths—quinine has reemerged as a major treatment.

Quinine's bitter taste is the basis for its use as a flavoring agent in tonic water and other beverages. For many decades, it was also used in nonprescription products for the treatment of nocturnal leg cramps, but in 1995, the **Food and Drug Administration** banned it for that purpose because of its questionable effectiveness and potential risks.

SEE ALSO Cinchona bark (1639), Alkaloids (1806), Quinidine (1914), Chloroquine (1947), Artemisinin (1972).

The female Anopheles mosquito lays 30–150 eggs every two to three days and needs human blood to nourish them. After the bite of the mosquito penetrates the skin, saliva containing chemicals enter the bloodstream and prevent the blood from clotting. Other chemicals reduce sensitivity to pain, rendering victims unaware of the bite and of the young malaria parasites being injected into their blood.

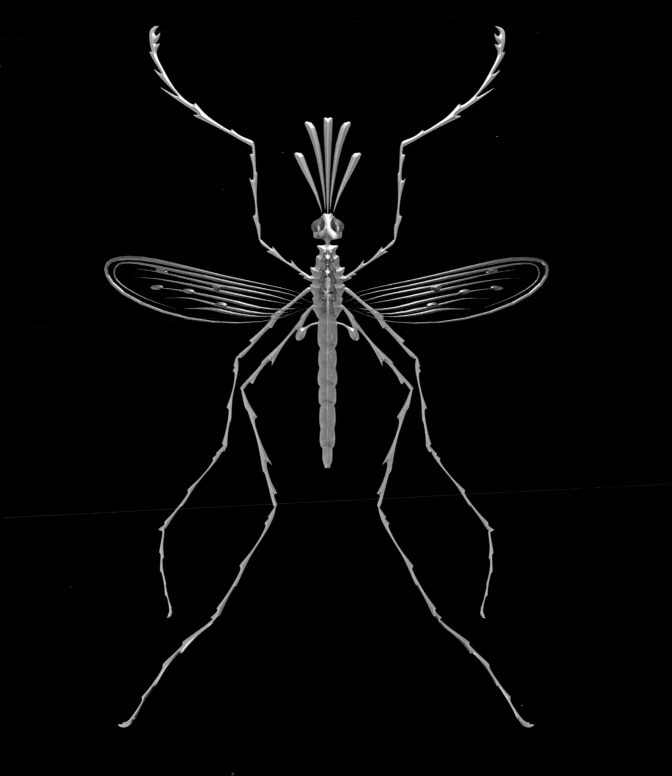

Atropine

Friedlieb Ferdinand Runge (1795–1867), Heinrich F. G. Mein (1799–1864)

Over many centuries, the deadly nightshade (*Atropa belladonna*) and Jimson weed (*Datura stramonium*), among other members of the *Solanaceae* family, have been used with benevolent or malevolent intent. Their effects can be largely attributed to atropine, first isolated in pure form from plants in 1831 by German pharmacist Heinrich F. G. Mein. Of all the drugs contained within this book, atropine is among the least recognized yet most important in early medicine. In addition to its poisonous and medicinal properties, it has also served as a chemical tool to better understand the nervous system and for cosmetic purposes. Plant extracts containing atropine were used by Cleopatra to widen the pupils of her eyes. In the nineteenth century, this effect was studied by the German chemist Friedlieb Ferdinand Runge, whose numerous contributions to chemistry include the discovery of caffeine.

Atropine has profound effects on many target sites, including the heart, involuntary (smooth) muscles in the intestines and eye, and glands associated with the secretion of saliva and sweat as well as those in the bronchioles and stomach. To understand how atropine exerts such diverse effects, it helps to know how it works. After a nerve is stimulated, it releases a **neurotransmitter**, which interacts with a specialized receptor site on its target tissue to bring about an effect. This effect may cause the heart to beat faster or slower, an involuntary muscle to contract or relax, or a gland to secrete a fluid.

Outside the brain, the most important neurotransmitter is acetylcholine, which regulates involuntary functions, such as heart rate and respiration, in the autonomic nervous system (ANS) and activates muscles. Atropine acts as an antagonist, blocking acetylcholine receptors and, hence, preventing acetylcholine from activating its target. Many medicines have atropine-like effects, which are responsible for their beneficial and adverse side effects.

An abbreviated catalog of atropine's current medical uses includes: application to the eye for ophthalmic examination and surgery; stimulation of the heart in cardiac arrest and heart block; application as an antidote in nerve-gas, insecticide, and mushroom poisoning; and reduction of excessive bowel movements and cramping. Newer atropine-like drugs are far more specific, thereby reducing undesirable side effects.

SEE ALSO Belladonna (1542), Alkaloids (1806), Scopolamine (1881), Drug Receptors (1905), Neurotransmitters (1920).

Atropine has been used in eye examinations to widen pupils but has been generally replaced by related drugs whose effects are not as long-lasting.

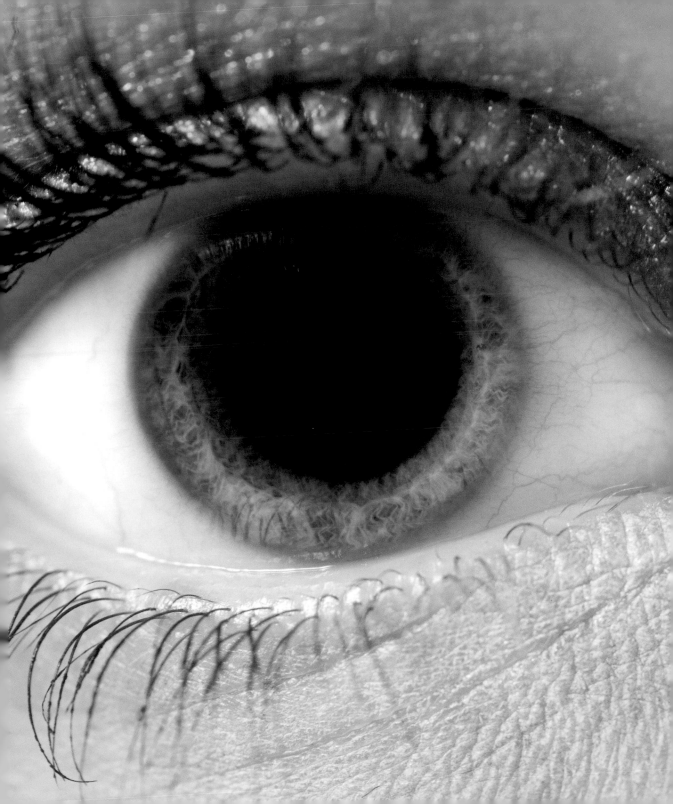

Codeine

Pierre-Jean Robiquet (1780–1840), **Friedrich Wilhelm Sertürner** (1783–1841)

Morphine was isolated from **opium** in 1806 by Friedrich Wilhelm Sertürner, an obscure German apprentice apothecary. Codeine was extracted from the same plant in 1832 by Pierre-Jean Robiquet, a highly distinguished French pharmacist and professor of chemistry at the École de Pharmacie in Paris. Although this was considered Robiquet's most significant scientific accomplishment, in 1805 he had identified the chemical structure of asparagine, the first amino acid; and in 1826 he had isolated the alizarin red dye from madder root.

Codeine, the second most important of the twenty **alkaloids** derived from the opium poppy, may be considered a diminutive first cousin of morphine. Relative to morphine, codeine is a less effective analgesic that produces less sedation and is less prone to abuse. However, codeine is no second-class drug. Codeine is the most commonly used **opioid** (morphine-like drug) in the world. Most codeine used for medical purposes is manufactured from morphine in laboratories and is usually taken by mouth alone or in combination with **aspirin** or **acetaminophen (paracetamol)** for relief of mild-to-moderate pain. Codeine is also an effective antitussive (cough suppressant) but has been largely supplanted by **dextromethorphan** (DM), a drug with fewer side effects and far lower abuse potential.

Codeine's similarity to morphine is not surprising, as codeine (a.k.a. 3-methyl-morphine) is converted in the body to morphine. However, 7–10 percent of the Caucasian population has a genetic defect that renders the enzyme responsible for the conversion nonfunctional, and for these individuals, codeine is ineffective at normal doses. Conversely, some 1–3 percent of whites and more than 25 percent of Ethiopians are born with an enzyme that is ultra-active in converting codeine to morphine. For them, normal doses of codeine can lead to a buildup of excessive levels of morphine, increasing the risk of toxicity.

SEE ALSO Opium (c. 2500 BCE), Alkaloids (1806), Morphine (1806), Heroin (1898), Aspirin (1899), Drug Metabolism (1947), Acetaminophen/Paracetamol (1953), Dextromethorphan (1958), Opioids (1973).

When codeine is used with other drugs in cough and cold products, it is often dissolved in flavored syrups in order to mask its unpalatable taste.

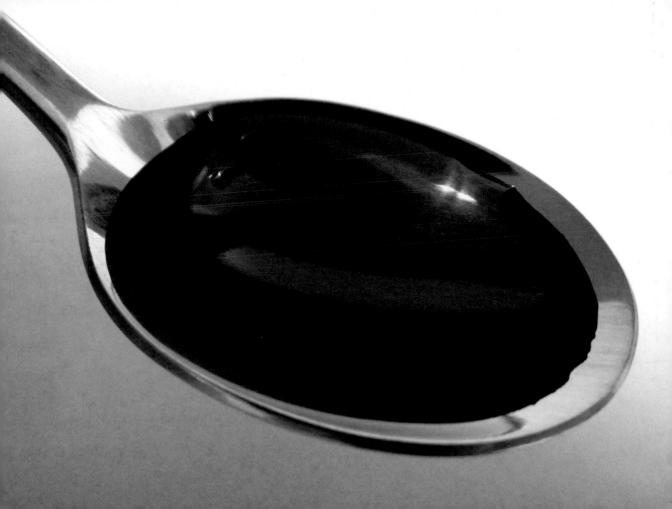

Medical Marijuana

William B. O'Shaughnessy (1808–1889)

Although marijuana (**cannabis**) has been used in medicine for thousands of years, its place as a drug in modern medicine has been the subject of intense debate. Among the earliest Western medical reports was one written in 1839 by William O'Shaughnessy, an Irish physician working in India. He noted that cannabis was nontoxic in animals and that it suppressed convulsions and relieved muscle spasms and pain in his patients. In 1912, the author of a leading textbook of therapeutics spoke with praise about cannabis's value in relieving cough, pain, menstrual cramps, and the tremors of Parkinson's disease, and in preventing migraine headaches. Other authors extolled its virtues for curbing the withdrawal symptoms of **alcohol** and **heroin** addiction. Over the years, however, more effective drugs became available for these purposes, and cannabis lost favor in the medical community.

In recent decades, marijuana has been the subject of renewed medical interest because of its very low toxicity. Among its most promising potential uses is relief of severe, debilitating nausea and vomiting caused by anticancer drugs, when other antiemetic drugs prove ineffective. It also stimulates appetite in AIDS patients who have experienced extreme weight loss. Other medical applications may include reduction in the eye-fluid pressure of glaucoma patients, relief of spasticity in patients with multiple sclerosis or spinal cord injuries, and suppression of pain that fails to respond to other drugs. Dronabinol (Marinol), a synthetic THC, and nabilone (Cesamet), a THC derivative, are available in several countries as orally active substitutes for cannabis, which is smoked and medically discouraged.

The recreational use of marijuana is illegal in most nations, but its medical use is legal in some countries. The **Food and Drug Administration** has not approved of the use of marijuana for medical purposes, although it is available for such use in approximately one-third of the United States. A conflict exists in the United States between the federal law making the possession of cannabis illegal and creating major impediments to testing its medical effectiveness, and state laws, which permit its use for selected medical conditions.

SEE ALSO Alcohol (c. 10,000 BCE), Cannabis (c. 3000 BCE), Heroin (1898), Food and Drug Administration (1906).

The medical marijuana logo consists of a caduceus with a Cannabis *leaf. The caduceus, with two intertwined snakes and wings, is commonly mistaken by medical and health organizations for the rod of Asclepius, the Greek god of medicine and healing, which has a single snake wrapped around a wingless staff.*

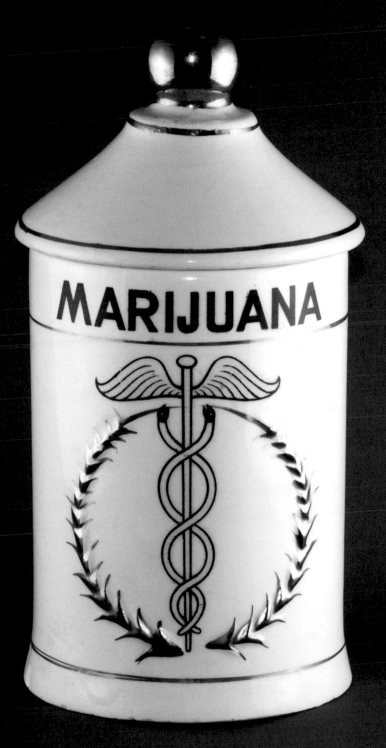

Nitrous Oxide

Joseph Priestley (1733–1804), **Humphry Davy** (1778–1829), **Horace Wells** (1815–1848)

THE FIRST ANESTHETIC. During the early decades of the nineteenth century, shortly after its discovery, nitrous oxide was the featured recreational drug at "laughing gas parties" in England. English chemist Joseph Priestley discovered this gas in 1776, two years after his far more significant finding of "dephlogisticated air" (oxygen). In 1798, during the course of his studies of the "medical powers of factitious airs and gases," the young chemist Humphry Davy sampled and, in the course of his studies, became addicted to the euphoric effects of nitrous oxide. Although he experienced the loss of sensation of pain (anesthesia) of a toothache after inhaling the gas, he failed to pursue its medical potential.

While attending an entertaining demonstration of laughing gas in Hartford, Connecticut, in December 1844, American dentist Horace Wells was astounded when an audience member, under its influence, fell and severely gashed his leg. Upon questioning by Wells, the man was apparently oblivious to pain. Seeing its possibilities, Wells had one of his own teeth painlessly extracted after inhaling the gas the following day.

Seeking a more prestigious audience to exhibit the phenomenon of anesthesia, Wells organized a demonstration at Boston's Massachusetts General Hospital in January 1845. It ended in failure when his subject awakened prematurely as his tooth was being removed, screaming in pain. Disheartened by the negative response of his medical witnesses, Wells drifted from dentistry. He experimented with **chloroform**, became mentally deranged, was arrested after throwing acid on two New York City streetwalkers, and finally ended his misery by committing suicide in 1848. Within days of his death, the Medical Society of Paris honored him as the discoverer of anesthesia, as did the American Dental Association in 1864 and the American Medical Association in 1872.

Dental interest in nitrous oxide was renewed in the 1860s and has persisted to this day. It has a slightly sweet odor and taste, is quite safe, acts quickly, produces a feeling of euphoria, and induces anesthesia while the patient remains conscious. When used alone, "laughing gas" is insufficient for use in surgical operations but is adequate in childbirth and for minor operative procedures.

SEE ALSO Ether (1846), Chloroform (1847), Novocain (1905).

A statue of Horace Wells—a Hartford, Connecticut, dentist credited with discovering the anesthetic effects of nitrous oxide—was erected 30 years after his 1844 discovery.

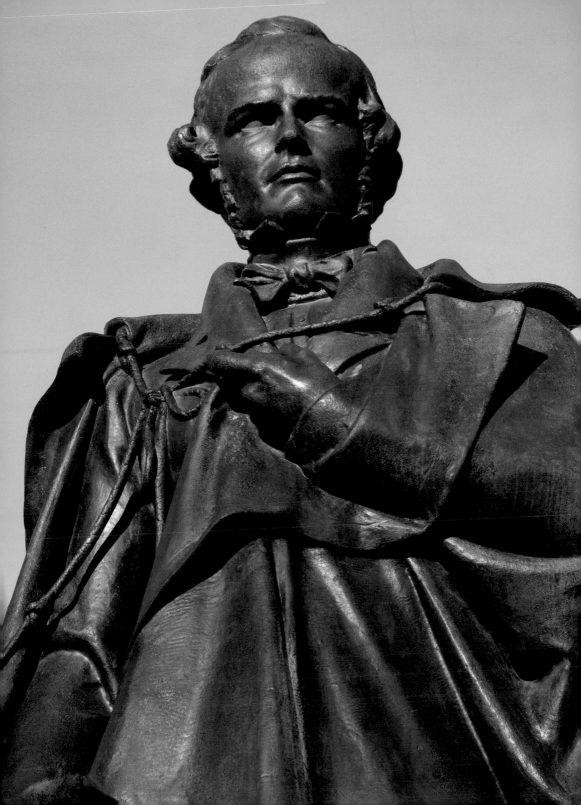

1846

Ether

Charles T. Jackson (1805–1880), **Oliver Wendell Holmes Sr.** (1809–1894), **Crawford W. Long** (1815–1878), **Horace Wells** (1815–1848), **Thomas Green Morton** (1819–1868)

THE FIRST SURGICAL ANESTHETIC. Upon witnessing the first public demonstration of ether's medical properties in 1846, surgeon Henry Bigelow proclaimed "I have seen something today that will go around the world." Medical historians are generally of a single mind that ether (also known as ethyl ether or diethyl ether) is one of the most significant drugs, but more than 150 years later they are still debating who should be credited with the discovery of surgical anesthesia.

Was it Crawford W. Long, a physician in rural Jefferson, Georgia, who after attending "ether parties" and witnessing its painkilling effects on injured partygoers, used it to painlessly remove two tumors from his patient's neck in 1842? Not realizing the importance of his discovery, Long never shared it in any publications. Was it Harvard Professor of Chemistry Charles T. Jackson, who accidentally anesthetized himself with ether? In response to an inquiry from his student William T. G. Morton, Jackson recommended substituting ether as an anesthetic for **nitrous oxide**. Was it William T. G. Morton, a student and partner of Horace Wells and a practicing Boston dentist? In 1846, in the "ether dome" (operating room) at Massachusetts General Hospital and using an anesthetic mask of his own design, Morton successfully anesthetized a patient with ether and painlessly removed a tumor from his neck. What about Connecticut dentist Horace Wells? First to publicly recognize the potential of anesthetics, he was unsuccessful in demonstrating the effectiveness of nitrous oxide.

Sadly, three of our protagonists experienced miserable ends in their quests to be recognized. Wells became mentally deranged and committed suicide in 1848. In his fruitless quest for a patent for "letheon" (ether) and a congressional award of $100,000, Morton destroyed his health and died penniless in 1868. Jackson spent the last seven years of his life in an insane asylum before dying in 1880. One thing that is not disputed: physician, Harvard medical professor, and author Oliver Wendell Holmes Sr. coined the terms *anesthesia* (Greek for the "absence of sensation") for the process of inducing an unresponsive state in a surgical patient, and *anesthetic* for the drug.

SEE ALSO Nitrous Oxide (1844), Chloroform (1847), Thiopental (1934), Propofol (1983).

In this early and simple approach to delivering ether and chloroform anesthesia, gauze was placed over the mesh portion of the mask and held in place by a wire spring. The device was placed over the patient's nose and mouth, and the liquid anesthetic was dripped onto the gauze to produce anesthesia.

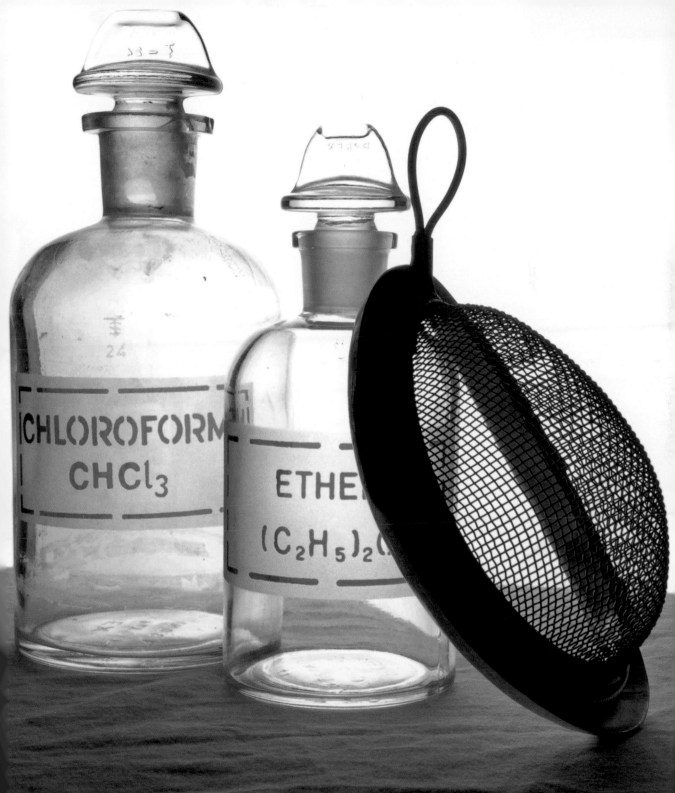

Chloroform

James Young Simpson (1811–1870), **John Snow** (1813–1858), **Robert Glover** (1815–1859)

THE QUEEN'S ANESTHETIC. In the year 1831, chemists working independently in New York, France, and Germany synthesized chloroform. In 1842, Robert Glover, an English physician, noted its ability to cause a loss of consciousness in dogs but overlooked its medical potential. Its medical application was, however, appreciated by James Young Simpson, a professor of midwifery at the University of Edinburgh and physician to Queen Victoria. In 1847, Simpson was looking for a nonexplosive substitute for **ether** that would be more pleasant to inhale, easier to administer to patients, and more rapid in producing its effects. In the course of sampling various liquid chemicals, he fell asleep after inhaling chloroform. Confident that he found a superior anesthetic, Simpson began to use chloroform in his obstetrics practice.

Resistance to the use of chloroform to attenuate the pain of childbirth did not come from the medical establishment questioning its safety or effectiveness; rather, the resistance came from the Church. The clergy cited Genesis 3:16, "I will greatly multiply thy sorrow and thy conception; in sorrow thou shalt bring forth children." Simpson rejoined with Genesis 2:21, "And the Lord God caused a deep sleep to fall upon Adam, and he slept; and He took one of his ribs, and closed up the flesh in its place." The Church's argument ended when chloroform was used to anesthetize Queen Victoria for the birth of Prince Leopold, her eighth child, in 1853, and Princess Beatrice, her ninth and last child, in 1857. The anesthetist was John Snow, who was also a pioneer in epidemiology, tracing the spread of an 1854 cholera epidemic in Soho. Chloroform proved to be much more popular in Europe than in the United States.

With mounting evidence of its potential to cause fatal abnormal heart rhythms and liver toxicity, chloroform fell into disfavor and obsolescence as a surgical anesthetic in the United States by the 1930s. This sweet-smelling, heavy liquid was formerly an ingredient in some toothpastes and cough syrups, but in 1976 it was banned from American consumer products. It continues to be used as a solvent in the pharmaceutical industry and in the synthesis of Teflon.

SEE ALSO Nitrous Oxide (1844), Ether (1846), Thiopental (1934).

The propriety of using anesthesia to reduce childbirth pain was long subject to theological dispute. After chloroform was successfully administered to anesthetize Queen Victoria—head of the Church of England—during childbirth in 1853, the matter was deemed settled and clerical opposition was silenced.

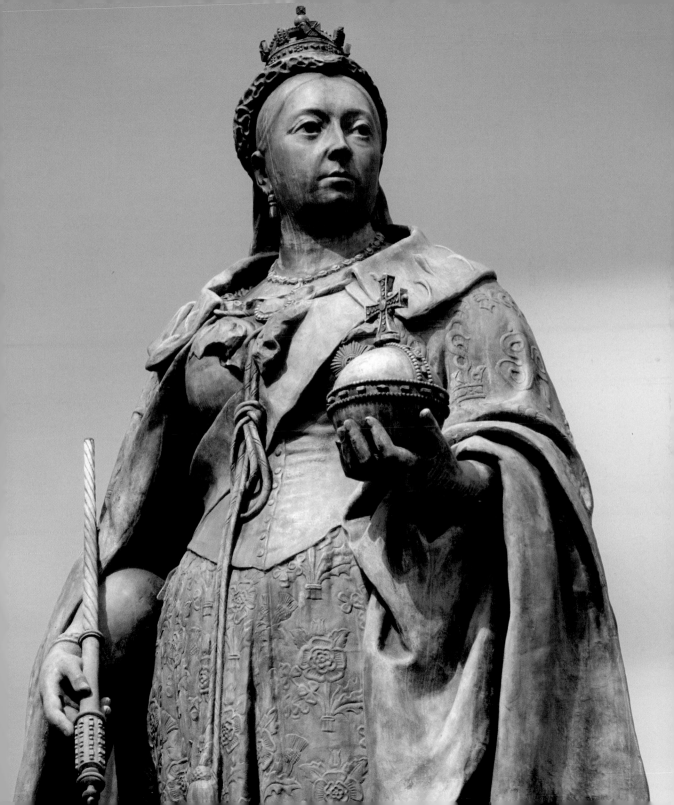

Curare

Sir Walter Raleigh (1552–1618), **Claude Bernard** (1813–1878)

FROM ARROWHEAD POISON TO OPERATING ROOM RELAXANT. Curare, the inspiration behind the "rare and untraceable poison" causing death in mystery novels, is a general term referring to a South American arrow poison. Long before Europeans arrived, indigenous people of the upper Amazon and Orinoco river basins were dipping arrows into crude extracts prepared from the bark of *Chondodendron* vines. Even a modest wound inflicted by an arrow or spear covered in curare caused respiratory failure or paralysis of voluntary muscles, thus preventing the hunted victim from escaping. Interestingly, eating the flesh was not hazardous to the hunter because the active chemical is absorbed very poorly after oral administration.

Sir Walter Raleigh brought curare to England in 1595, and for centuries it remained the subject of experimental studies—one of which was of groundbreaking significance. Claude Bernard, a French physiologist considered among the giants of science, championed the application of the scientific method to experimental medicine. In experiments conducted in 1850 at the Sorbonne in Paris, Bernard demonstrated that curare caused paralysis of voluntary muscles by acting not on the nerve or on the muscle but rather at the neuromuscular junction between the nerve and the muscle. This finding—among the most important in physiology and pharmacology—was the linchpin in subsequent studies demonstrating that nerves released chemicals (**neurotransmitters**) that activate muscle contraction.

The highly variable content of the curare extracts tested in clinical studies during the late nineteenth and early twentieth centuries yielded inconsistent results. More purified extracts of curare were first used medically in the 1930s to relax muscles in patients with tetanus and to soften the effects of shock treatments on patients with psychiatric and seizure disorders. Isolated in 1935, **tubocurarine**, curare's active chemical, was first used with surgical anesthetics in the early 1940s as a skeletal muscle relaxant but has since been largely replaced by safer and more rapid-acting drugs.

SEE ALSO Neurotransmitters (1920), Tubocurarine (1935), Succinylcholine (1951).

New Granada is the title of an 1818 map of northwestern South America prepared by Scottish cartographer John Pinkerton (1758–1826). The map is accompanied by ethnographic commentary on the indigenous tribes, including "Gaberres: Inventors of the Curare, the most active poison hitherto known."

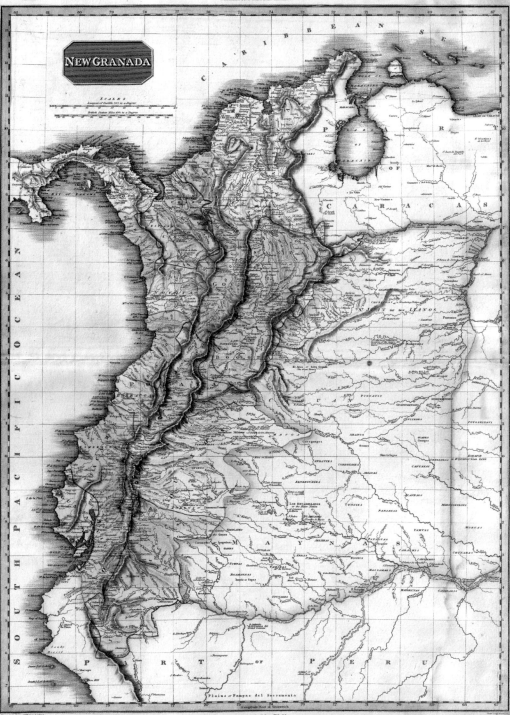

New Granada

SCALES

Bromides

Charles Locock (1799–1875), **Antoine Jérôme Balard** (1802–1876)

In 1826, Antoine Jérôme Balard, professor of chemistry at the University of Montpellier in France, discovered the element bromine in seawater. Potassium bromide, an ionic compound (salt), gained medical attention in 1857 when Queen Victoria's physician Charles Locock reported on its effectiveness in "blunt[ing] or suspend[ing] sexual desire or power." (Then, the prevailing medical thinking held that masturbation was a cause of epilepsy.)

SEIZURE RELIEF AT A PRICE. Potassium bromide was the first drug found to control (but not cure) tonic-clonic (grand mal) epileptic seizures. As the dose of bromide is gradually increased over a period of six to eight weeks, seizure control improves—at the price of mental and physical lethargy, slow and confused thinking, and impaired memory and speech. It was generally believed at the time that seizure control was inextricably linked to depression, but drowsiness was far less a problem with **phenobarbital** and was absent with phenytoin (**Dilantin**), two safer and more effective antiepileptic drugs. Potassium bromide has long ceased to be used in humans, although it remains a first choice for treating epilepsy in dogs (but not cats), used either alone or with phenobarbital.

When taken over many months as a sedative or for epilepsy, symptoms of bromism may unexpectedly make their appearance. Among these are skin rashes indistinguishable from acne, gastrointestinal disturbances, and behavioral and neurological aberrations. The latter include hallucinations, delirium, and mania, which are sometimes misdiagnosed as symptoms of mental disease.

From 1891 to 1975, sodium bromide was readily available as effervescent granules to be mixed into water in a product called Bromo-Seltzer. In numerous older films and plays, characters in distress called for a "bromo" to treat their hangovers. **Acetaminophen/paracetamol** replaced the bromide ingredient in 1975, but the time-honored Bromo-Seltzer brand remains for the relief of pain with heartburn, indigestion, or upset stomach. Thanks to the drug's sedative effects, "bromide" has been used to describe a boring statement that promotes sleepiness.

SEE ALSO Phenobarbital (1912), Dilantin (1938), Acetaminophen/Paracetamol (1953), Valproic Acid (1967).

Perhaps the most famous of all epileptics, Fyodor Dostoyevsky (1821–1881) described seizures and symptoms in at least four of his twelve novels (including The Idiot *and* The Brothers Karamazov*)—depictions likely based on his own experiences.*

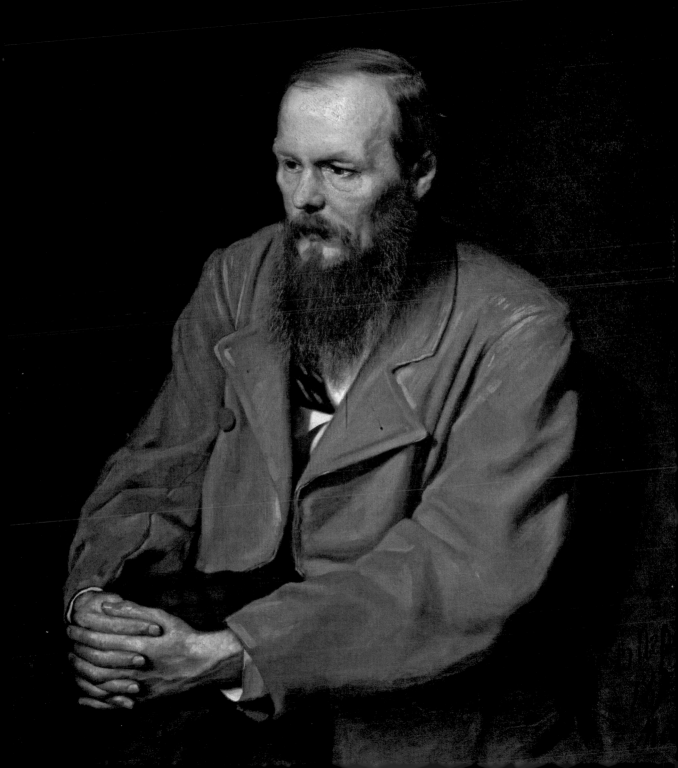

Phenol

Ignaz Philipp Semmelweis (1818–1865), Joseph Lister (1827–1912)

Two major drug-related advances propelled surgery forward in the middle of the nineteenth century: The first was the discovery of the general anesthetics **ether** and **chloroform** (1846–1847), which extended the range of the surgeon's scalpel from rapidly performed crude amputations to extended operations involving internal organs. The next major advance was the reduction of fatal postoperative complications, particularly after childbirth.

Childbed (puerperal) fever was such a common cause of death that many women wisely believed it safer to have midwives deliver their babies at home than to give birth at teaching hospitals. Medical students commonly traveled directly from pathology labs to maternity wards, where they performed vaginal examinations on expectant mothers without pausing to wash their hands. After the Hungarian-born obstetrician Ignaz Philipp Semmelweis insisted that his students and assistants disinfect their hands in a chlorine solution before administering to expectant mothers, the incidence of childbed fever precipitously fell in his Viennese hospital. Nevertheless, the medical establishment rejected his classic 1861 monograph, *The Etiology, Concept, and Prophylaxis of Childbed Fever.* This, coupled with personal and financial losses, led to his mental deterioration and commitment to an asylum, where he died within weeks from either a beating by an attendant or, ironically, from sepsis originating in a hand wound.

Joseph Lister, by contrast, was lionized for extending the teachings of Semmelweis. In 1867, while a professor of surgery at the University of Glasgow, Lister instructed his assistants to use phenol (carbolic acid) solutions to wash their hands and surgical instruments before operating and to bathe their patients' incisions after operating. He was, thus, a pioneer in promoting the use of antiseptics—chemicals that kill bacteria—and later the modern preventative approach of asepsis.

Lister may not be a household name for his surgical advances, but he is remembered via the antiseptic mouthwash Listerine, which first appeared on the market in 1914. The product, marketed to "kill germs that cause bad breath," contains antiseptics, ethanol (**alcohol**), and flavoring agents but—despite its namesake—no phenol. Phenol is damaging to the skin and has long been replaced by far safer antiseptics.

SEE ALSO Ether (1846), Chloroform (1847), Hexachlorophene (1961).

After the introduction of general anesthesia, the next major challenge for the advancement of surgery was the control of postoperative infections, which claimed 50–80 percent of surgical patients. Adoption of Lister's use of phenol and his principles of antiseptic surgery reduced the death rate from infection to virtually zero.

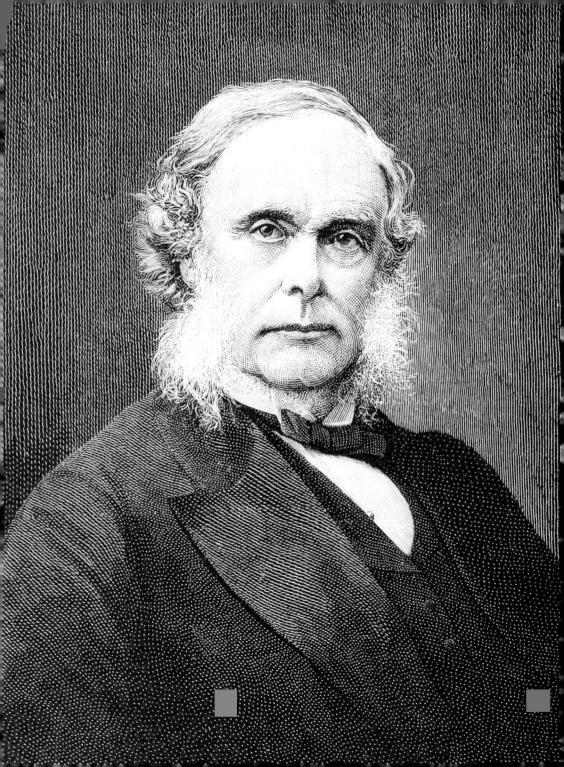

Chloral Hydrate

Justus von Liebig (1803–1873), Oskar Liebreich (1839–1908)

Devotees of film noir and mysteries know that the main ingredient in the infamous "knockout drops" or "Mickey Finn" is chloral hydrate. As the story goes, after the chemical is surreptitiously slipped into an alcoholic beverage, the unsuspecting victim drinks it, loses consciousness, and awakens hours later—robbed, kidnapped, or date-raped.

The distinguished German chemist Justus von Liebig first synthesized chloral hydrate in 1832 at the University of Giessen, which was renamed in his honor after World War II. Known as the Father of the Fertilizer Industry, he is far better known for discovering that nitrogen is an essential plant nutrient. In the late 1860s, Oskar Liebreich, a German pharmacologist at Berlin University, discovered that, in the presence of alkali, chloral hydrate breaks down into **chloroform** and formic acid. Liebreich speculated that the same reaction might occur in the body, and that the body's release of chloroform would produce a sedative effect. The results were right but the theory was wrong: Chloral hydrate produces sleep but not because it forms chloroform in the body.

Introduced into medicine in 1869, chloral hydrate rapidly became a very widely used, relatively safe hypnotic (sleep-producing) drug. In the 1869 hypnotic market, chloral hydrate's primary rivals were **alcohol**, **opium**, and **cannabis**. From a historic perspective, it was among the first synthetic drugs developed exclusively in the laboratory and not obtained from a plant or an animal source.

In the twentieth century, **barbital** and other barbiturates—and, later, **Librium** and related benzodiazepines—displaced chloral hydrate. It continues to be used, albeit to a very limited extent, as a hypnotic and to calm patients before surgery. Chloral hydrate can be deadly when combined with alcohol, other depressants, or **opiates**—it may have played a role in the deaths of two blonde bombshells: Marilyn Monroe in 1962 and Anna Nicole Smith in 2007. Their mysterious deaths are consistent with the film-noir tradition.

SEE ALSO Alcohol (c. 10,000 BCE), Cannabis (c. 3000 BCE), Opium (c. 2500 BCE), Chloroform (1847), Barbital (1903), Phenobarbital (1912), Nembutal and Seconal (1928), Librium (1960), Rohypnol (1975), Ambien (1992).

Franscisco Goya's Caprichos *plate no. 43 (1799) bears the inscription, "The dream of reason brings forth monsters."*

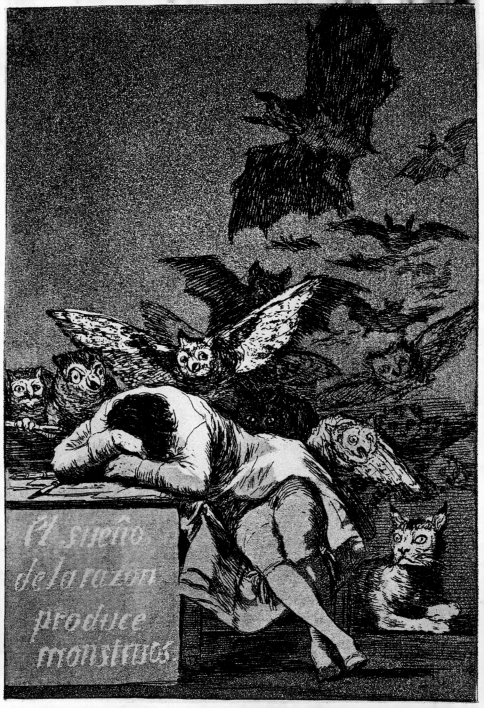

El sueño de la razon produce monstruos.

Digitoxin

Oswald Schmiedeberg (1838–1921)

Medicinal plants may contain dozens of chemicals—some that are biologically active and potential drugs, others that are toxic, and still others that lack activity. Depending on the vagaries of growing and collecting such plants, the quantities of the contained chemicals may vary, complicating their doses when parts of the plants are used as drugs. Throughout the nineteenth century, considerable effort was expended to extract and isolate pure active chemicals from plant and animal sources.

Oswald Schmiedeberg studied medicine in Dorpat, Estonia, and in 1872 was appointed professor at a newly established institute of pharmacology in Strasbourg. There he researched the most important drugs and poisons of the era, one of which was **digitalis**. In 1875, the "father of modern pharmacology," isolated the glycoside (sugar-containing compound) digitoxin from digitalis leaves. Over the years, other glycosides were isolated from digitalis, most notably digoxin (Lanoxin) in 1930. These glycosides were formerly widely used to treat congestive heart failure and abnormal heart rhythms.

Digitalis has no monopoly on heart glycosides. Ouabain (G-strophantin), a digoxin-like glycoside, is obtained from the seeds and bark of the *Strophanthus* and *Acokanthera* plants of tropical Africa. Tribesmen of eastern Africa have used ouabain-containing extracts to prepare arrow poisons that can kill a hippopotamus. Ouabain was formerly used to treat heart disorders but is now a research tool used to study the movement of ions across cell membranes.

In addition, the bufotoxins are a group of digitoxin-like compounds found in toad skin and have been applied to dart tips used in blowpipes for hunting by the Choco Indians of Panama and Colombia. Toad poisoning has been reported in humans and animals, with symptoms resembling digitalis-induced ventricular fibrillation. Since the early 1990s, several deaths in New York have been associated with ingestion of an illegal nonprescription aphrodisiac made from toad venom.

SEE ALSO Herbs (c. 10,000 BCE), Digitalis (1775), Propranolol (1964).

During his forty-six years as professor at the University of Strasbourg in France, Oswald Schmiedeberg, who had discovered digitoxin, trained more than 150 pharmacologists. At the time of his death, more than forty academic chairs were held by his students.

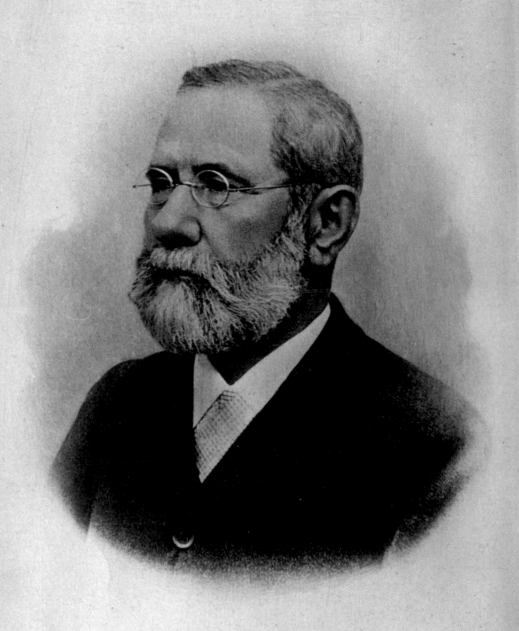

O. Schmiedeberg

Physostigmine

Robert Christison (1797–1882), **Ludwig Laqueur** (1839–1909), **Thomas Fraser** (1841–1920), **Mary Walker** (1888–1974)

TRIAL BY BEAN. Physostigmine, the first effective drug found for the treatment of glaucoma in 1875, has a far earlier history in trials for witchcraft in West Africa. The accused was compelled to ingest seeds of the Calabar bean to assess guilt. If the ingestion was slow and hesitant, symptoms of poisoning appeared as evidence of guilt. By contrast, innocent individuals would presumably eat the beans rapidly, which caused them to vomit and purge the poison from their bodies.

A professor of materia medica, Robert Christison of Edinburgh first scientifically sampled the beans in 1855 and almost died as a result. In 1863, his distinguished pupil Thomas Fraser tested extracts of the bean on many body tissues and organs, including the pupil, and proposed its use in ophthalmology. The following year, the active chemical in the bean, physostigmine (an **alkaloid**, also termed *eserine* after the West African designation of Calabar bean) was isolated. In 1875, Ludwig Laqueur, a German ophthalmologist who suffered from glaucoma, showed physostigmine to be effective in treating the disease.

In glaucoma (a leading cause of vision loss and blindness in adults older than forty), increased pressure within the eye damages the optic nerve. Physostigmine increases the outflow of aqueous humor from the eye, thereby reducing the intraocular pressure. In recent decades, many more longer-acting drugs that cause fewer adverse effects have replaced physostigmine as an eye ointment.

In 1934, the Scottish physician Mary Walker discovered that an injection of physostigmine could temporarily restore muscle strength to patients with myasthenia gravis, but it was replaced with the more effective **neostigmine** a year later. Organophosphate nerve gases such as **tabun and sarin**—the most deadly chemical warfare agents—act in a manner similar to physostigmine.

SEE ALSO Alkaloids (1806), Neostigmine and Pyridostigmine (1935), Tabun and Sarin (1936), Diamox (1953), Timoptic (1978).

Physostigmine treats glaucoma by reducing intraocular pressure. Here, illustrations of the eye are exhibited in Brockhaus and Efron Encyclopedic Dictionary, *published in Imperial Russia between 1890 and 1907.*

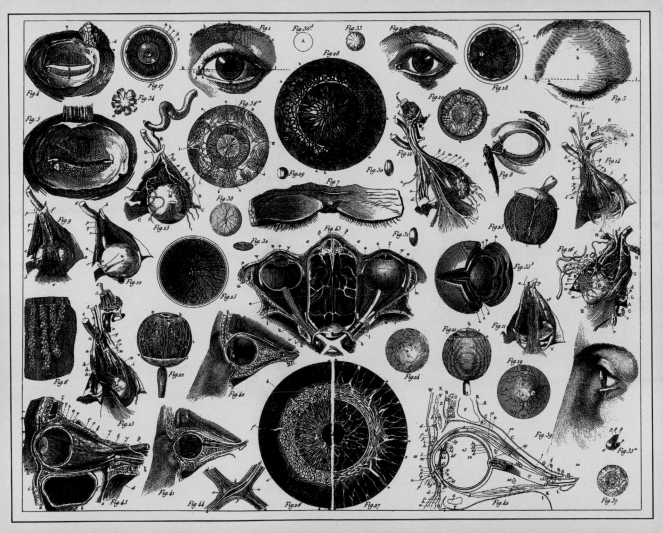

Fig.1 Fig.36' Fig.33 Fig.2
Fig.4 Fig.17 Fig.28 Fig.20 Fig.18 Fig.5
Fig.5 Fig.34 Fig.36° Fig.12 Fig.8 Fig.14
Fig.13 Fig.38 Fig.29 Fig.30 Fig.23
Fig.9 Fig.10 Fig.32 Fig.43 Fig.31 Fig.35° Fig.16
Fig.25 Fig.35°
Fig.6 Fig.22 Fig.40 Fig.24 Fig.21 Fig.11 Fig.19 Fig.39
Fig.13 Fig.41 Fig.44 Fig.26 Fig.27 Fig.42 Fig.35° Fig.37
Fig.45

Nitroglycerin

Ascanio Sobrero (1812–1888), **Alfred Nobel** (1833–1896)

Ascanio Sobrero, a chemistry professor at the University of Turin, first prepared nitroglycerin in 1847. He observed that the liquid was extremely dangerous to handle because of its explosive properties and that inhalation caused an intense, throbbing headache. Over the next three decades, the future of nitroglycerin took two significant, divergent paths—one medical, and the other for construction and armaments.

A number of British physicians observed that nitroglycerin rapidly terminated the intense chest pain of angina, and, following the publication of a systematic study in 1879, the drug was adopted for routine medical use. Prepared in sublingual tablets, it reliably relieves the crushing chest pain within one to two minutes of being placed under the tongue. To this day, nitroglycerin (medically renamed glyceryl trinitrate to dissociate itself from the explosive) and related nitrates are used to prevent and treat angina.

Swedish chemist Alfred Nobel, also at the University of Turin, found that when nitroglycerin was mixed with inert ingredients, it could be handled more safely. In 1867, he patented this mixture *Dynamite*, which, with its subsequent improvements and variations, was widely adopted in construction, mining, and armament industries.

Rapid development of tolerance is an issue with nitroglycerin. When used on a regular basis for angina, it becomes less effective, but side effects also become less intense. For industrial workers using nitroglycerin in the manufacture of explosives, the development of tolerance is fortunate. During their first days of employment, new workers often experience severe headaches and a drop in blood pressure. Tolerance is rapidly acquired but also rapidly lost if the worker is away from the job for even a few days, so, to prevent this loss, workers rub nitrates on their clothing.

Likely feeling guilty that his products were responsible for widespread death and destruction, upon Nobel's death, he established prizes in his name, which were to be awarded annually, beginning in 1901, for the "greatest benefit on mankind" in chemistry, physics, the medical sciences, literature, and peace.

SEE ALSO Propranolol (1964).

Alfred Nobel made his fortune by mixing the highly explosive nitroglycerin with inert ingredients, molding this safer-to-handle mixture into short sticks and wrapping it in paper—a patented product he called Dynamite. *This poster (c. 1895), an advertisement for the Aetna Dynamite Company of New York, was drawn by Edward Penfield (1866–1925), the leading American illustrator of the era and the "Father of the American Poster."*

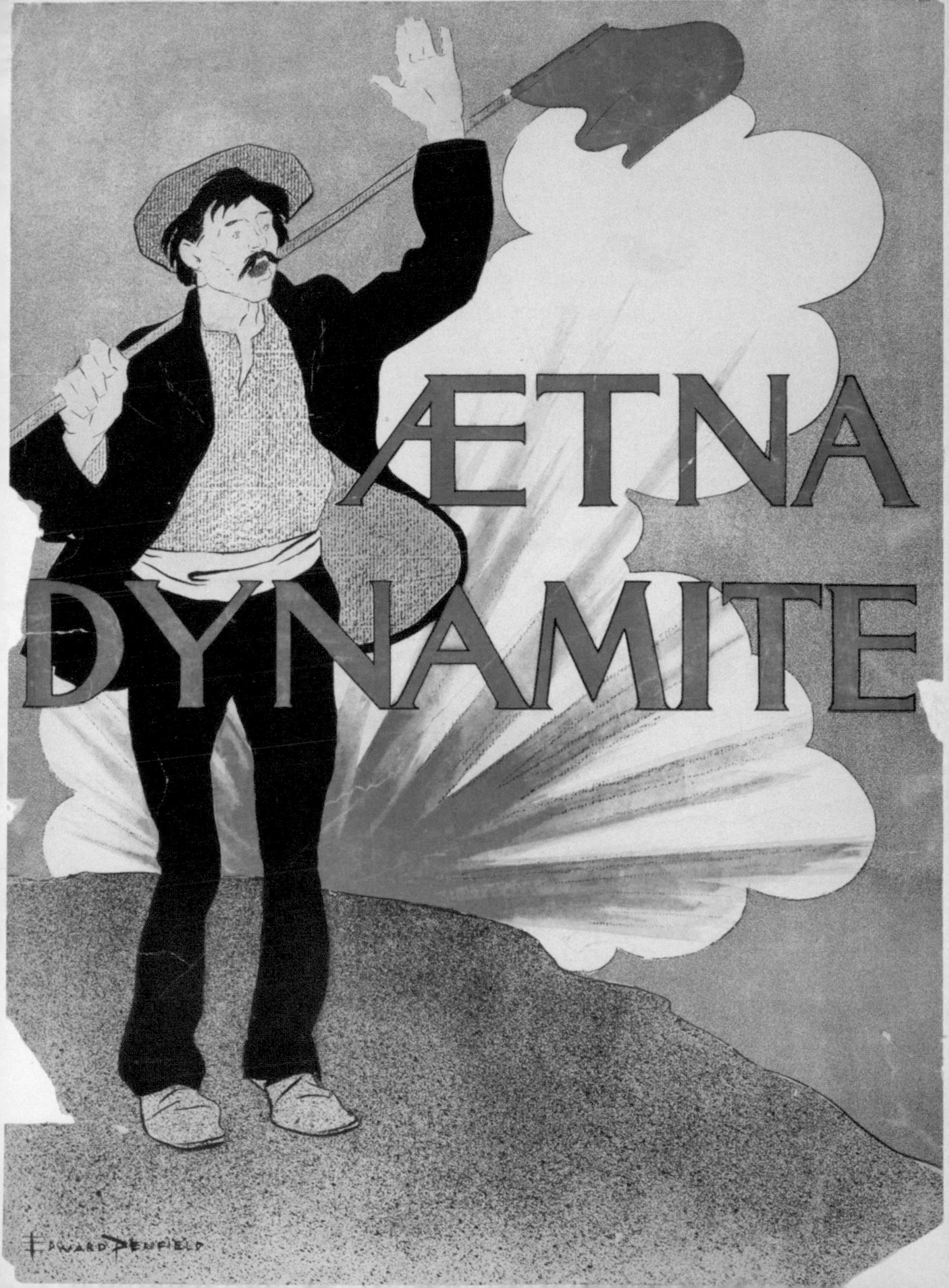
ÆTNA
DYNAMITE
EDWARD PENFIELD

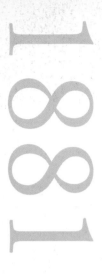

Scopolamine

Scopolamine or hyoscine is an **alkaloid** obtained from plants of the *Solanaceae* or potato family, most notably **belladonna**. Its effects on the body are very similar to those of its first cousin, **atropine**, but scopolamine has far more pronounced effects on the brain that have served as the basis for its many uses over the years.

During World War II, it was of obvious military importance to find drugs useful for the prevention of motion sickness, in order to maintain the combat-readiness of troops traveling by sea or air. In controlled studies of drugs, scopolamine was found to be most effective in averting the dizziness, nausea, and vomiting associated with violent trips of short (four- to six-hour) duration. Today, a scopolamine-containing patch (Transderm-Scop) is available. When placed behind one ear, it provides anti-motion sickness protection for 72 hours. As is the case with other anti-motion sickness drugs, scopolamine is most effective when used to prevent and not to relieve an unpleasant mid-trip event.

For the first six decades of the twentieth century, scopolamine was administered in combination with morphine to produce "twilight sleep" for obstetrical anesthesia. This drug combination produces marked drowsiness without the loss of consciousness and without pain or unpleasant recollection of the traumas of childbirth. It fell into disfavor because these drugs often greatly depressed the newborn's nervous system and erased the mother's experience of childbirth.

Other bygone medical uses of scopolamine that capitalized upon its anticholinergic effects on the brain included the treatment of Parkinson's disease and as an ingredient in nonprescription sleep-aid products. Scholarly analysis provides evidence that extracts of belladonna were among the major ingredients in **witches' flying ointments** that were generously applied to the body. High doses of scopolamine can produce hallucinations, which may have produced sensations that simulated flying and those associated with attending and participating at a Sabbat or Black Mass.

SEE ALSO Witches' Flying Ointments (1456), Belladonna (1542), Atropine (1831).

During adaptation to weightlessness, some one-half of space travelers experience "space sickness," a condition related to motion sickness. Scopolamine has been used for decades to effectively prevent motion sickness and is commonly used as a transdermal patch placed behind the ear.

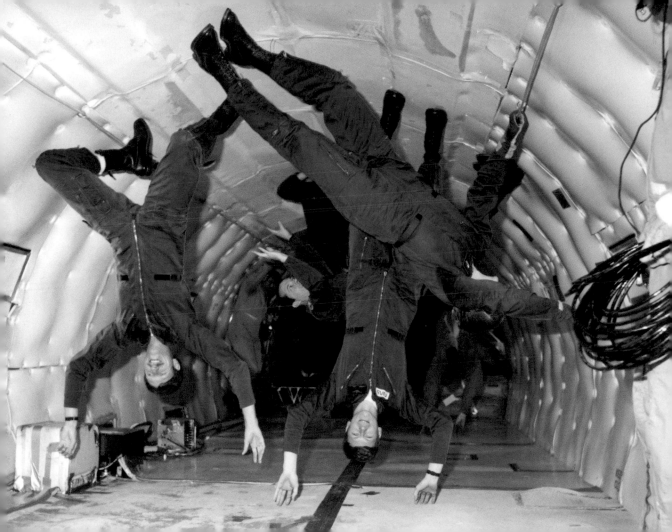

Paraldehyde

Vincenzo Cervello (1854–1918)

Paraldehyde was first synthesized in 1829 and later introduced into medicine by the Italian physician Vincenzo Cervello in 1882. Along with the **bromides** and **chloral hydrate**, it was among the first few effective sleep-producing drugs. Barbiturates such as **barbital** and **phenobarbital**, which first appeared early in the twentieth century, proved to be far easier to administer and more agreeable to take, in turn displaced the older drugs. Paraldehyde is still used, although hardly achieving blockbuster sales.

Paraldehyde is a colorless liquid, with a strong characteristic odor and a burning, highly disagreeable taste. Within minutes after its ingestion, irritating the throat and stomach on the way down, its fusel oil odor permeates the breath and persists for an entire day. About 30 percent of the dose is eliminated from the body in the exhaled, odorous air.

Recipients must be in bed when taking paraldehyde, because it induces sleep within ten to fifteen minutes. It is occasionally used in children to treat status epilepticus, a potentially life-threatening condition in which seizures persist for more than thirty minutes. At an earlier time, until the appearance of **Librium**-related benzodiazepines in the 1960s, paraldehyde was used to calm highly agitated hospitalized alcoholics undergoing withdrawal, including delirium tremens (DTs).

Paraldehyde's effects are similar to alcohol, but it is far more powerful in its ability to induce sleep. Notwithstanding paraldehyde's odor and taste, it has been abused. After being given paraldehyde to treat their alcoholism, some alcoholics may prefer it. Vivid auditory and visual hallucinations have been reported after paraldehyde's abrupt withdrawal.

Many medical supporters over the years have advocated its continued use, but with the introduction of safer, more effective, and certainly more palatable alternatives, its eventual demise was inevitable. Paraldehyde is still used in resin manufacture, as a preservative, and in other processes as a solvent.

SEE ALSO Bromides (1857), Chloral Hydrate (1869), Barbital (1903), Phenobarbital (1912), Librium (1960).

The drunkard in Flemish painter Adriaen Brouwer's The Bitter Tonic *(c. 1635) would have been a good candidate for paraldehyde when experiencing alcohol-withdrawal symptoms.*

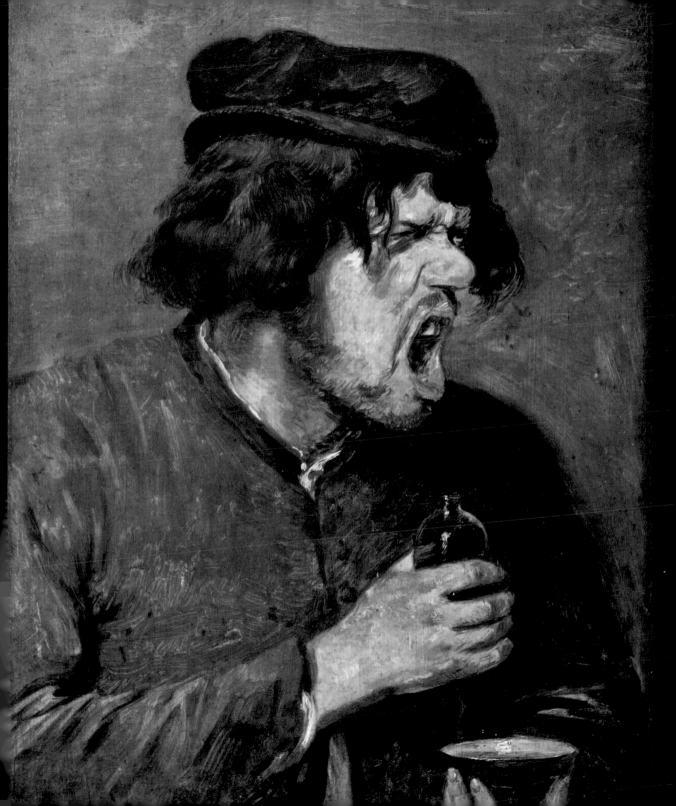

Cocaine

Albert Niemann (1834–1861), **Sigmund Freud** (1856–1939), **Carl Koller** (1857–1944)

In 1860, Albert Niemann, a chemistry graduate student at Göttingen University, published his doctoral dissertation, which described the isolation of cocaine from **coca** leaves and the numbness it caused when applied to his tongue. By 1880, reports of cocaine's miraculous properties abounded. It was purported to cure **morphine** and **alcohol** addiction, tuberculosis, and even impotency. The young Viennese physician Sigmund Freud used cocaine in an attempt to cure a friend of morphine addiction; he succeeded in transferring the friend's addiction to cocaine.

In 1884, Freud's colleague, the Austrian ophthalmologist Carl Koller, discovered cocaine's very potent local anesthetic effects on the eye. For the first time, it was possible to perform eye operations on a fully conscious patient. The medical community immediately embraced the significance of Koller's report, but their enthusiasm was tempered by reports of its abuse. In 1905, the nonaddicting synthetic local anesthetic **Novocain** replaced cocaine.

The abuse potential of cocaine is among the strongest of all behaviorally active substances. Cocaine produces intense stimulation and euphoric excitement, coupled with complete self-confidence in the user's mental and physical capabilities. These effects result from dopamine activation in the brain's reward center and persist for fifteen to thirty minutes. With high-dose or long-term use, extreme anxiety, paranoid feelings of persecution, and tactile hallucinations (cocaine bugs) may occur. Toxic doses can cause heart arrhythmias, potentially resulting in heart failure.

Many users develop dependence on cocaine. After abrupt drug stoppage, the user typically "crashes," experiencing depression, exhaustion, and craving for more of the drug—feelings that may persist for months. Cocaine addiction is very difficult to treat, with more than 95 percent of addicts relapsing.

Cocaine is difficult to give up, but not impossible, as exemplified by such notable former users as Robert Downey Jr., Jerry Garcia, Elton John, Stephen King, Robin Williams, and my childhood hero, Sherlock Holmes. Some sources state that Robert Louis Stevenson wrote *The Strange Case of Dr. Jekyll and Mr. Hyde* in six cocaine-fueled days.

SEE ALSO Alcohol (c. 10,000 BCE), Coca (1532), Morphine (1806), Novocain (1905), Methamphetamine (1944), Xylocaine (1948), Crack Cocaine (1986).

Between 1884 and 1887, Freud (shown in this 1926 photograph) was thought to have taken cocaine. He strongly advocated its use as a stimulant, as an analgesic, and as a treatment for mental disorders. After his failed attempt to cure his friend's morphine addiction with cocaine, however, he no longer promoted this treatment.

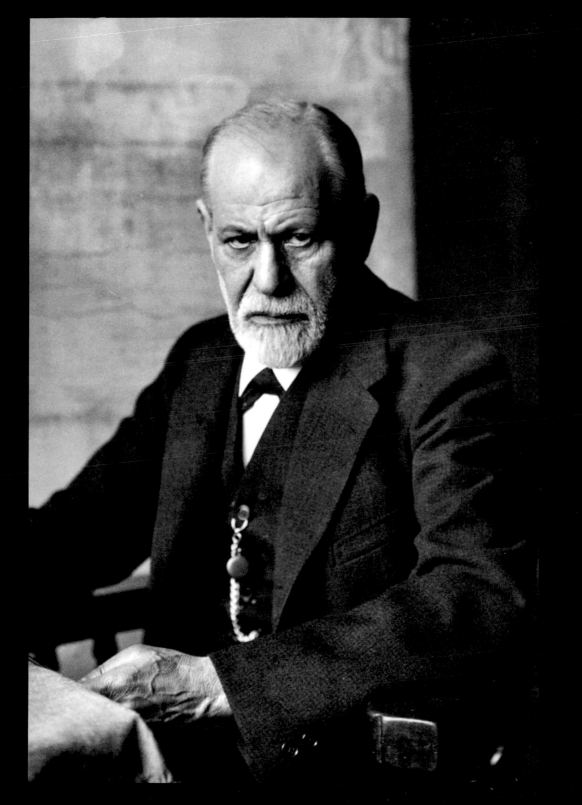

Theophylline

Albrecht Kossel (1853–1927)

CAFFEINE'S COUSIN. Coffee and tea, the two most commonly consumed hot beverages worldwide, contain two very closely related **alkaloids**: **caffeine** and theophylline. Caffeine was first isolated from coffee in 1819. Theophylline was extracted and isolated from tea in 1888 by the German physiological chemist Albrecht Kossel (1853–1927), who was awarded the 1910 Nobel Prize in Physiology or Medicine for his studies on the protein and nucleic acid chemistry of cells.

Caffeine and theophylline are chemical cousins of the xanthine family. They share the same biological effects, although not with the same intensity. Caffeine is a strong nervous-system stimulant, while theophylline is far less so. By contrast, theophylline is much more active than caffeine in relaxing and widening the bronchi to facilitate breathing and in promoting urine output (diuretic effect).

Theophylline first appeared in medicine in 1902 for use as a diuretic, and it continued to be used for many decades until it was replaced in the 1950s by the far more effective and safer **Diuril**-related drugs. In the early 1920s, laboratory studies in animals demonstrated theophylline's effects on the bronchioles, leading to its use three decades later for the treatment of bronchial asthma and chronic obstructive pulmonary disease (COPD). Theophylline and closely related aminophylline continue to be used as antiasthmatic drugs, although such inhaled steroids as beclomethasone and such long-acting bronchodilators as **albuterol/salbutamol** are more effective, cause fewer heart problems, and are far less irritating to the stomach.

In addition, very importantly, approximately 318 drugs interact with theophylline, 47 of which interact significantly. Theophylline elevates the blood level of some of these drugs, increasing the risk of adverse effects, while lowering the blood level of others, hence reducing their effectiveness.

SEE ALSO Tea (c. 2737 BCE), Coffee (c. 800), Alkaloids (1806), Caffeine (1819), Diuril (1958), Albuterol/ Salbutamol (1968).

Albrecht Kossel's primary scientific research and fame were based on determining the relationship between the chemistry of cellular components (in particular, the nucleus) and their biological function.

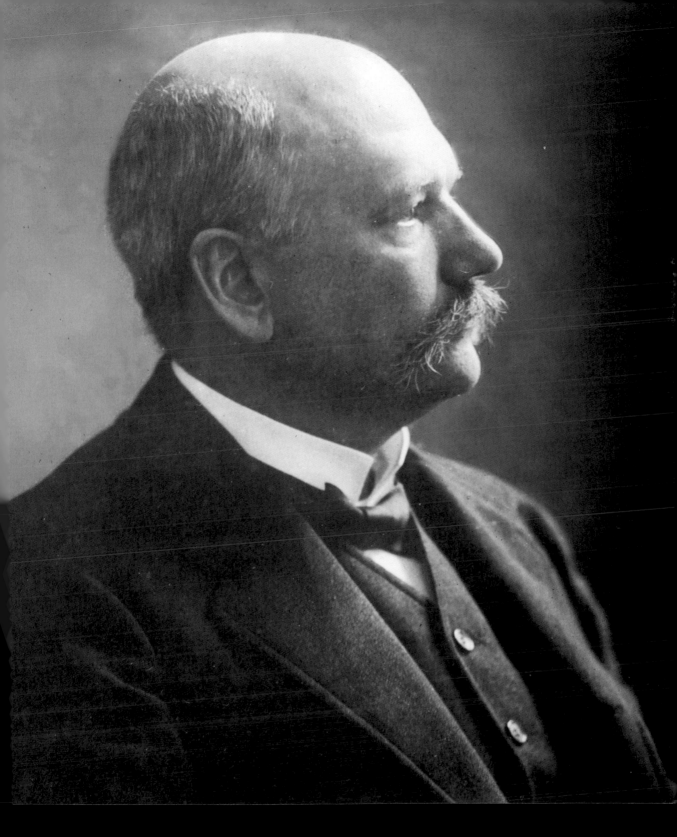

Mescaline

Arthur Heffter (1859–1925)

The mind-altering effects of **LSD**, a synthetic drug, were first discovered in Switzerland in 1943, but some sources suggest that Native Americans living in the southwestern United States used the peyote cactus, a plant with LSD-like effects, 5,700 years ago. The peyote cactus, *Lophophora williamsii* is a dome-shaped, spineless cactus, indigenous to the deserts of Mexico and southwestern Texas. It played a major role in the religious rituals of the Aztecs and other Mexican Indians in the pre-Columbian period and was used medicinally. The upper portion of the cactus was sliced into discs and allowed to dry to form "mescal buttons," which were soaked in the mouth, rounded by hand into a ball, and swallowed.

Over the years, the Native American peyote users migrated northward into the Great Plains region of the United States. During the 1880s, members of the Peyote Religion joined together to form the Native American Church of North America, which has a current membership of 250,000. They have fused their beliefs in Jesus and the Bible with the traditions of Native Americans, and view peyote as the sacrament when taking Communion.

In 1990, the Supreme Court ruled that states can specifically permit the use of peyote (an illegal drug) for religious rituals. Conversely, states, if they choose, can prosecute Native American Church members for using peyote for sacramental purposes, and such individuals cannot invoke freedom of religion as a defense.

Arthur Heffter, a German pharmacologist and chemist, first isolated mescaline—peyote's active chemical, to which its hallucinogenic effects are attributed—in 1897. Vivid descriptions of mescaline's effects appear in the writings of Aldous Huxley in *Doors of Perception* (1953) and of Hunter S. Thompson in *Fear and Loathing in Las Vegas* (1972)—descriptions that include visual hallucinations seen in vivid color and episodes of synesthesia, a mixing of senses, such as "seeing" music in colors or "hearing" a painting as music. Users also report deep insights into reality or communion with gods.

SEE ALSO LSD (1943).

In addition to its use for religious purposes, peyote has been used by Native Americans to treat pain associated with childbirth and toothaches, as well as fever, skin conditions, diabetes, and blindness.

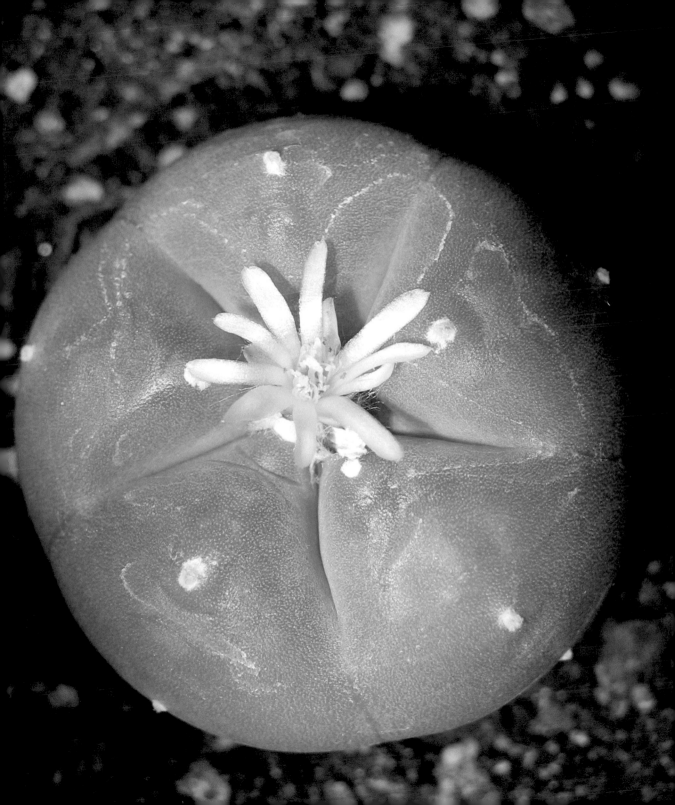

Heroin

Heinrich Dreser (1860–1924)

For the German F. Bayer & Company, the world's first pharmaceutical powerhouse, 1898 and 1899 were outstanding years. In those years, head of pharmacology Heinrich Dreser launched **aspirin**, which for many decades was the most widely used drug in the world. Heroin (from the German *heroisch* or "heroic") also appeared as a cough suppressant and a purported nonaddicting substitute for **morphine** that could cure morphine addiction. At this time, tuberculosis and pneumonia were leading causes of death, and the market for a drug to calm a cough was significant.

Heroin sales were impressive, but within a year or two, the first reports of heroin addiction began appearing. Unbeknownst to Bayer, heroin (diacetylmorphine) is rapidly broken down into morphine when taken by mouth, and the acetyl derivative of morphine promotes its rapid entry into the brain. In 1924, the manufacture, distribution, and sale of heroin were banned in the United States, but not in the United Kingdom, where diamorphine continues to be used legally, by injection, for the relief of severe pain. Moreover, in select European cities, heroin can be prescribed for the treatment of heroin addicts. (In the United States, **methadone** and buprenorphine are primary substitutes.)

Heroin is synthesized from morphine, which is isolated from the **opium** poppy. Considered the **opioid** most subject to abuse, heroin can be injected, smoked, or snorted. Users report an initial short-lived euphoria or "rush," followed by a period of tranquility, which may persist for several hours. Repeated use leads to the development of tolerance, necessitating the use of higher doses, and physical dependence, as evidenced by withdrawal effects when its use is reduced or stopped. Overdose can result in death from respiratory failure.

Heroin use has been well publicized among musicians and was reportedly a factor in the deaths of Kurt Cobain, Jim Morrison, and Sid Vicious. Users have included Charlie Parker, Billie Holiday, Ray Charles, Lou Reed (who wrote the song "Heroin," sung by The Velvet Underground, in 1964), David Bowie, and Jerry Garcia.

SEE ALSO Opium (c. 2500 BCE), Morphine (1806), Aspirin (1899), Methadone (1947), Opioids (1973), OxyContin (1996).

Heroin, initially introduced as a safer substitute for morphine, soon became synonymous with the most negative aspects of drug addiction and has long been judged among the most dangerous drugs to both the user and society. Here a woman is preparing her heroin for a syringe to keep up with her addiction.

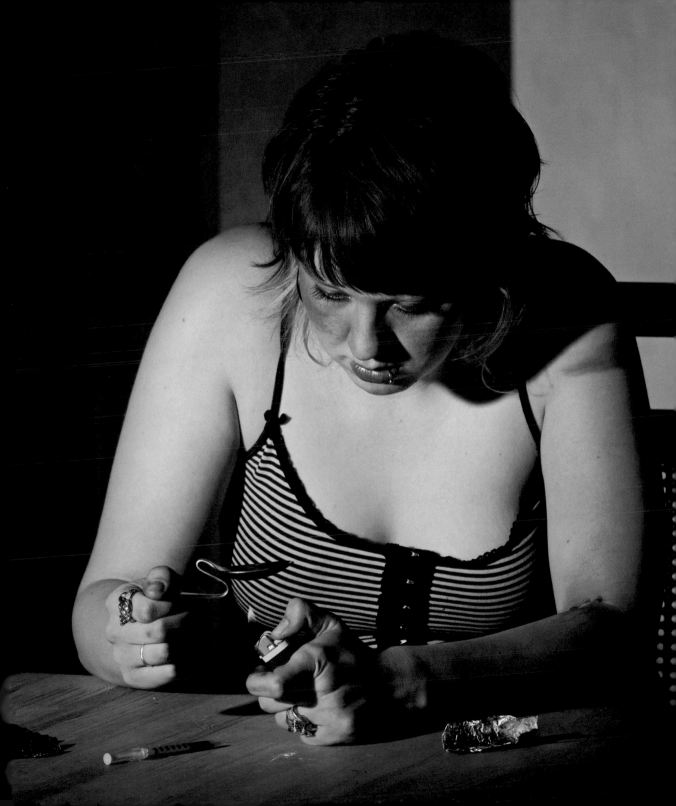

Aspirin

Heinrich Dreser (1860–1924), **Arthur Eichengrün** (1867–1949), **Felix Hoffmann** (1968–1946), **John Vane** (1927–2004)

Aspirin is one of the cheapest, most readily available, and widely used drugs in the world for the reduction of fever and relief of pain and inflammation. It is also routinely used as a "blood thinner" to prevent clots, reducing the risk of heart attack and stroke. Regular aspirin use may also reduce the risk of several cancers and Alzheimer's disease—claims that are not yet substantiated.

Aspirin, a product introduced into medicine in 1899, transformed F. Bayer & Company from a small German dye company to an international pharmaceutical and chemical giant. But who at Bayer was responsible for aspirin's discovery? The principal claimants were Felix Hoffmann, Heinrich Dreser, and Arthur Eichengrün. Hoffmann, the chemist who synthesized aspirin in 1897, is generally acknowledged as aspirin's discoverer. He later said that he prepared it as a substitute for the sodium salicylate his father was taking for rheumatism. Dreser was responsible for the pharmacological evaluation of new chemicals at Bayer but lacked initial interest in testing aspirin. After his **heroin** pet project had begun to show signs of failure, however, he became aspirin's champion and authored an early paper on its effectiveness—omitting reference to Hoffmann and Eichengrün. Eichengrün, the director of pharmaceutical research, aggressively promoted the secret testing of aspirin by Berlin physicians, even when actively discouraged by upper management.

Recent evidence suggests that Eichengrün, and not Hoffmann, should receive credit for aspirin's discovery. Before his death in 1949, Eichengrün claimed that he directed Hoffmann to synthesize acetylsalicylic acid, although Hoffmann was unaware of why. Moreover, Eichengrün did not challenge Hoffmann's 1934 claim to be the discoverer because, as a Jew in Nazi Germany, he needed to maintain a low profile.

Not in dispute was the trade name *Aspirin* for acetylsalicyclic acid, with *a* representing *acetyl* and *spirin* representing *Spiraea ulmaria*, the former name of a plant from which salicylic acid is derived. Seven decades after the release of aspirin, John Vane, at the University of London, determined how aspirin works: All its major effects can be attributed to its ability to inhibit the synthesis of prostaglandins, which play a major role in pain, fever, and inflammation.

SEE ALSO Heroin (1898), Acetaminophen/Paracetamol (1953), Plavix (1997), Enbrel, Remicide and Humira (1998).

From the time of its introduction, aspirin has been called a wonder drug. Reports of new medical applications continue to appear far beyond those promoted in this 1923 French advertisement.

Migraines, Névralgies, Rhumatismes

Demandez à
votre Pharmacien

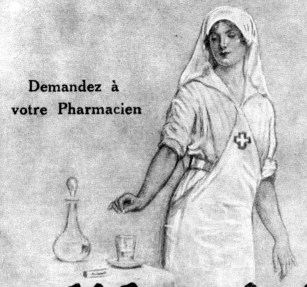

l'Aspirine
"USINES du RHÔNE"

En TUBES de 20 COMPRIMÉS

LABORATOIRE des PRODUITS USINES du RHÔNE
21, Rue Jean Goujon, PARIS

Epinephrine/Adrenaline

George Oliver (1841–1915), **Edward Schafer** (1850–1935), **Jockichi Takamine** (1854–1922), **Walter Bradford Cannon** (1871–1945)

Epinephrine/adrenaline has attracted the enthusiastic interest of scientists and the medical community for more than a century. It was the first hormone isolated in pure crystalline form and quickly played an important role in medical clinics and operating rooms. Notable physiologists focused attention on its protective functions when stress and danger confront the body.

In the mid-1890s, George Oliver and Edward Schafer, working at University College, London, determined that injections of adrenal gland extracts increased blood pressure in animals to an extent not previously seen. Not surprisingly, attempts were made in various laboratories to isolate the chemical responsible for this powerful response. Credit for the successful purification of epinephrine (alternatively called adrenaline in the United Kingdom and British Commonwealth) belongs to Jockichi Takamine, a Japanese American chemist. In 1901, Takamine assigned his patented process to Parke, Davis & Company, which marketed it as Adrenalin and made Takamine extremely wealthy.

Within a few years, epinephrine/adrenaline was widely used for the emergency treatment of acute asthmatic attacks, heart failure, sudden and severe drops in blood pressure, and bronchial asthma. In operating rooms, this drug is applied to the skin and mucous membranes to control superficial bleeding by shrinking blood vessels. When combined with local anesthetics, it extends their duration of action. Many of these therapeutic applications continue to be of value in contemporary medical practice.

Walter Cannon, an illustrious American physiologist at Harvard Medical School studied in detail the role of epinephrine/adrenaline in our "fight or flight" response to fear and extreme stress. Cannon initially published his findings in 1915 and popularized them in his 1932 book *The Wisdom of the Body*. Mediated largely by epinephrine/adrenaline, these "fight or flight" responses—including increases in heart rate and blood pressure, redirection of blood flow to voluntary muscles, enhanced breathing efficiency, and increased blood glucose to provide energy—have all permitted us to survive.

SEE ALSO Percorten (1939), Albuterol/Salbutamol (1968), Ephedra/Ephedrine (1994).

This illustration from Gray's Anatomy (1870) depicts the adrenal (suprarenal) gland sitting as a cap atop the kidney. The adrenal gland consists of two distinct structures: the outer adrenal cortex, which secretes such hormones as cortisol (hydrocortisone) and aldosterone, and the inner adrenal medulla that produces epinephrine (adrenaline) and norepinephrine.

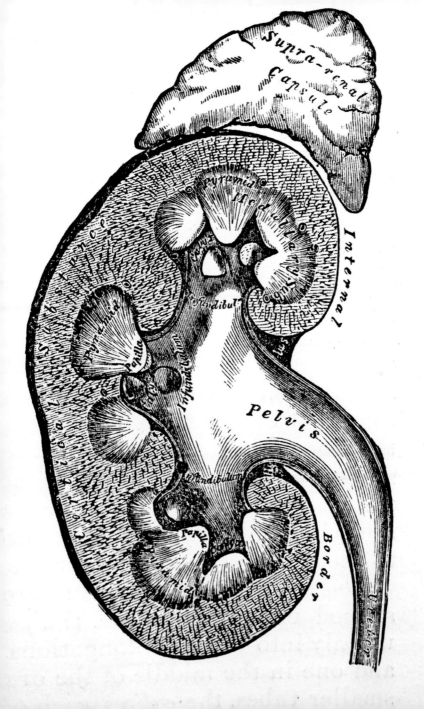

Phenolphthalein

The use of herbs to facilitate bowel movements probably represents one of the very earliest internal uses of drugs to correct a medical problem. An obsession with the frequency and consistency of bowel movements has survived antiquity and is very much with us today—whether motivated by the desire to remain healthy, to deal with a medical problem, or to follow a weight loss program.

Before the twentieth century, when the causes of disease were not well understood and the practice of medicine was based on relief of symptoms, a wide assortment of drugs were used to deal with recalcitrant bowels. Textbooks of the day contained extensive drug classifications and included such terms as *aperient*, *laxative*, *purgative*, *cathartic*, and *drastic*. Our contemporary books have happily truncated this list to four, based on how the drugs facilitate bowel movements.

One reliable source states that more than 700 different laxative preparations were available in the United States in the early 1970s. The best-selling laxatives of that time contained phenolphthalein, the same acid-base indicator you used in your chemistry laboratory. As a drug, it was the active ingredient in (chocolate-coated) Ex-Lax, as well as Feen-A-Mint, Correctol, and Carter's Little Liver Pills. Phenolphthalein's laxative properties were discovered quite by accident in 1902, after the Hungarian government ordered that it be added to wines to detect adulteration. Those who excessively imbibed the wine experienced diarrhea. The result was a new laxative that was colorless, tasteless, dependable, perceived to be safe, and pleasant to use.

After more than ninety years of successful use, phenolphthalein's drug days came to an abrupt end when, in 1996, it was shown to cause cancer in laboratory animals. Products containing phenolphthalein were hastily removed from the shelves, but they reappeared shortly thereafter, bearing their familiar time-honored names, but with another drug as their active laxative ingredient. It's the trade name that sells, not the active ingredient.

SEE ALSO Patent Medicine (1623).

A 1919 French advertisement not only promoted Jubol to relieve constipation but also to assuage vertigo, hemorrhoids, indigestion, and migraine headaches. Note the diligent workers cleaning out the intestinal cavity.

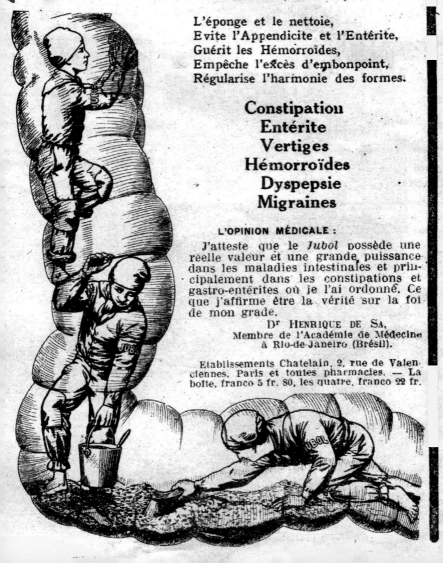

Barbital

Adolf von Baeyer (1835–1917), **Josef von Mering** (1849–1908), **Emil Fischer** (1852–1919)

MOTHER OF ALL OF BARBITURATES. Adolf von Baeyer went to a Munich tavern on December 4, 1864, St. Barbara's Day, to celebrate. He had successfully synthesized malonylurea, which—likely in honor of St. Barbara—he termed barbituric acid. He could not have realized at the time how significant his finding would be to the practice of medicine.

Barbital, the first barbituric acid derivative, was introduced into therapy as a sleep-producing and antiseizure barbiturate in 1903 by the German chemist Emil Fischer and physician Josef von Mering. An etymological controversy surrounds the derivation of barbital's trade name Veronal. Perhaps it was based on the Latin word *verus* (*truth*), an allusion to barbital being the true hypnotic. Then again, it might have referred to the Italian city of Verona, a peaceful vacation spot for von Mering.

Before barbital, there were the **bromides** (1857), **chloral hydrate** (1869), and **paraldehyde** (1882). After its appearance, barbital enjoyed widespread use for a decade until the appearance of **phenobarbital** (Luminal) in 1912, a drug that continues to be prescribed today. More than 2,500 derivatives of barbituric acid have been synthesized over the years, and about fifty of these were used for anxiety, insomnia, anesthesia, and seizure disorders. Barbiturates differ primarily with respect to their time of onset and their duration of action. Interestingly, the British refer to barbital as *barbitone*, preferring the suffix *-one* to the standard American and international barbiturate suffix of *-al*.

Barbiturates continued to be very widely used until the 1950s, when **Librium**, **Valium**, and related benzodiazepines appeared. The benzodiazepines were more specific, had fewer side effects and reduced potential to be abused, and were safer when taken in excessive doses, accidentally or intentionally.

Both Fischer and Baeyer were awarded Nobel Prizes in Chemistry, but not for their work on barbituric acid or barbiturates. Fischer significantly advanced our understanding of proteins and received the Prize in 1902 for his work on the chemistry and synthesis of sugars and purines. Among his many other accomplishments, Baeyer received the 1905 Prize for his synthesis of the indigo dye used in blue jeans.

SEE ALSO Bromides (1857), Chloral Hydrate (1869), Paraldehyde (1882), Phenobarbital (1912), Nembutal and Seconal (1928), Thiopental (1934), Librium (1960), Valium (1963).

Barbital and related barbiturates were initially promoted for producing restful and natural sleep. Research demonstrated that these drugs disrupted normal sleep patterns, however, leading to insomnia and disturbed sleep when abruptly stopped after long-term usage.

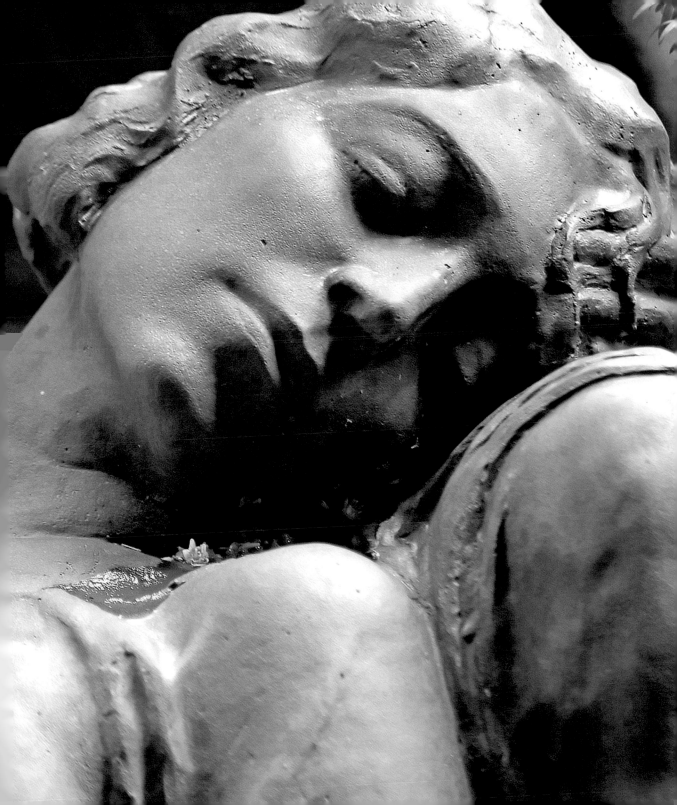

Atoxyl

David Livingstone (1813–1873), Paul Ehrlich (1854–1915)

European exploration and colonization of much of the world began in the late fifteenth century, but it was not until almost 400 years later that attention focused on the neglected interior of the African continent. The attraction of rich, untapped natural resources outweighed the challenges of deserts, jungles, hostile people, and unique, devastating diseases.

COMBATING SLEEPING SICKNESS. African sleeping sickness, or trypanosomiasis, has long been a significant health problem in the hot and humid regions of central and southern Africa. The disease is caused by several species of trypanosomes—spindle-shaped protozoa with trailing flagella—and transmitted by the bite of the tsetse fly. The primary victims are humans and domesticated cattle, and they invariably die in a state of profound drowsiness within months if not treated.

One of many sleeping-sickness epidemics occurred in the Congo region from 1896 to 1906 and claimed some 300,000 to 500,000 human lives. This episode served as an impetus for European medical scientists to develop an effective treatment and coincided with the early years of treating infectious diseases with synthetic chemicals.

In 1858, the Scottish medical missionary and African explorer David Livingstone—immortalized by the *New York Herald* correspondent Henry Stanley's supposed greeting, "Dr. Livingstone, I presume?"—proposed using Fowler's solution (potassium arsenite) for the treatment of sleeping sickness. In 1905, the more effective and safer organic arsenic compound Atoxyl was found useful. Atoxyl failed to live up to its benign name, however, causing blindness via damage to the optic nerve. In the early 1920s, the Atoxyl derivative tryparsamide was developed at the Rockefeller Institute, and when used in combination with suramin (Bayer 205; Germanin), it remained the treatment of choice for sleeping sickness for four decades.

While seeking safer and more effective organic arsenic compounds than Atoxyl for sleeping sickness, Paul Ehrlich redirected his efforts and discovered arsphenamine (**Salvarsan**) in 1910, the first cure for syphilis.

SEE ALSO Salvarsan (1910).

The medical missionary–explorer David Livingstone was among the first Westerners to travel across the African continent—a journey impeded by the prevalence of malaria, dysentery, and sleeping sickness, for which he recommended Fowler's solution, an inorganic precursor to the organic arsenical, Atoxyl. In his well-publicized writings, he actively supported the abolition of slavery.

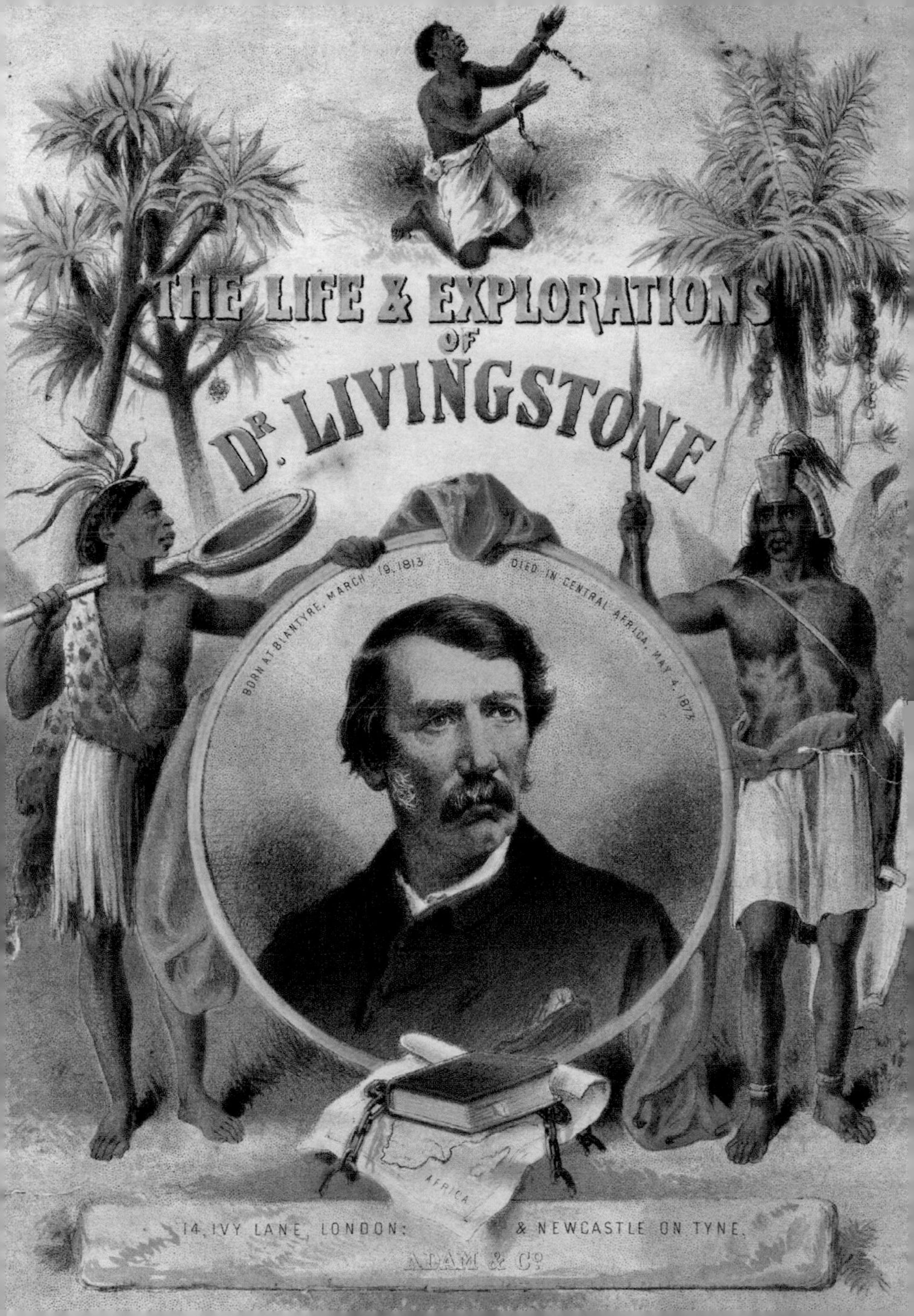

THE LIFE & EXPLORATIONS
OF
DR. LIVINGSTONE

BORN AT BLANTYRE, MARCH 19, 1813

DIED IN CENTRAL AFRICA, MAY 4, 1873

AFRICA

14, IVY LANE, LONDON;   & NEWCASTLE ON TYNE.
ADAM & CO.

Novocain

Alfred Einhorn (1856–1917)

Novocain is so ingrained in our drug vocabulary that it needs little explanation. When visiting dentists, we are told that we will first be given a "shot of Novocain to numb the tooth." Although it's highly unlikely that we are getting the "real" Novocain, we are getting a first cousin that acts in a similar manner. Nevertheless, for more than a hundred years, *Novocain* has remained a synonym for a *local anesthetic*—a drug that causes a loss of sensation of pain in a restricted or localized site, without altering consciousness.

Cocaine, a naturally occurring chemical isolated from the **coca** leaf, was the first local anesthetic, introduced in 1884. It was highly effective but toxic, causing a number of fatalities and addictions—a limitation recognized within a few short years. In 1892, German chemist Alfred Einhorn, a professor at the University of Munich, began his search for a safer alternative that was not subject to abuse. After multiple attempts at finding a suitable chemical, in 1905 Einhorn discovered the first injectable local anesthetic, procaine, which was given the trade name *Novocain*.

After Novocain is injected, it rapidly gains access to the bloodstream and is rapidly inactivated by the enzyme cholinesterase. Hence, it is usually given in combination with **epinephrine/adrenaline**, which constricts blood vessels in order to prolong the time Novocain will continue to act and to reduce the likelihood that large amounts will enter the circulatory system and cause toxicity. Unlike cocaine, Novocain is ineffective when applied topically.

Following the appearance of Novocain, hundreds of potential local anesthetics have been synthesized, which by convention end in *-caine*. Some two dozen have been marketed for use by injection or local application and occasionally both. Procaine remained the primary local anesthetic until 1948, when **Xylocaine**—a superior drug that can be applied topically or injected—was introduced.

SEE ALSO Coca (1532), Cocaine (1884), Epinephrine/Adrenaline (1901), Xylocaine (1948).

This painting by Johann Liss (c. 1597–1631), based on a copper engraving by Lucas van Leyden (1494–1533), depicts a medieval dentist removing a tooth—without the benefit of Novocain.

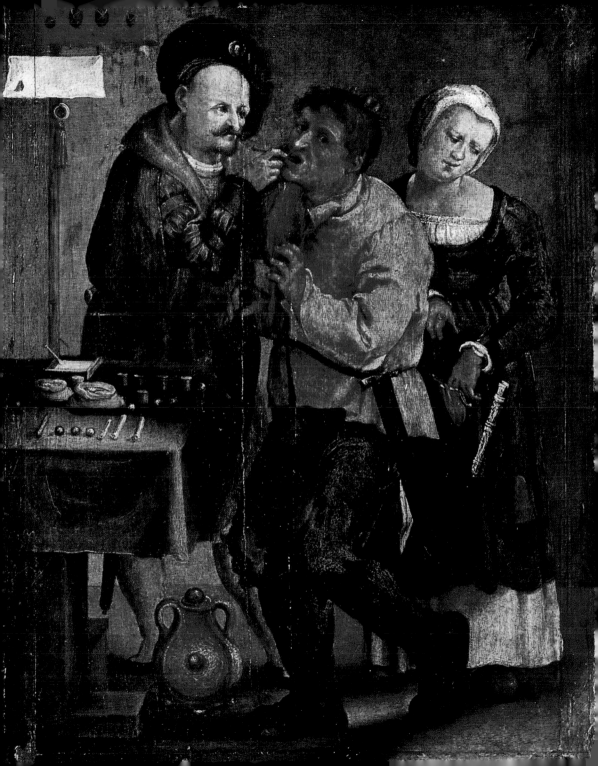

Drug Receptors

John Newport Langley (1852–1925), **Paul Ehrlich** (1854–1915)

How do drugs produce their effects on the heart or brain? Drugs do not work by uniformly affecting these organs but rather by acting on specific sites called receptors, located in or on the surface of cells. The concept of receptors emerged in the early twentieth century from studies by the English physiologist John Newport Langley and the German microbiologist and chemist Paul Ehrlich. Drugs can produce their effects by acting on many different kinds of receptors, which can, in turn, cause muscle contraction, gland secretion, or mood alteration.

Although a somewhat gross oversimplification, we can envision the interaction of a receptor and drug to be analogous to a lock and key. Just as the correct key fits the keyhole and opens the lock, the "correct" drug binds to a receptor and initiates a response. Further, very similar keys can sometimes open the same lock, and very similar drugs can produce a comparable response. The specific nature of that response differs depending upon where in the body the receptor is located.

Some keys perfectly fit, while others are close enough to fit the keyhole but not close enough to open the lock. An agonist is a drug that perfectly fits the receptor to produce a response. Other drugs called antagonists less perfectly attach to the receptor, and not only fail to produce a response but also prevent the agonist from acting. Receptors were designed in our bodies to interact with natural agonists, such as **neurotransmitters** or hormones.

There are more than fifty different receptor and sub-receptor types. Drugs that interact with multiple receptor types are likely to produce multiple effects, desirable and undesirable. Over the years, drugs have become increasingly selective in their ability to interact with specific receptors.

SEE ALSO Neurotransmitters (1920), Opioids (1973).

The interaction of a drug and a given receptor is analogous to a lock and key.

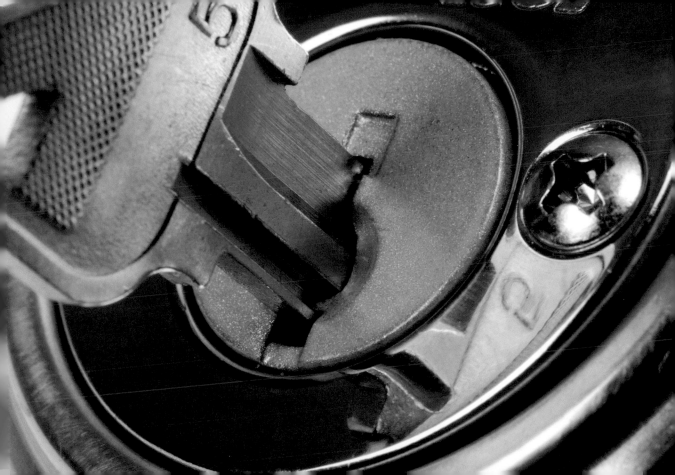

Pure Food and Drug Act

Theodore Roosevelt (1858–1919), Samuel Hopkins Adams (1871–1958), Upton Sinclair (1878–1968)

Many of the best-selling **patent medicines** available at the turn of the twentieth century claimed to not only benefit but actually "cure" a range of medical problems, including cancer, infertility, tuberculosis, epilepsy, and "female complaints," to name very few. Although they contained secret formulas, none contained "harmful" ingredients—or so claimed testimonials or the creative pens of manufacturers. Two monumental works by American activists destroyed these long-held myths and led to the passage of the first federal legislation enacted to protect the public from unsafe medications—the Pure Food and Drug Act, which President Theodore Roosevelt signed into law in 1906.

Upton Sinclair's 1906 novel *The Jungle* was written with the intent of exposing the meat-packing industry and the exploitation of its workers. The revolting and grossly unsanitary conditions Sinclair described in the preparation of meat products succeeded in catching the public's attention. In October 1905, the first of an eleven-article series titled "The Great American Fraud," authored by the investigative reporter Samuel Hopkins Adams, appeared in *Collier's Weekly*. In these articles, which were reprinted the following year as a book, Adams exposed the false claims patent medicine manufacturers made for their products and the harmful and even dangerous nature of their ingredients.

The rapidly enacted Pure Food and Drug Act prohibited adulterated and misbranded foods and drugs and destroyed the cloak of secrecy concealing the presence of potentially harmful and habit-forming patent medicines. Although the act did not outlaw the inclusion of **alcohol**, **morphine**, **opium**, **cocaine**, or **cannabis** in nonprescription products, products containing these substances had to disclose their presence and amounts. To some, Adams may be better known as the author of "Night Bus," a short story that served as the basis for the 1934 film (and winner of five major Academy Awards) *It Happened One Night*, starring Clark Gable and Claudette Colbert.

SEE ALSO Alcohol (c. 10,000 BCE), Cannabis (c. 3000), Opium (c. 2500 BCE), Patent Medicine (1623), Morphine (1806), Cocaine (1884), Food and Drug Administration (1906), Federal Food, Drug, and Cosmetic Act (1938), Kefauver-Harris Amendment (1962).

This 1909 advertisement was rather restrained when compared to others of the period. Malt Rainier tonic, a liquid extract of malt and hops, claimed to provide the user with "new vigor and strength in every drop."

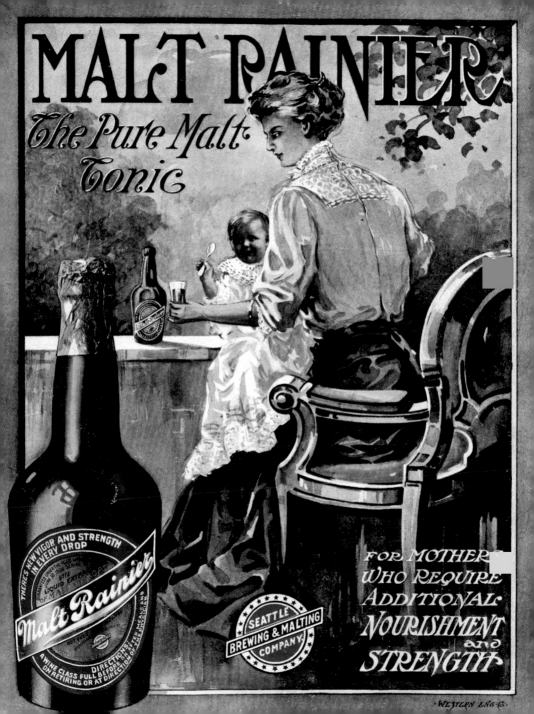

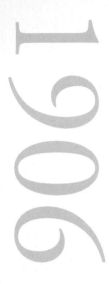

Food and Drug Administration

Harvey Washington Wiley (1844–1930)

American consumers had little federal protection against misbranded and adulterated foods and drugs before the twentieth century. The **Pure Food and Drug Act** of 1906, which led to the establishment of the Food and Drug Administration (FDA), was intended to correct this deplorable situation and has served as a model for the decentralized, newly renamed European Medicines Agency, as well as comparable agencies around the world.

The FDA's origins go back to 1883, when Harvey Washington Wiley was appointed chief chemist of the U.S. Department of Agriculture's Division of Chemistry (later Bureau of Chemistry). Wiley's efforts, coupled with published works by literary muckrakers, heightened public awareness of the hazards in the food-and-drug marketplace, and in 1906, the USDA Bureau of Chemistry—renamed the Food and Drug Administration in 1930—was charged with examining and testing all food and drug products. Early efforts were focused upon removing unsafe patent medicines from the market and preventing misleading drug claims. The **Federal Food, Drug, and Cosmetic Acts** of 1938 and 1962 authorized the FDA to require that manufacturers provide evidence for the safety and effectiveness of their new drugs before marketing.

The FDA regulates 25 percent of consumer expenditures in the United States. Thus, manufacturers, legislators, patient advocacy groups, and the media attempt to influence FDA policies and decisions. Points of contention include the speed of drug approval (not fast enough for manufacturers and some patient groups); removal of potentially dangerous dietary supplements and previously approved drugs from the market; regulation of the dietary supplement industries; appointment of FDA advisory committee members based on political considerations; and the legalization of **medical marijuana**.

While there is far from international agreement on all FDA decisions and drug approvals, their rigorous standards for evaluating drug safety, effectiveness, and purity remain the "gold standard" in the pharmaceutical regulatory world.

SEE ALSO Patent Medicines (1623), Medical Marijuana (1839), Pure Food and Drug Act (1906), Federal Food, Drug, and Cosmetic Act (1938), Thalidomide (1957), Kefauver-Harris Amendment (1962), Dietary Supplements (1994).

The approval process primarily involves balancing drug effectiveness with its potential adverse effects and risks. What constitutes an acceptable risk is relative and depends on the severity of the medical condition (minor vs. life threatening). Often, scientists and clinicians differ in their assessment of evidence supporting benefits and risks and whether, in the final analysis, the drug should be approved for marketing.

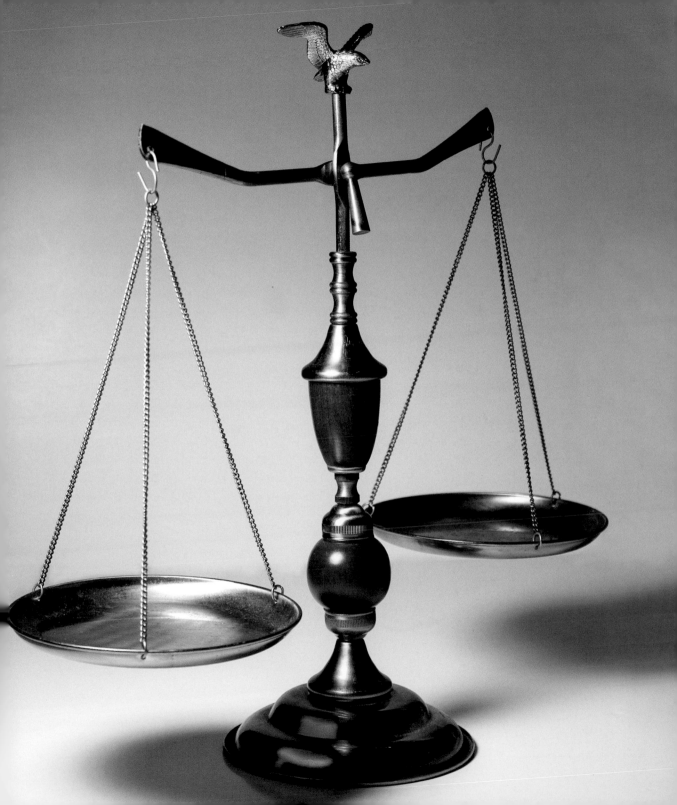

Oxytocin

Vincent du Vigneaud (1901–1978)

Some 100 years ago, extracts prepared from the posterior pituitary gland were first used to induce labor and stop uterine bleeding after delivery—effects attributed to oxytocin, a drug that continues to be employed for these purposes in childbirth. In 1928, scientists at Parke, Davis & Company separated oxytocin from vasopressin, another hormone in the gland. In 1953, at Cornell Medical College in New York, the American biochemist Vincent du Vigneaud isolated pure oxytocin, which he found contained nine amino acids. For synthesizing the first peptide hormone, du Vigneaud was awarded the 1955 Nobel Prize in Chemistry.

Synthetic oxytocin produces the same effects as the natural hormone. Before childbirth, oxytocin is released from the posterior pituitary gland, a pea-size structure located at the base of the brain. This hormone plays a key role in causing dilation of the uterus (stage 1 of labor) and contraction of the muscles of the uterus, leading to expulsion of the fetus and placenta (stages 2 and 3). To induce labor, oxytocin (Pitocin) is slowly injected intravenously.

Oxytocin is also involved in nursing. During breast-feeding, the infant's suckling stimulates oxytocin release, which causes mammary glands to contract and excrete milk during the "milk let-down" process.

The role of oxytocin in enhancing human sexual behavior remains the subject of scientific inquiry. Some reports suggest that oxytocin levels are elevated and may play a role in the sexual arousal of both men and women and in orgasm in women. Oxytocin may also promote bonding between individuals, mother and baby, and adult couples, increasing trust and decreasing fear.

SEE ALSO Ergotamine and Ergonovine (1925).

The naturally occurring hormone oxytocin is involved in many aspects of maternal behavior, including childbirth and nursing, and it may even promote bonding between mother and baby.

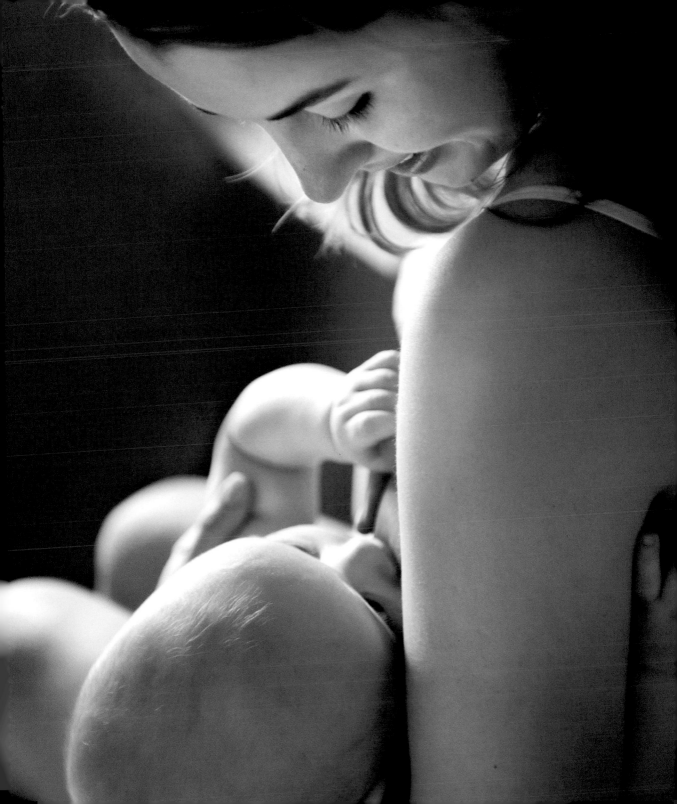

Salvarsan

Paul Ehrlich (1854–1915), Sacachiro Hata (1873–1938)

Paul Ehrlich was one of the outstanding biomedical scientists of the twentieth century, distinguishing himself through significant discoveries in pharmacology, the chemistry of drugs, bacteriology, pathology, and immunology, including his "side-chain theory" of antibody formation, for which he received the 1908 Nobel Prize. His discoveries of **Atoxyl** for sleeping sickness and, more important, Salvarsan for syphilis, established his reputation as the Father of Chemotherapy.

German-born and medically trained, Ehrlich spent the first twenty years of his scientific career investigating the selective staining of cells and tissues by dye substances. He noted that some cells were stained, while others remained colorless, and he was the first to stain the tuberculosis-causing microbe, permitting its visualization for diagnostic purposes. He postulated that drugs interact with selective chemical groupings on cells, which he termed *receptors*.

IN SEARCH OF THE MAGIC BULLET. These studies led Ehrlich to theorize that drugs could be selectively toxic to infectious-disease-causing microbes and harmless to the patient. Seeking such a "magic bullet" and working with his Japanese colleague Sacachiro Hata at the Georg-Speyer-Haus Institute in Frankfurt, he tested hundreds of organic arsenic-containing compounds to discover a cure for syphilis. A major public health scourge that had afflicted Europe for at least four centuries, syphilis was previously treated with highly toxic mercury for the duration of a patient's lifetime.

The 606th of these chemicals, arsphenamine or Compound 606, proved to be highly effective against the syphilis-causing microbe. It required multiple injections and often caused serious adverse effects; thus, it was not quite the "magic bullet" Ehrlich had envisioned. The drug, marketed as Salvarsan, appeared 1910, and two years later his improved compound Neosalvarsan was released, remaining the primary treatment for syphilis until **penicillin** became available at the end of World War II.

Ehrlich's discovery of Salvarsan and the initial opposition he encountered before its medical acceptance (incited, in part, by anti-Semitism) are depicted in the classic 1941 film *Dr. Ehrlich's Magic Bullet*, with Edward G. Robinson in the title role.

SEE ALSO Atoxyl (1905), Drug Receptors (1905), Penicillin (1928).

Congenital syphilis can become a severe and chronic disease that affects the cardiovascular and neurological systems and causes abnormalities in the lower leg, as depicted in this late 1930s poster. Salvarsan and related drugs continued to be used for the treatment of syphilis until 1944.

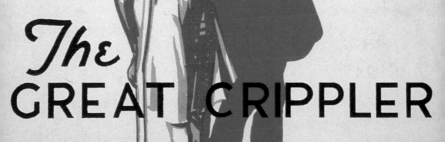

The
GREAT CRIPPLER

SYPHILIS

PRODUCED FOR TOWN OF HEMPSTEAD HEALTH DEPT. BY FEDERAL ART PROJECT NASSAU CO. W.P.A.

Phenobarbital

Alfred Hauptmann (1881–1948)

The barbiturates were the most versatile nervous system depressants available during the first half of the twentieth century. Unlike the **bromides**, **paraldehyde**, and **chloral hydrate** that preceded them, the degree of central-nervous-system depression produced by barbiturates can be controlled by the dose. Small doses calm and produce sedation, higher doses induce sleep, and still higher doses produce surgical anesthesia. Beyond these doses—and particularly when washed down with **alcohol**—barbiturates are all too effective in causing irreversible coma.

Phenobarbital, a long-acting barbiturate introduced in 1912 under the trade name Luminal, was initially marketed for sedation and to induce sleep. That same year, German psychiatrist and neurologist Alfred Hauptmann administered phenobarbital to his epileptic patients to enable them (and him) to sleep through the night. It worked, and much to his surprise, they experienced far fewer seizures during the daytime. Moreover, unlike the bromides—the principle antiseizure drugs at that time—phenobarbital did not cause excessive sedation. It was the most effective drug available for tonic-clonic (grand mal) seizures until 1938, when **Dilantin**, a far less sedating drug, displaced it.

Phenobarbital has low toxicity and continues to be used at a very low cost, but it can modify the effects of other drugs taken at the same time. By increasing the activity of many enzymes—biological catalysts that chemically convert drugs into products that are generally less active and more readily removed from the body—phenobarbital can reduce the plasma concentration and effectiveness of such drugs as oral contraceptives, the blood thinner **warfarin**, and certain antidepressants.

A MASS SUICIDE DRUG. Heaven's Gate, a California-based doomsday religious cult that believed they had to evacuate the earth in March 1997 as quickly as possible, used phenobarbital to assist them in their exit strategy. Under the direction of their spiritual leader, Marshall Applewhite, thirty-nine followers committed suicide by ingesting a mixture of phenobarbital and applesauce or pudding, followed by vodka. To ensure the completion of their deadly mission, they placed plastic bags over their heads.

SEE ALSO Alcohol (c. 10,000 BCE), Bromides (1857), Chloral Hydrate (1869), Barbital (1903), Dilantin (1938), Warfarin (1940), Librium (1960), Valproic Acid (1967).

Despite suffering from epilepsy most of his life, Grover Cleveland Alexander (1887–1950) was one of major league baseball's greatest players, pitching for the Phillies, Cubs, and Cardinals between 1911 and 1930. His epileptic seizures were often mistaken for heavy-drinking behavior, and the film The Winning Team (1952), *with Ronald Reagan portraying Alexander, never mentions his epilepsy.*

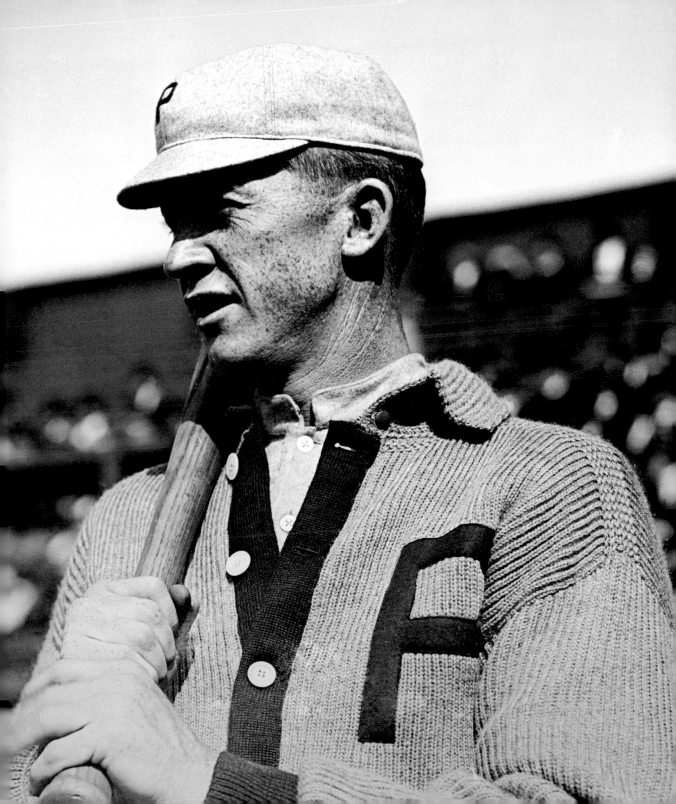

Quinidine

Karl-Friedrich Wenckebach (1864–1940)

The **cinchona bark** of Peru and its active chemical **quinine** are most commonly associated with malaria. However, eighteenth-century reports described how quinine also corrected heart problems in malaria sufferers who experienced abnormal heart rhythms. In 1912, a Dutch merchant who sought assistance in ridding himself of atrial fibrillation visited the eminent Dutch cardiologist Karl-Friedrich Wenckebach. In this condition, the upper heart chambers (the atria) are beating too fast and causing palpitations. Wenckebach professed an inability to help. The patient returned the following morning with a regular heartbeat, explaining that he took quinine, which benefited him on business trips to countries in which malaria was common. Wenckebach tried quinine in some patients, with disappointing results, and shared these findings in his 1914 book on arrhythmias.

Wenckebach's account inspired the German physician Walter Frey to compare the effects of quinine and quinidine, another naturally occurring **alkaloid** in cinchona bark, on his patients with atrial fibrillation. Frey's 1918 report showed the superiority of quinidine, leading to its widespread use for a variety of heart rhythm disorders.

Quinidine continues to be used for the treatment of a wide range of arrhythmias and has been joined by almost twenty other antiarrhythmic drugs over the years. Based on their rather complex mechanisms of action, these drugs have been categorized into four major classes, several subclasses, and a fifth "miscellaneous" class.

While most arrhythmias neither interfere with the heart's ability to pump blood nor present a health risk, some can be life threatening. "Pharmacophiles" note that the use of antiarrhythmic drugs is declining; they can worsen existing arrhythmias and even cause new ones. Moreover, new nondrug approaches, such as artificial pacemakers, defibrillators, and surgical procedures, are more effective and are now the preferred treatments. In short, drugs are not always the first and best means of treating medical disorders.

SEE ALSO Cinchona Bark (1639), Alkaloids (1806), Quinine (1820), Xylocaine (1948), Propranolol (1964).

The electrocardiogram (ECG) is used to measure heart rhythm disorders and monitor the effectiveness of quinidine and other antiarrhythmic drugs. This compact, portable monitoring device has evolved from Einthoven's very cumbersome laboratory apparatus first used in 1903.

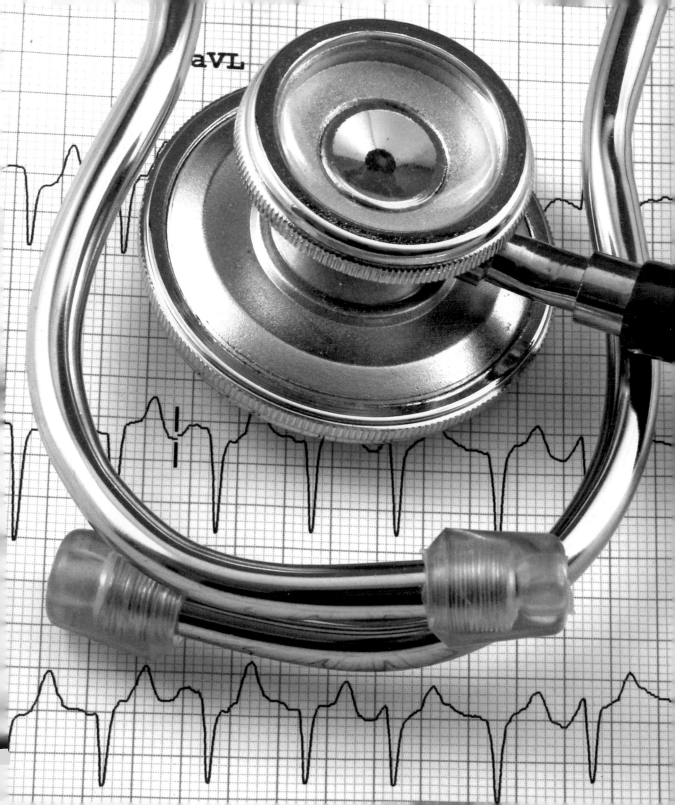

Thyroxine

William Gull (1816–1890), **George Redmayne Murray** (1865–1939), **Edward Calvin Kendall** (1886–1972)

The thyroid gland, which lies under the skin just below the Adam's apple, was first described in 1656. Its function and larger size in women remained the subject of speculation—some overtly sexist—throughout the greater part of the nineteenth century. In 1873, English physician William Gull first showed an association between the gland's atrophy and the symptoms of sluggish thyroid function, or hypothyroidism. English physician George Redmayne Murray followed up on Gull's findings and, in 1891, successfully treated hypothyroidism with injections of sheep thyroid extract. Thyroxine, the thyroid gland's principal hormone, was isolated in pure form at the Mayo Clinic in 1914 by the American chemist Edward Kendall, who later received the 1950 Nobel Prize for his work on **cortisone**.

KEEPING THE BODY'S FURNACE BURNING. The thyroid gland is primarily involved in regulating the metabolism of most tissues, increasing the rate at which calories are burned and heat is produced, and it plays a critical role in the growth and development of the brain, in particular. The gland actively concentrates iodine obtained from food and water and becomes enlarged, producing a "goiter," in iodine's absence. The typical hypothyroid adult is overweight, sluggish, with cold and dry skin and a low rate of metabolism—and, thus, is very sensitive to cold. If iodine deficiency is not diagnosed in newborns, permanent mental retardation (cretinism) can result.

Hypothyroidism is by no measure a rare condition. It affects some 200 million people worldwide and 3 percent of the North American population, although many of these individuals go undiagnosed. A dietary deficiency is its most common cause in many developing countries but is rare in countries in which iodine is added to table salt or diets are rich in seafood. Other causes include an autoimmune disorder, exposure to radioactive iodine, or surgical removal of the gland.

Regardless of the cause, natural or synthetic thyroid hormones, when taken for a lifetime, provide excellent relief of symptoms, although they do not produce a cure. The variety of available products includes extracts of the beef or pork gland and the much-preferred levothyroxine (**Synthroid**), a synthetic preparation of thyroxine.

SEE ALSO Radioiodide (1946), Cortisone (1949), Synthroid (1997).

Among roughly one hundred suspected perpetrators of the Whitechapel murders of eleven women in London from 1888 to 1891, Dr. William Gull, a pioneer in treating thyroid disease, was identified as Jack the Ripper in a number of films and books. His candidacy for this infamous role is no stronger than that of other contenders, however.

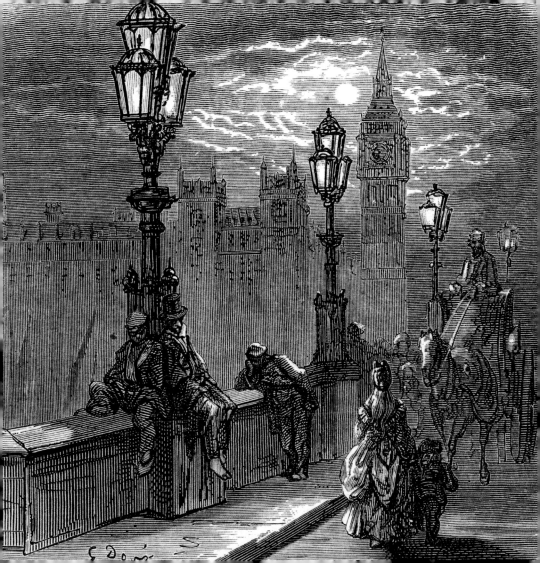

Heparin

William Henry Howell (1860–1945), **Jay McLean** (1890–1957), **Gordon Murray** (1894–1976), **Charles Best** (1899–1978)

Heparin's journey from discovery to clinical use was long, tortuous, and controversial. In 1916, Jay McLean, a second-year medical school student working in the laboratory of William Henry Howell, a distinguished Professor of Physiology at Johns Hopkins University, isolated an anticoagulant from a dog liver. Two years later, Howell isolated another distinct anticoagulant from the liver and named it heparin (from Greek *hepar*, or *liver*).

Although Howell's heparin was impure and caused toxic reactions, its promise was recognized. Starting in the late 1920s, Charles Best (of **insulin** fame) and members of his laboratory at the University of Toronto set out to purify it—a method not accomplished until 1936. In 1937, Gordon Murray, one of Canada's most famous surgeons, first used heparin to prevent clotting in veins and in kidney-dialysis machines.

Heparin, which retards the ability of blood to clot in blood vessels, is used during open-heart surgery, bypass surgery, kidney dialysis, blood transfusions, and pregnancy. Medically used heparin is prepared from the lungs of cattle and intestines of pigs. Although heparin and related anticoagulants are colloquially referred to as "blood thinners," they do not thin the blood or dissolve blood clots. Rather, they prevent clots from becoming larger and blocking the flow of blood in blood vessels, which can have lethal consequences.

The anticoagulant effects of heparin begin almost immediately after being injected and continue for several hours. Heparin is a medical "double-edged sword": It can be lifesaving, but if not used at correct doses and monitored carefully, potentially fatal bleeding can occur. This danger was highlighted in 2007, when the twelve-day-old twins of the actor Dennis Quaid were mistakenly given 1,000 times the recommended dose with near-fatal results.

Credit for the discovery of heparin has shifted over the years and currently remains a subject of active debate among medical historians. Before the 1940s, Howell was overwhelmingly lauded for this honor. After Howell's death in 1945, McLean aggressively campaigned in national lectures and published articles that it was *he* who discovered, or at least co-discovered, heparin.

SEE ALSO Aspirin (1899), Insulin (1921), Warfarin (1940), Plavix (1997), Pradaxa (2010).

William Henry Howell (1860–1945) had a career-long passion for the physiology of blood coagulation. This research led to the 1916 discovery of heparin, a substance naturally circulating in the blood that inhibits coagulation within blood vessels. Howell's studies in the 1930s were instrumental to the introduction of heparin into clinical practice for the treatment of life-threatening clotting disorders.

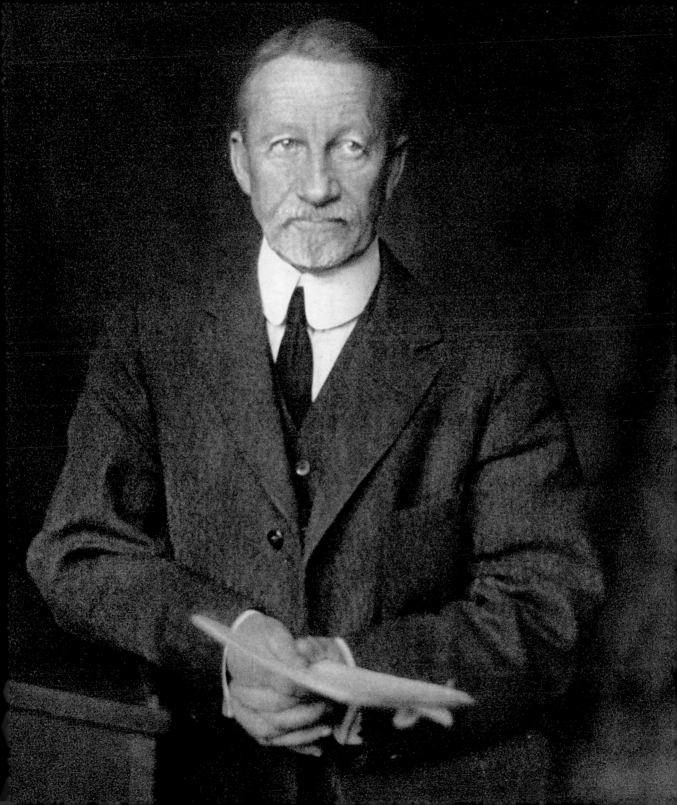

Neurotransmitters

Otto Loewi (1873–1961)

When nerves are stimulated, they are able to increase or decrease the activity of their target cells, which include muscles, glands, and the heart. At the turn of the twentieth century, scientific protagonists were at odds explaining how the message was carried from a nerve to a target cell across the synapse—a small but real space between them. This so-called soup versus spark controversy asked, Were messages carried chemically or electrically?

Proof of a chemical messenger came to the German physiologist-pharmacologist Otto Loewi in a dream on the evening before Easter Sunday in 1920. He awoke, scribbled some notes derived from his nocturnal inspiration, and returned to sleep. Upon awakening in the morning, he was unable to decipher his notes. Happily, the same dream recurred the following morning at 3:00 a.m. This time, he rushed to his laboratory at the University of Graz in Austria and, using two beating frogs' hearts, showed how fluid from a stimulated heart caused another heart to beat more rapidly. Loewi was awarded the 1936 Nobel Prize in Physiology or Medicine—money he used to buy his way out of Austria after Hitler's 1938 invasion.

How Nerves Talk. In addition to Loewi's first established neurotransmitter, acetylcholine, some of the several dozen other messengers include norepinephrine, dopamine, serotonin, glycine, GABA, and glutamate. These chemicals are synthesized and stored in specific nerve cells and released across a synapse in response to an electrical impulse, binding to a specific receptor on another nerve or target cell. The neurotransmitter-receptor interaction can trigger an increase or decrease in the activity of the target cell, causing contraction or relaxation of a muscle, secretion from a gland, changes in heart rate, and alterations in behavior. The effects of the neurotransmitter are then terminated in several different ways.

Neurotransmitters play a critical role in physiology and behavior, underlying physical and mental disorders and aberrations. Not surprisingly, a wide range of drugs can mimic the effects of naturally occurring neurotransmitters as well as increasing or decreasing the effects of neurotransmitters at their receptor sites.

SEE ALSO Drug Receptors (1905), Neostigmine and Pyridostigmine (1935), Reserpine (1952), Tofranil and Elavil (1957), Monoamine Oxidase Inhibitors (1961), Propranolol (1964), Levodopa (1968), Opioids (1973), Tagamet (1976).

The brain neurotransmitter dopamine is synthesized, stored, and released from a nerve ending, interacting with specific dopamine receptor sites after crossing a synapse.

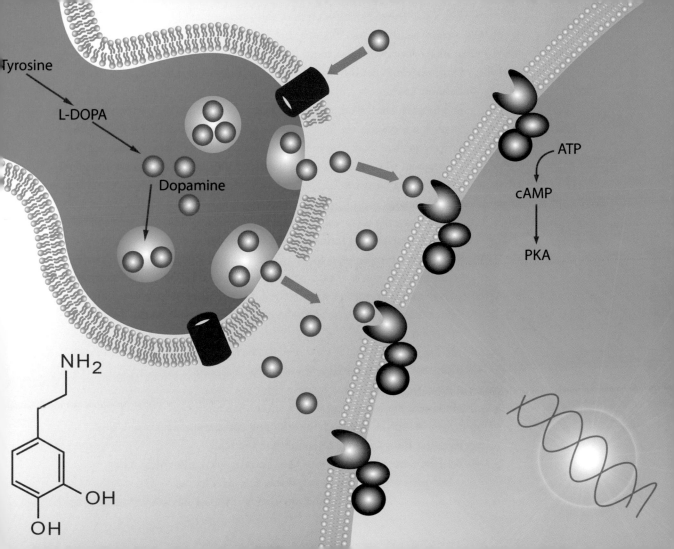

Tyrosine

L-DOPA

Dopamine

NH_2

OH

OH

ATP

cAMP

PKA

Merbaphen

Alfred Vogl (1895–1973)

What began as a problematic treatment for syphilis became a highly significant therapy for life-threatening heart disease. The use of inorganic mercury salts, such as mercurous chloride (**calomel**), for syphilis and to promote urine output (diuresis) dates back to Paracelsus in the sixteenth century. However, these drugs were questionably effective but unquestionably toxic.

Merbaphen, which contained mercury in a very complex organic combination, made its first appearance in medicine in 1912 for the treatment of syphilis. In 1919–20, Alfred Vogl, an American medical student at the Wenckeback Clinic in Vienna, observed that after a syphilitic patient was injected with merbaphen, urine output increased many-fold. He then gave merbaphen to a syphilitic patient with advanced heart failure, a condition in which the heart inadequately pumps blood, leading to a voluminous accumulation of body fluids. Whereas this patient had failed to respond to the existing diuretics, merbaphen produced profound fluid loss that restored his heart function.

Reflecting back on his discovery thirty years later, Vogl wrote, "We were convinced that we had witnessed the greatest [hu]man-made diuresis in history . . . we scurried about in search of more patients on whom to test our discovery. We were repeatedly able to reproduce these miraculous results, causing deluges at will, to the delight of the patients and ourselves."

While merbaphen (Novasural) produced dramatic effects, it was painful when injected and capable of causing kidney damage. In 1924, mersalyl (Salyrgan), an equally effective but less toxic would-be anti-syphilis drug, replaced it. Other organic mercurial compounds followed. For more than three decades, the mercurial diuretics enjoyed an undisputed reputation as the most powerful and consistently effective diuretics for removal of excessive fluid and sodium buildup in the body.

These benefits came at a heavy price. Mercurial diuretics sometimes lost effectiveness and were capable of causing kidney and liver toxicity—and, most ominously, sudden death within minutes after being injected. Far safer drugs appeared in the 1950s.

SEE ALSO Calomel (1793), Salvarsan (1910), Diuril (1958), Lasix (1966).

Syphilis is caused by the spiral-shaped bacterium Treponema, *which is spread by sexual contact or transmitted from an infected pregnant woman to her child.*

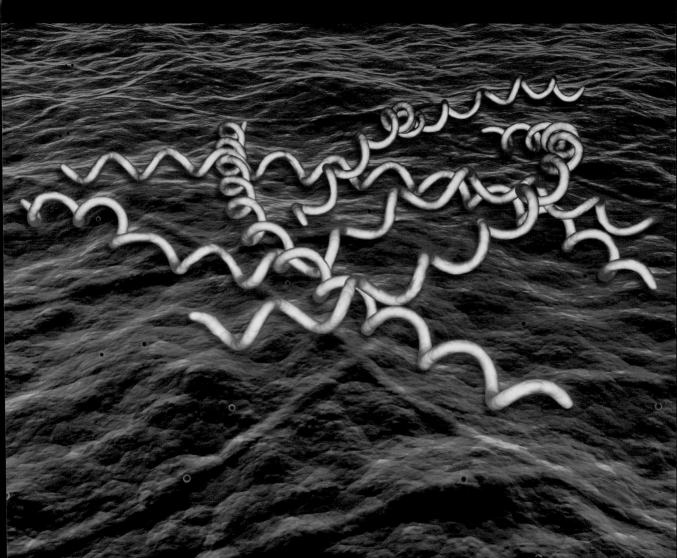

Carbon Tetrachloride

James Young Simpson (1811–1870)

HAMMERING THE HOOKWORM. It may be difficult for the contemporary reader to believe that carbon tetrachloride, now vilified as an environmental hazard, was used internally for the treatment of hookworm infections. The hookworm is an intestinal parasite, located primarily in tropical and subtropical climates worldwide, that infects some 600 million to 1.3 billion people. Walking barefoot on hookworm egg–contaminated soil can prompt an infection. The eggs penetrate the skin, travel to the intestine, and cause anemia.

Several years after James Simpson introduced **chloroform** for use as a surgical anesthetic in 1847, he studied the anesthetic effects of carbon tetrachloride, a chemical very similar to chloroform (CCl_4 versus $CHCl_3$). Although extremely powerful as an anesthetic, because of its toxicity it proved unsatisfactory and was set aside as a drug for the next seven decades.

In 1921, Maurice Hall, Zoology Chief at the U.S. Department of Agriculture, reported that carbon tetrachloride was 100 percent effective in eradicating hookworms from dogs. He proposed that it be used in humans, and it lived up to clinical expectations. Within a score of years, however, the effective-but-less-toxic tetrachloroethylene had replaced it.

Carbon tetrachloride had a far greater and more long-lasting impact in the industrial sector than as a drug. Nonflammable, noncorrosive, readily available, and very inexpensive, it was formerly used as a flame-extinguishing chemical in fire extinguishers, a dry-cleaning solvent, a spot-cleaning fluid, a starting material in the synthesis of chlorofluorocarbon (CFC) refrigerants, as well as a nail-polish remover.

The established toxic effects caused by inhaling carbon tetrachloride vapors in poorly ventilated settings led to its disuse in the 1990s. Early symptoms of high-level exposure included behavioral effects, loss of consciousness, and respiratory or heart failure. More common, however, were the damaging effects on the liver and kidneys after repeated exposure to the chemical.

SEE ALSO Chloroform (1847), Praziquantel (1972).

Hookworm infections have no symptoms. The most serious consequences of the infection are anemia and protein deficiency at the site where the worm attaches to the inner wall of the intestines. In children, the loss of iron and proteins can slow growth and can cause mental retardation.

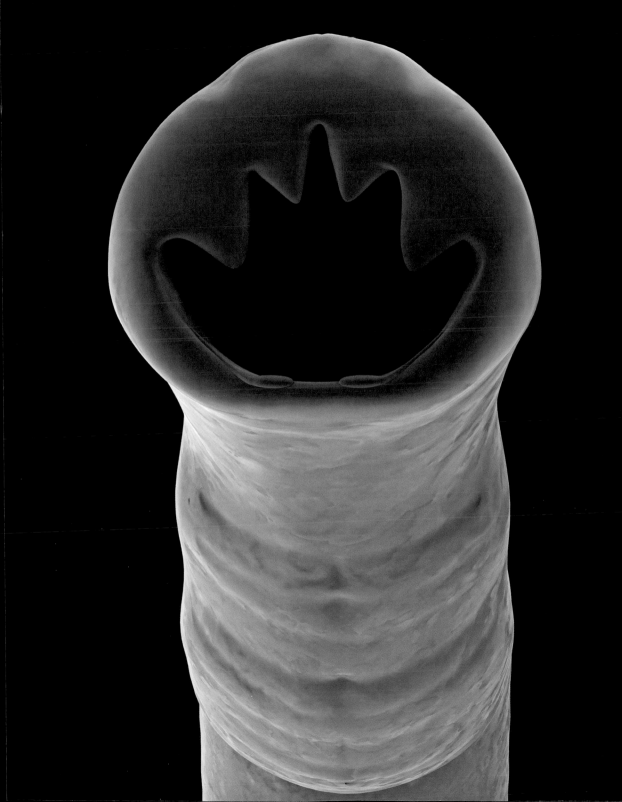

Insulin

John J. R. MacLeod (1876–1936), **Frederick G. Banting** (1891–1941), **James B. Collip** (1892–1965), **Charles H. Best** (1899–1978), **Frederick Sanger** (b. 1918)

The basic details surrounding the discovery of insulin and its impact on the treatment of diabetes are widely accepted. To whom credit should be bestowed remains a subject of controversy.

Descriptions of patients experiencing extreme thirst and copious urination date back thousands of years, and in the first century, this condition was termed *diabetes* (Greek for *siphon*). In the 1670s, the diabetic's urine was found to contain sugar, and in 1889, the pancreas's role in the disease was identified.

Canadian surgeon Frederick Banting persuaded University of Toronto professor of physiology John J. R. MacLeod to let him use McLeod's laboratory and ten dogs in 1921, while the professor was vacationing. Banting enlisted the assistance of Charles Best, who was waiting to enter medical school. They extracted the sugar-lowering principle from one dog's pancreas and then administered it to and successfully treated another severely diabetic dog. After returning, MacLeod offered Banting some helpful advice, extended his time in the lab, and paid him a modest salary.

Within months, in early 1922, injections of this same extract saved the life of fourteen-year-old diabetic Leonard Thompson. Chemist James Collip helped to improve extraction and purification techniques, and several dozen children were successfully treated shortly thereafter. In record time, the 1923 Nobel Prize in Physiology or Medicine was awarded to Banting and MacLeod, but Best was conspicuously overlooked. Banting rightly viewed this oversight as a travesty and split half his prize money with Best. McLeod, in turn, shared his award with Collip. That year, Eli Lilly began the commercial production of insulin. To control the blood-sugar levels of diabetics, there are four basic types of insulin, which differ based on how rapidly they start and stop working.

Less controversial was the granting of the 1958 Nobel Prize in Chemistry to Frederick Sanger for determining the amino acid sequence of the insulin molecule. Insulin's importance transcends diabetes. This use of estrogen to alleviate the symptoms of menopause is called hormone replacement therapy, a concept developed with the use of insulin to replace a deficient hormone in diabetics.

SEE ALSO Insulin Shock Therapy (1927), Premarin (1941), Human Insulin (1982).

A high-power microscopic view of an islet of Langerhans. These islets, which number about one million in a healthy adult pancreas, are responsible for the production of insulin. In type 1 diabetes, an autoimmune process selectively destroys the islets.

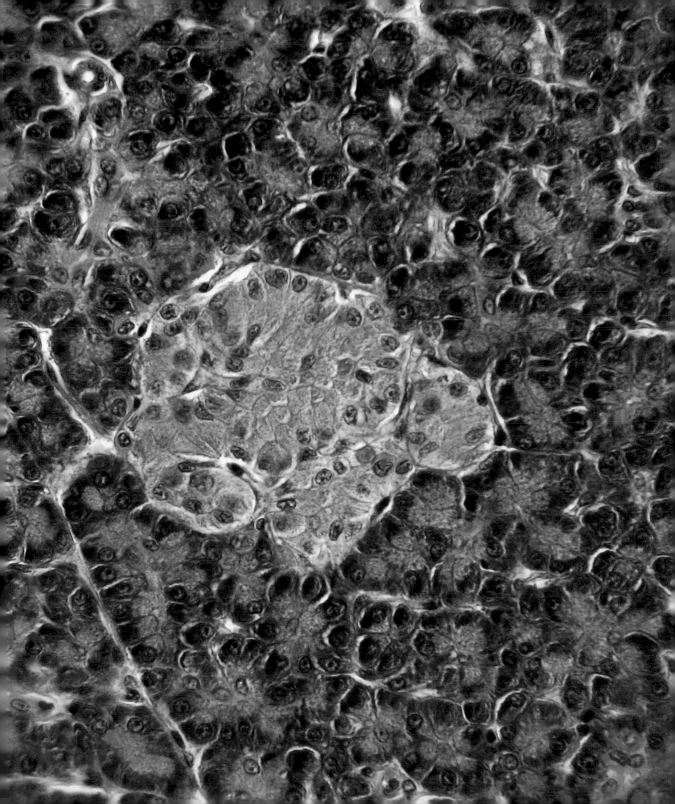

Hexylresorcinol

Phenol, the first *antiseptic*—a drug used to kill microbes on the skin and surgical instruments—appeared in 1867. It was effective but rather indiscriminate in its ability to destroy living cells, both of bacteria and of patients. Moreover, it was a preferred drug for committing suicide.

Over the years, chemists set to work to find derivatives that would be more active (that is, be active at lower concentrations) than phenol and also less toxic and less irritating to the patient's skin. Hexylresorcinol was one such drug, and it continues to be used today, albeit with less frequency, in first-aid antiseptics, mouthwashes, and sore-throat products.

Bacteria, of course, reside not only on the surface but also inside the body. As many women are aware, many bacteria like to take residence in the bladder, resulting in urinary tract infections. In 1924, Veander Leonard at Johns Hopkins School of Hygiene and Public Health proposed the use of hexylresorcinol as a urinary antiseptic, an antibacterial drug that selectively concentrates in the urinary tract.

An *Evening Post* article on April 17, 1926, praised hexylresorcinol: "Dr Leonard believes, the span of life can be lengthened. 'Disease germs no longer remain entrenched in the human body, but can be cast out, one and all.'" Notwithstanding this optimistic assessment, the appearance of the far more effective sulfa drugs and mandelic acid in the 1930s displaced hexylresorcinol for the treatment of urinary tract infections.

During the 1930s, hexylresorcinol was reintroduced to the medical world. Here, it had its greatest impact as an anthelmintic, a drug used for the treatment of worm infections. Unlike most other anthelmintics, it is effective against many different varieties of worm infections, including hookworm, roundworm, tapeworm, whipworm, and pinworm. Although not the best choice for treating any single type, it is useful because of its ability to treat mixed worm infections and its relatively low toxicity.

SEE ALSO Phenol (1867), Carbon Tetrachloride (1921), Praziquantel (1972).

This cross-section is of Ascaris roundworm, the largest and most common parasitic worm in humans. Human Parasitic Diseases Sourcebook estimates that one-quarter of the human population is infected by this worm.

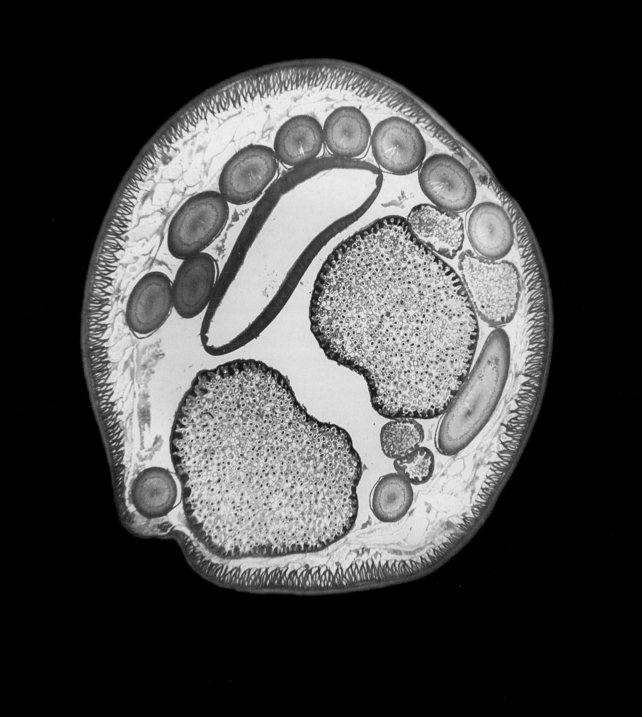

Ergotamine and Ergonovine

Henry Hallett Dale (1875–1968), **Arthur Stoll** (1887–1971), **Albert Hofmann** (1906–2008)

Ergot has a fascinating history dating back to the Middle Ages, so it is not surprising that during the early years of the twentieth century, Nobel Prize–winning pharmacologist Henry Hallett Dale was attracted to explore its pharmacological properties. Ergot extracts contain a virtual gold mine of unstudied **alkaloids** produced by the fungus *Claviceps purpurea*, a contaminant of rye and other grains. In 1917, Swiss biochemist Arthur Stoll became director of pharmacological research at Sandoz (now Novartis) in Basel. His job was to identify active chemicals from natural sources, and the first that he tackled was ergot.

MIGRAINE AND CHILDBIRTH DRUGS. Stoll isolated ergotamine in 1920 and ergonovine in 1935, the latter contemporaneously with other research groups in England and the United States. Ergotamine, ergonovine, and their closely related cousins have had two primary medicinal uses—namely, the treatment of migraine headaches and postpartum bleeding.

The anti-migraine effects of ergotamine are complicated and complex. Migraine headaches are associated with the pulsation (constricting, then widening) of arteries in the brain. Ergotamine may act by opposing this widening. Its ability to stop an attack after an injection is dramatic, but when used too often, in higher doses, or in very sensitive individuals, it can produce signs of ergotism—historically referred to as St. Anthony's fire—including gangrene affecting the extremities.

Midwives have given extracts of ergot for hundreds of years to cause contractions of the uterus to hasten labor; stillborns often resulted. Ergonovine is now used postpartum and after abortions to decrease bleeding and to promote shrinkage of the uterus.

Both ergotamine and envonovine are chemically lysergic acid derivatives. While studying their chemistry, Albert Hofmann, a colleague of Stoll at Sandoz, developed lysergic acid diethylamide (**LSD**), discovering its psychedelic effects in 1943.

SEE ALSO Alcohol (c. 10,000 BCE), Ergot (1670), Alkaloids (1806), LSD (1943), Imitrex (1991).

Ergot, the natural source of ergotamine, has been used in childbirth for hundreds of years to stimulate labor contractions. This terra-cotta statuette from South America depicts a woman giving birth.

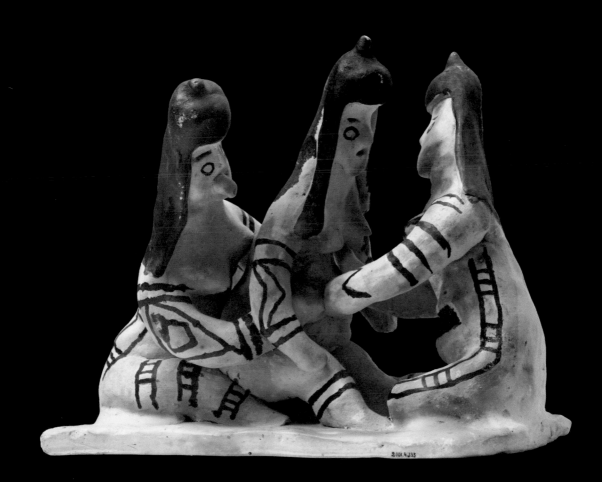

Insulin Shock Therapy

Manfred J. Sakel (1900–1957)

What do the following notables have in common?: James Forrestal (first U.S. Secretary of Defense), John Nash (mathematician, Nobel Prize winner, *A Beautiful Mind*), Vaslav Nijinski (ballet dancer extraordinaire), Zelda Fitzgerald (novelist, wife of F. Scott). All received insulin shock therapy for treatment of their mental disorders.

To be both safe and effective for treatment of diabetes mellitus, the proper dose of **insulin** must be administered. If the dose is too low, elevated blood-sugar levels are not brought down, and the diabetic condition is not controlled. Too much insulin causes blood sugar levels to fall precipitously, causing coma and convulsions.

In 1927, the Polish neurophysiologist-neuropsychiatrist Manfred Sakel, working in Vienna, was using insulin to relieve the anxiety and agitation of patients undergoing narcotic withdrawal. When, on occasion, an inadvertently excessive insulin dose was given, the patients experienced coma and convulsions. Sakel reasoned that by blocking a weakened nerve cell by inducing a coma with insulin, the nerve would conserve energy and restore its normal function, thus enabling the schizophrenic patient to recover. It was later understood that the benefits of insulin shock therapy (also referred to as insulin coma therapy) resulted from the coma and not the "shock."

Sakal's report that up to 88 percent of his schizophrenic patients improved was particularly impressive, considering the other potentially dangerous treatment options available in the mid-1930s. These included electroconvulsive shock therapy, Metrazol-induced convulsions, and psychosurgery (usually a frontal lobotomy).

The worldwide psychiatric community enthusiastically embraced the "Sakel technique." Typical courses of therapy in specialized facilities entailed up to sixty coma episodes. As with many drug discoveries, the initial excitement was tempered by later reports showing far less favorable results, a high incidence of remissions to the schizophrenic state, adverse effects, and even deaths in 1–10 percent of patients. The appearance of the antischizophrenic drugs Thorazine and **Haldol** in the 1950s contributed to the virtual demise of insulin coma therapy by the 1970s.

SEE ALSO Insulin (1921), Chlorpromazine (1952), Haldol (1958), Clozapine (1989).

Vaslav Nijinsky (1890–1950), photographed here during a 1912 performance of Scheherazade, *was a Russian-born ballet dancer celebrated for his spectacular leaps and sensitive interpretations as a choreographer. When, at the age of twenty-nine, he was diagnosed with schizophrenia, his career essentially ended. He spent the rest of his life in psychiatric hospitals and asylums being treated with insulin shock therapy, among other antipsychotic modalities.*

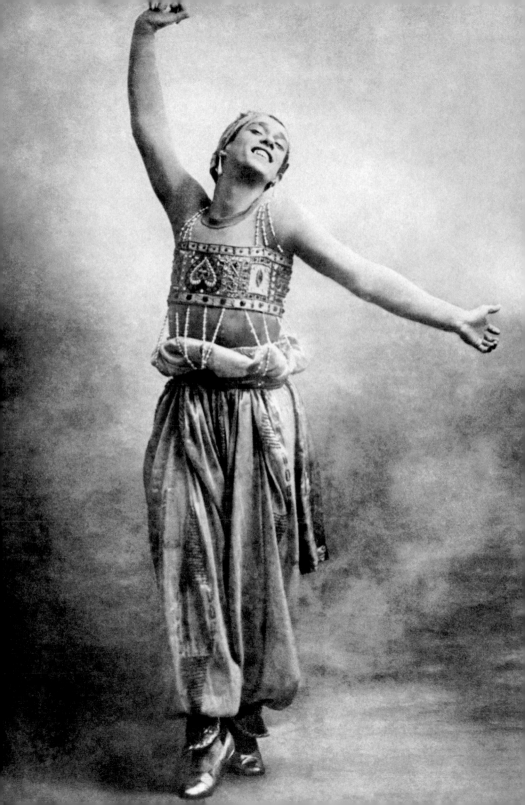

Thimerosal

1927

Is there an association between thimerosal in vaccines and autism? Although the biomedical community and the courts in the United States have rejected this assertion, they have not convinced many vocal and well-intentioned parents that such a link does not exist. What is thimerosal (better known internationally as thiomersal), why has it been included in vaccines, and what is the current status of the controversy?

Thimerosal (Merthiolate) is an antibacterial and antifungal antiseptic, containing almost 50 percent mercury, which since 1927 has been applied to the skin. Since the 1930s, it has been added to multidose vials of some vaccines as a preservative to prevent their accidental microbial contamination. Mercury is a nerve poison. As a precautionary measure, in 1999, the Centers for Disease Control and Prevention (CDC) strongly encouraged vaccine manufacturers to reduce or eliminate thimerosal at the earliest possible date and, with few exceptions, this has been done in the United States, Canada, and Europe.

In its 2004 report, the National Academy of Science's Institute of Medicine (IOM), incorporating data from Europe, concluded that no causal relationship exists between thimerosal-containing vaccines and autism. Medical groups in North America and Europe, the World Health Organization, and Autism Speaks support this position. Moreover, the medical community has expressed concern that while the dangers of thimerosal were speculative, there are far greater dangers of contracting such serious infectious diseases as measles, whooping cough, and bacterial meningitis if parents refuse the use of vaccines for their children or for influenza during pregnancy.

Parent groups, scientists, and personal-injury lawyers support a thimerosal-autism link by pointing to mercury health warnings, an increase in the number of vaccinations, and a dramatic ten-fold increase in the number of autism cases between 1996 and 2007.

In 1986, a "Vaccine Court" was established to protect vaccine makers from state-court lawsuits and provide funds to compensate parents of children who were injured by a vaccine. Whereas the U.S. Vaccine Court has failed to support claims by concerned parents, in 2010 a British medical panel backed the claim of a link between a vaccine and seizures in a child. The jury remains out.

SEE ALSO Smallpox Vaccine (1796), Polio Vaccine (1954), Gardasil (2006).

A number of parent groups have argued that thimerosal added to vaccines to prevent microbial contamination is responsible for autism in their children. This puzzle-patterned ribbon symbolizes autism awareness.

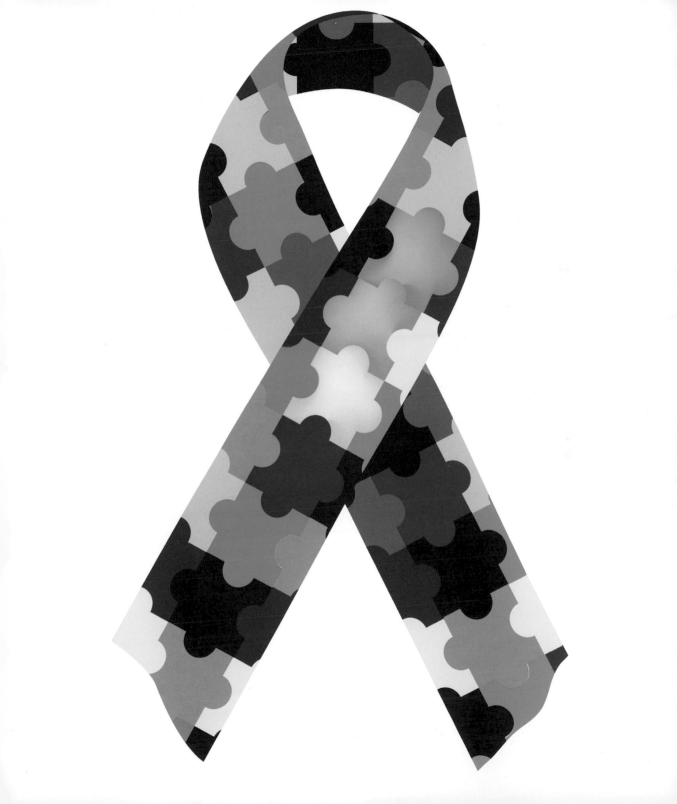

Penicillin

Alexander Fleming (1881–1955), **Howard Florey** (1898–1968), **Ernst Chain** (1906–1979)

The discovery of penicillin G marked the start of the antibiotic epoch. It is estimated to have saved some 100 million lives. The antibiotic also decreased syphilis deaths by more than 98 percent from 1940 to 1975. Not surprisingly, penicillin is considered by many (including this author) to have been the most significant drug ever discovered.

During his years serving in the British Royal Army Medical Corps on the Western Front in France during World War I, Alexander Fleming observed that more troops died from infected wounds than from battle injuries. After the war, the Scottish-born Fleming returned to his alma mater, St. Mary's Hospital in London, where he devoted the remainder of his career to research in bacteriology.

Returning to his far-less-than meticulous laboratory after a summer holiday in 1928, he detected an unwanted guest, an airborne fungus, inside a lab dish in which he was growing staphylococci. Such contamination was nothing new, but Fleming astutely observed that bacterial colonies were absent in places where the green mold grew. Fleming tested extracts of the mold, *Penicllium notatum*, and found that it killed some disease-causing bacteria (Gram-positive) but not others (Gram-negative), and it was not toxic to his test animals. He published his findings in the *British Journal of Experimental Pathology* in 1929. The response of the scientific community was a deafening silence!

The significance of Fleming's findings was better appreciated a decade later, when ominous war clouds were descending on England. Working at Oxford, Australian pathologist Howard Florey and German refugee biochemist Ernst Chain isolated and purified penicillin G from the mold (something Fleming was unable to do), reconfirmed its antibacterial properties, and were instrumental in getting the antibiotic produced in mass quantities for wartime use. The three were awarded the 1945 Nobel Prize for Physiology or Medicine, and Fleming was selected as one of *Time* magazine's "100 Most Important People of the Century."

Newer penicillin derivatives are more effective by mouth, capable of withstanding inactivation by the bacteria-producing enzyme penicillinase, and able to kill a wider range of disease-causing bacteria. Some 100 drugs are now available to treat a wide assortment of microbial infections, yet penicillin remains one of the safest and most effective.

SEE ALSO Calomel (1793), Salvarsan (1910), Benemid (1951), Ampicillin (1961).

Alexander Fleming's discovery of penicillin has been universally acclaimed. He received the highest honors, awards, and honorary professorships from the world's leading societies and universities.

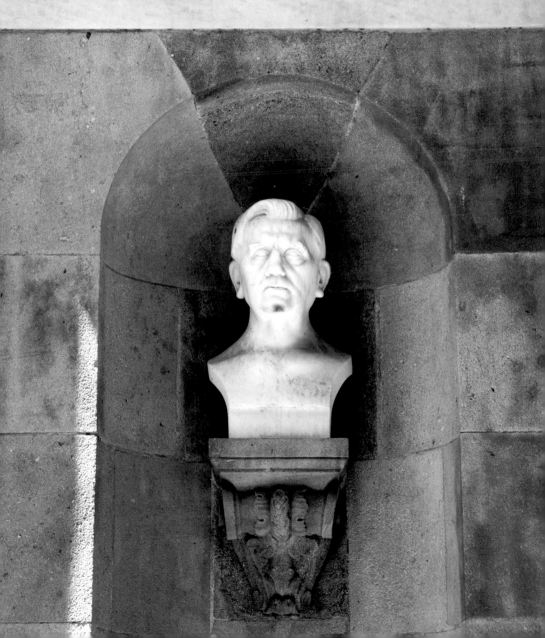

BARCELONA
A SIR
ALEXANDER FLEMING

Nembutal and Seconal

The barbiturates enjoyed almost unchallenged rivalry for the relief of anxiety and insomnia after the introduction of **phenobarbital** in 1912. Among the most widely used of the dozens of barbiturate-like drugs were Nembutal and Seconal, both synthesized in 1928. Marketed by Abbott Laboratories and Eli Lilly, respectively, these barbiturates have also been used for the treatment of seizures and insomnia and to calm patients before surgery.

With the appearance of **Librium** and other benzodiazepines in the 1960s and 1970s, the medical popularity of the barbiturates Nembutal (pentobarbital) and Seconal (secobarbital) declined. Notwithstanding the effectiveness of the barbiturates, the benzodiazepines possessed a number of distinct advantages: they were more focused in their effects, safer when taken in overdoses, effective over extended periods, and less subject to abuse. The popularity of the barbiturates was further marred because of their nonmedical use for recreation, suicides, and euthanasia.

With street names such as yellow jackets and red devils referring to the colors of their respective capsules, Nembutal and Seconal have been used recreationally to get "high." In Jacqueline Susann's novel (1966) and film *Valley of the Dolls* (1967), one of the "dolls" is Seconal, used by a number of characters as a sleep aid and by one for suicidal purposes.

These drugs have caused or contributed to the death of a number of high-visibility individuals, including movie star Marilyn Monroe (1962), blues and jazz singer Dinah Washington (1963), actor and entertainer Judy Garland (1969), guitarist Jimi Hendrix (1970), and playwright Tennessee Williams (1983).

DRUG FOR DEATH TOURISTS. Pentobarbital has long been used for animal euthanasia and is the preferred drug for unassisted or physician-assisted suicide—a practice legal in several states, most notably Oregon, and European countries such as the Netherlands. While the sale of this drug is carefully controlled in the United States, "death tourists" can readily purchase it in pet shops in Tijuana and other Mexican cities.

SEE ALSO Chloral Hydrate (1869), Barbital (1903), Phenobarbital (1912), Librium (1960), Valium (1963), Ambien (1992).

For more than three decades, the barbiturates Nembutal and Seconal were widely used for the treatment of insomnia. In the 1960s, these drugs assumed greater notoriety for their non-medical recreational use and for their contribution in high-visibility suicides.

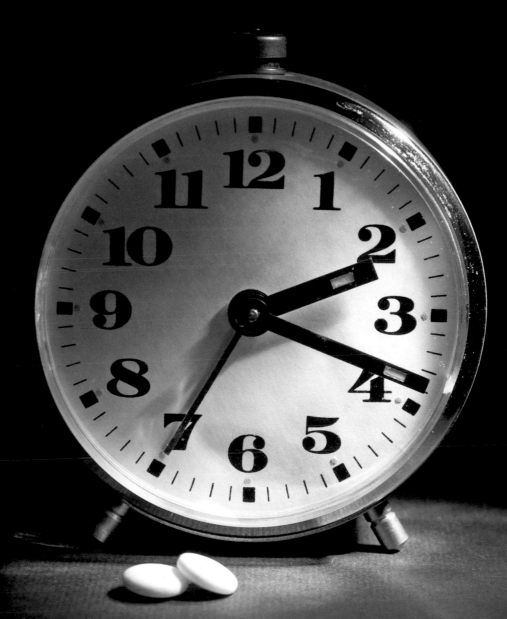

Estrone and Estrogen

Edgar Allen (1892–1943), **Edward Doisy** (1893–1986)

Removal of the ovaries has long been associated with atrophy of the uterus and the loss of sexual function. Transplanting pieces of ovaries prevents these wasting effects in adult animals and stimulates the development of the uterus in immature animals. During the early decades of the twentieth century, interest centered on the secretions from such ductless or endocrine glands as the ovaries. In 1923, biologist Edgar Allen and biochemist Edward Doisy, working at St. Louis University School of Medicine, found active principles released into the urine from the ovaries of pregnant and nonpregnant women.

In 1929, Doisy isolated one such chemical—the first purified female hormone from the class of compounds collectively called estrogens—which he named theelin, later renamed estrone. In 1935, estradiol, the most active estrogen, was isolated from the ovaries. These were followed by the semisynthetic, orally active ethinyl estradiol (1935), one of the two primary ingredients in **Enovid** and other oral contraceptives. In 1938, the first laboratory-prepared estrogen, **diethylstilbestrol** (DES), was introduced, whose use to prevent miscarriages was later associated with an increased risk of cancers of the breast and vagina. The most notable estrogen—and the best-selling drug in the United States in the 1990s—was **Premarin** (1941), a mixture of estrone and other natural estrogens obtained from *pregnant mare urine* (hence its trade name). For more than seventy years, Premarin has been used to treat the symptoms of menopause.

Our first thoughts of estrogen typically concern its role as the female sex hormone required for the development of reproductive organs, such as the vagina and uterus, its role in the development and support of the secondary sex characteristics, including the breasts and distribution of body fat, and its critical contribution to the menstrual cycle. Estrogen also has a number of nonsexual physiological effects, such as increasing bone formation, elevating HDL (good) cholesterol, and lowering LDL (bad) cholesterol. Estrogen derivatives are used to treat prostate cancer, and antiestrogen drugs, such as **tamoxifen**, are employed for breast cancer.

SEE ALSO Diethylstilbestrol (1938), Premarin (1941), Enovid (1960), Tamoxifen (1973).

Estrogen is one of two female sex hormones that play an important role in preparing a woman's body for pregnancy. Under its influence, the walls of the uterus increase in size and, on approximately day fifteen of the menstrual cycle, ovulation occurs in anticipation of the ovum (egg) being fertilized by a sperm cell.

Ovarian Cycle

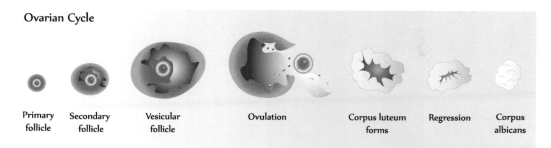

Primary follicle

Secondary follicle

Vesicular follicle

Ovulation

Corpus luteum forms

Regression

Corpus albicans

Uterine Cycle

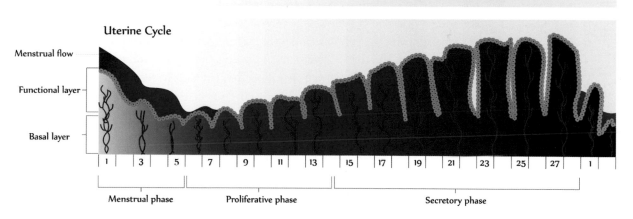

Menstrual flow

Functional layer

Basal layer

1 3 5 7 9 11 13 15 17 19 21 23 25 27 1

Menstrual phase

Proliferative phase

Secretory phase

Amphetamine

Lazãr Edeleanu (1861–1941), Gordon Alles (1901–1963)

In 1887, Lazãr Edeleanu, a Romanian graduate student at the University of Berlin, synthesized amphetamine. Four decades later, while searching for a substitute for the anti-asthmatic drug ephedrine, the American pharmacologist-chemist Gordon Alles rediscovered amphetamine and transferred the drug to Smith, Kline and French Laboratories (now GlaxoSmithKline), which recognized and exploited its considerable market potential during the 1930s.

Its first medical application was the Benzedrine inhaler, intended to treat nasal congestion and later used as a source of amphetamine for recreational purposes. Amphetamine's stimulant properties led to its 1935 use for the treatment of narcolepsy, a disorder characterized by multiple, uncontrollable periods of sleep during normal waking hours. Within the next few years, amphetamine (Dexedrine) was found to treat attention deficit hyperactivity disorder (ADHD) by calming and improving children's ability to concentrate.

Used by both Allied and Axis combatants, amphetamine assumed a nonpartisan role during World War II and subsequent wars. Post–World War II witnessed the widespread abuse of the amphetamines (in particular, **methamphetamine** or "speed") in Japan, Sweden, and the United States. The drug's capacity to increase mental and physical performance and to elevate the mood has led to its widespread use in recreation and athletic competition, and its antifatigue effects were capitalized on by students cramming before exams and by cross-country commercial truck drivers.

From a commercial perspective, amphetamine's most significant and lucrative use has been for weight loss. Amphetamine and related drugs reduce the activity of the feeding center in the hypothalamus, decreasing food intake. The most impressive weight losses occur during the first six-to-eight weeks, diminishing thereafter. To overcome this drug tolerance, some users increase their dosage, which may lead to amphetamine dependence—a scenario poignantly portrayed in the film *Requiem for a Dream* (2000).

SEE ALSO Methamphetamine (1944), Ritalin (1955), MDMA/Ecstasy (1976), Crack Cocaine (1986), Ephedra/Ephedrine (1994), Weight-Loss Drugs (2010), Smart Drugs (2018).

Of amphetamine's many uses as a drug, by far the most common has been to depress the appetite. This man's considerable weight loss is not typical. After its daily use for several months, amphetamine loses its effectiveness, commonly leading to a rebound increase in body weight.

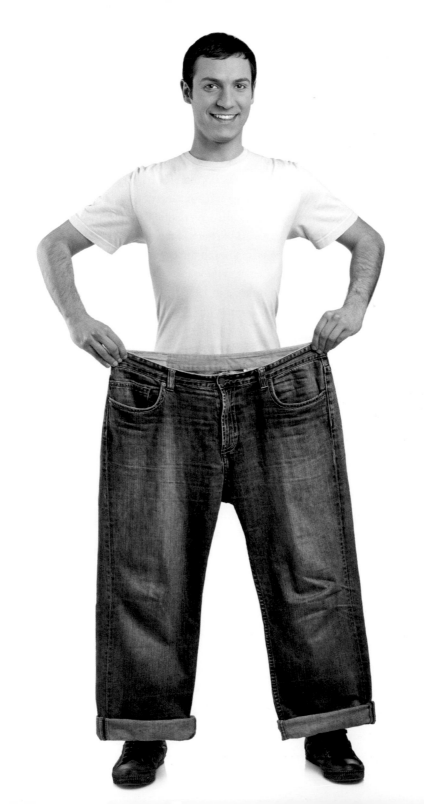

Progesterone and Progestin

George Corner (1889–1981), **Willard Allen** (1904–1993), **Carl Djerassi** (b. 1923), **Frank Colton** (1923–2003)

THE PREGNANCY HORMONE. To appreciate the use of progestins (synthetic progesterone-like drugs), we should first sketch the normal role of progesterone. During the second half of the menstrual cycle, after ovulation has occurred, progesterone promotes changes in the endometrium (lining of the uterus), preparing it for the arrival and attachment of a fertilized egg. It also decreases contractions of the uterus, providing a peaceful environment for the fertilized egg during pregnancy. If the egg is not fertilized, levels of progesterone and estrogen drop sharply, resulting in endometrium breakdown and menstruation.

Progesterone was first isolated in 1933 by George Corner and Willard Allen at the University of Rochester. Because it was rapidly inactivated after oral use, it had to be administered by injection to treat menstrual disorders and infertility and to prevent miscarriages; furthermore, it was very expensive. Ethisterone, the first orally active progestin, was prepared in 1938 in Berlin at Schering AG and marketed in the United States in 1945 as Pranone.

The major breakthrough came in 1951, when chemist, novelist, and playwright Carl Djerassi synthesized norethisterone (Norlutin) at Syntex in Mexico City, using the inexpensive and inedible Mexican yam as a starting material. The following year, Frank Colton at Searle synthesized norethynodrel. These inexpensive, orally active progestins were initially used to treat menstrual disorders and endometriosis. Of far greater importance, progestins inhibit ovulation and have been used alone (mini-pill) and in combination with estrogen in **Enovid** and other hormonal contraceptives, which are available as pills, injections, patches, and IUDs.

Premarin (conjugated estrogens) has long been used to treat the distressing symptoms of menopause. When used alone, it provides the deficient estrogen but also increases the risk of heart attack, stroke, and uterine cancer. The addition of a progestin may reduce this risk.

As noted, during pregnancy progesterone subdues contractions of the uterus. **Mifepristone** (RU-486, Mifeprex, Mifegyne), an anti-progesterone drug, blocks these quieting effects, resulting in a medical abortion.

SEE ALSO Estrone and Estrogen (1929), Premarin (1941), Enovid (1960), Mifepristone (1988), 17P/Progesterone Injections and Gel (2003).

The uterus in the female reproductive tract is the target site of progesterone, a hormone that promotes changes in its lining (endometrium) in preparation for pregnancy.

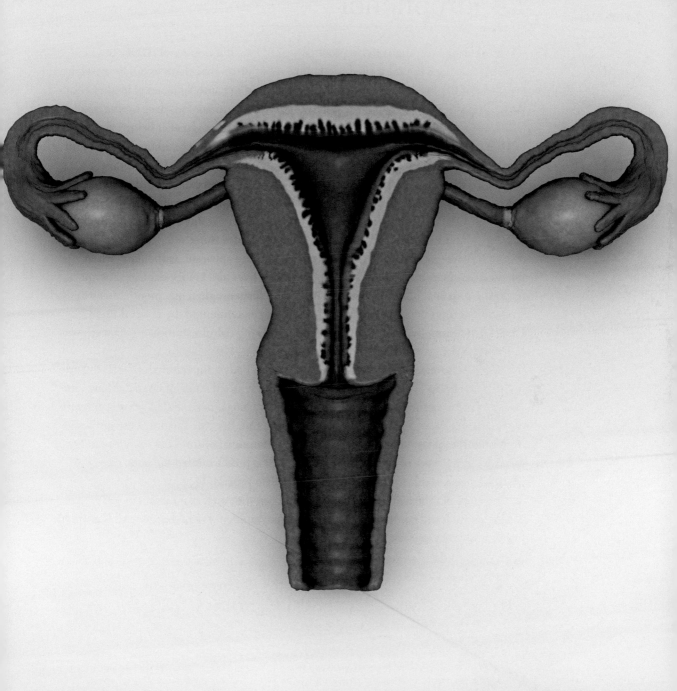

Dinitrophenol

Of all the drugs ever marketed to produce weight loss, dinitrophenol (DNP) has undoubtedly been the most effective. Unlike other drugs that claim to produce weight loss without the need to diet or exercise, DNP is said to cause fat losses of ten to twelve pounds (4.5–5.5 kg) in eight days. Why, then, isn't this miraculous drug on the market?

During World War I, French munitions workers lost weight after being exposed to DNP, used in the manufacture of explosives. In 1933, a paper authored by Stanford University researchers appeared in *Journal of the American Medical Association* describing that test subjects taking relatively low DNP doses experienced steady weight loss over a three-month period without suffering any apparent significant side effects. That year, DNP appeared on the market, and over the next three years, some 100,000 persons used it for weight reduction in the United States alone.

With widespread use, DNP's toxic effects became apparent, particularly when the dose was increased. These problems included liver and kidney damage, allergic reactions, and fatal blood disorders. When taken for more than one month, an estimated 1 percent of users developed cataracts. Before the enactment of the **Federal Food, Drug, and Cosmetic Act** (1938), the **Food and Drug Administration** was powerless to remove this dangerous drug from the market.

A major adverse effect involving a steep rise in body temperature has been linked to the mechanism by which DNP works. DNP increases the rate of fat metabolism by 20–30 percent for the first twenty-four hours after a single dose, and by 50 percent with repeated daily doses, as long as the drug is continued. Because the drug "uncouples" oxidation from phosphorylation, the increase in fat metabolism is not used for energy to carry out the work of cells. Rather, excess heat is produced that the body cannot effectively lose, resulting in marked rises in body temperature.

Because of its toxicity, DNP was banned from the American market in 1939. Nevertheless, it still continues to be used by bodybuilders as a fat-burner and is available through Internet sales for weight reduction.

SEE ALSO Amphetamine (1932), Food and Drug Administration (1906), Federal Food, Drug, and Cosmetic Act (1938), Weight-Loss Drugs (2010).

Increases in the dose of the weight-loss drug dinitrophenol produce an increase in the rate of fat metabolism, which leads to a steep rise in body temperature—up to and exceeding 40 degrees Celsius (104 degrees Fahrenheit). This thermometer records a temperature of 38.8 degrees Celsius (101.8 degrees Fahrenheit).

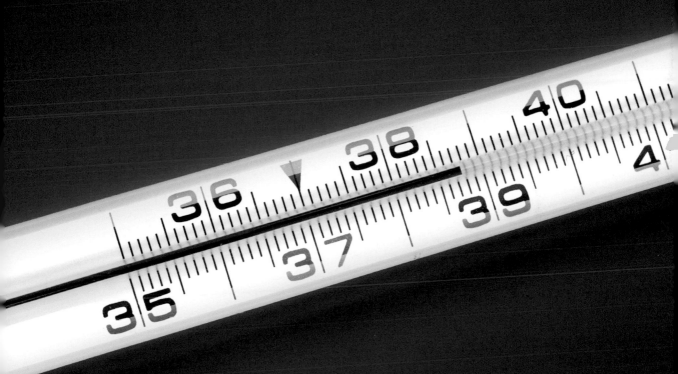

Thiopental

Ralph Waters (1883–1979), John Lundy (1894–1973)

The use of "truth serums" or "truth drugs" to extract information from unwilling informants goes back thousands of years. The first of these drugs was **alcohol**, in the form of wine. Drunken individuals certainly talk a great deal but don't necessarily divulge guarded secrets or even tell the truth. So, too, with thiopental. From the 1920s until the 1960s, police departments and the CIA used it to extract confessions. In 1963, the United States Supreme Court ruled that confessions induced under truth serums were unconstitutionally coerced and, therefore, inadmissible. The call for the use of truth serums in "ticking-bomb" terrorist threats has been renewed since 9/11. In a similar vein, psychiatrists have used thiopental and amobarbital in narcotherapy or narcoanalysis sessions designed to bring repressed memories or thoughts to conscious awareness.

Thiopental was initially developed and has had its most important use in general anesthesia. Imagine a patient lying on an operating room table, anxiously waiting to lose consciousness before a surgical procedure begins. The general anesthetic inhaled through a face mask causes a state of unpleasant excitement lasting for several minutes before the patient loses consciousness.

Clearly, there was a need to develop an anesthetic, given intravenously, that would markedly speed unconsciousness. The first barbiturate, **Barbital** (Veronal), and later amobarbital (Amytal) and hexobarbital (Evipal), did not prove satisfactory. Based on successful clinical studies by Ralph Waters at the University of Wisconsin–Madison and John Lundy of the Mayo Clinic, thiopental (Pentothal) was introduced in 1934 as the first ultra-short-acting barbiturate anesthetic.

After an IV thiopental injection, consciousness is lost within 20–60 seconds and regained about 10 minutes after its administration is terminated. Unfortunately, thiopental produces a hangover that persists for up to 36 hours. **Propofol**, an anesthetic developed in 1983, had more agreeable postoperative effects, and thiopental faded from view.

SEE ALSO Alcohol (c. 10,000 BCE), Ether (1846), Chloroform (1847), Barbital (1903), Lethal Injection (1977), Propofol (1983).

La Bocca della Verità (the Mouth of Truth) *carved in marble, is located in the portico of the Church of Santa Maria in Rome. Used as a lie detector since the Middle Ages, it was believed that if one lied while holding one's hand in the sculpture's mouth, the hand would be bitten off. Bocca made a cameo appearance in the film* Roman Holiday *(1953).*

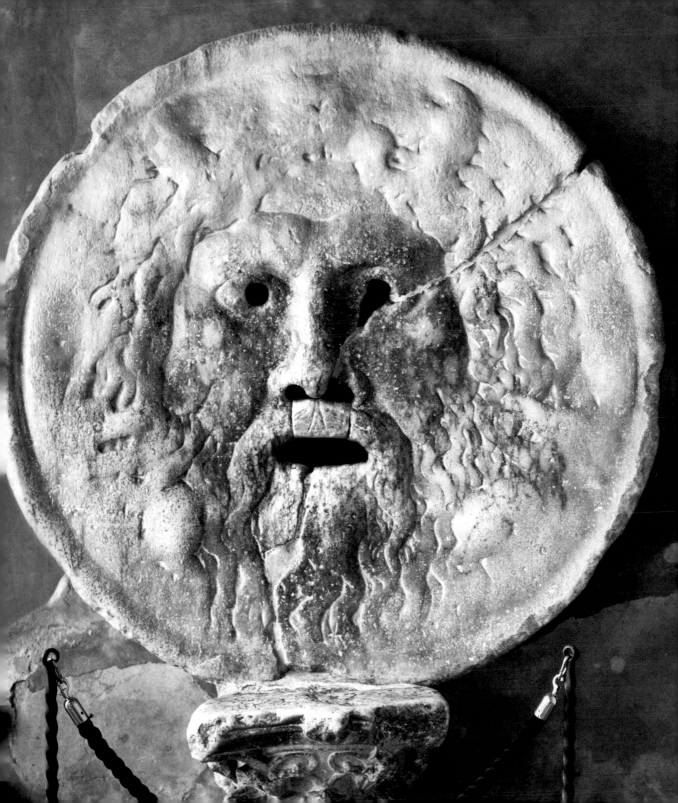

Tubocurarine

Harold King (1887–1956)

Extracts of **curare** were long used as arrow poisons for hunting by the indigenous people of the upper Amazon and Orinoco river basins of South America. Curare's profound effects captured the interest of scientists who sought to better understand the mechanisms underlying nerve-muscle interactions, as well as physicians who saw its clinical potential for muscle relaxation and the treatment of seizure disorders.

Preparation of curare extracts—along with the plant and animal ingredients and the magical, religious rituals that accompanied their fabrication—were a carefully guarded secret. Researchers collected samples of curare and classified and identified them based on the three types of containers in which they were stored and transported from South America. The contents of each container type came from a common region and were more homogeneous. However, the variable nature and composition of the extracts impeded clinical trials until 1935, when Harold King, a chemist at London's National Institute for Medical Research, isolated curare's active **alkaloid** from materials transported in bamboo tubes (hence, the name tubocurarine).

In 1942, tubocurarine was first used to relax the voluntary muscles of the abdominal and thoracic walls. When administered with surgical anesthetics and pain-relieving drugs, lower (and safer) doses of these anesthetics were needed to render the patient unconscious, oblivious to pain, and relaxed, thus reducing the stress of the operative procedure for both the patient and the surgeon. The use of such a drug combination is referred to as balanced anesthesia. Tubocurarine was also used to control spastic disorders involving voluntary muscles, such as tetanus.

Tubocurarine causes a number of undesirable side effects and acts for an inordinately long time (one to two hours), which delays the ability of the patient to breathe unassisted after the conclusion of the operation. Safer drugs that act for more abbreviated periods, such as atracurium (Tracrium) and **succinylcholine** (Anectine), have since replaced it.

SEE ALSO Alkaloids (1806), Curare (1850), Succinylcholine (1951).

This Amazonian woman's blowgun or blowpipe, propelling a curare-coated dart, is particularly effective for hunting such arboreal animals as monkeys and birds.

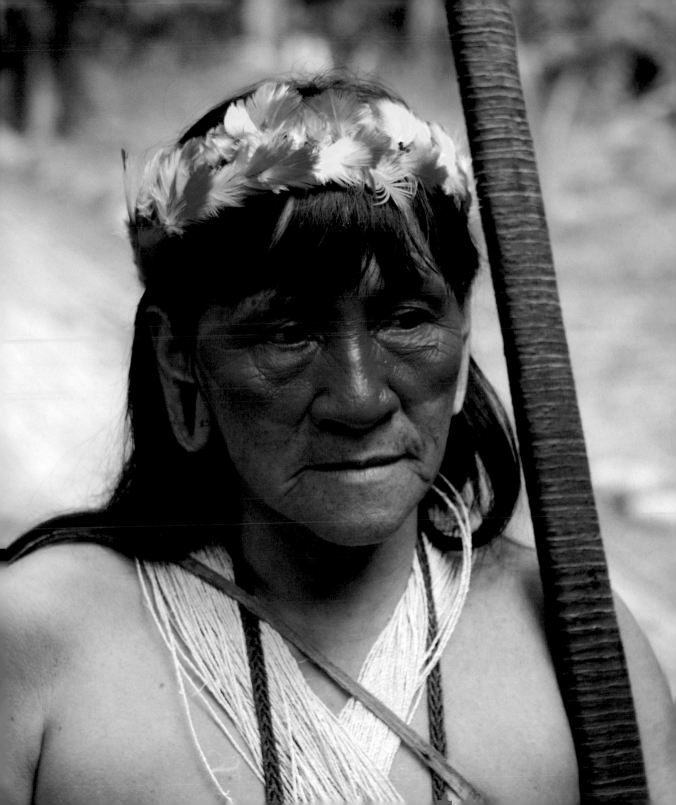

Prontosil

Ernest Fourneau (1872–1949), **Gerhard Domagk** (1895–1964)

Before the 1930s, the medical world believed that only infections caused by protozoa were sensitive to chemotherapeutic agents. **Penicillin** was the subject of an obscure laboratory report and not yet a medicine. In 1931, Gerhard Domagk, Director of Experimental Pathology at IG Farben in Germany, initiated a screening program to discover a drug effective against a wide range of bacterial infections. The most promising of these chemicals was Prontosil, a red dye first synthesized in 1908 that was intended for use in fiber products.

Testing of Prontosil in humans and animals proved very encouraging, but Domagk withheld publishing his results for patent-protection reasons. One of the first successesful treatments involved his six-year-old daughter Hildegarde, who was experiencing life-threatening streptococcal septicemia (blood poisoning) after pricking her finger on an embroidery needle in 1935. Far more visible, and capturing the 1936 headlines in the United States, was news that Prontosil cured President Franklin Delano Roosevelt's son, Franklin Jr., who had developed near-deadly complications caused by a streptococcal throat infection.

Prontosil was ineffective against bacteria in a test tube, but when administered to animals and humans infected with the same bacteria, its antibacterial effects became evident. In 1935, scientists at the Pasteur Institute in Paris, working under the very distinguished French medicinal chemist Ernest Fourneau, showed that in living organisms the inactive Prontosil is converted to **sulfanilamide**, an active antibacterial drug. Realizing that the simple sulfanilamide molecule was responsible for the effects, chemists synthesized more than 5,000 derivatives; more than a score of these sulfas have proved useful in medicine.

In 1939, the Nobel Award Committee bestowed the Nobel Prize in Physiology or Medicine upon Domagk for his discovery of the antibacterial effects of Prontosil. Unfortunately for Domagk, Hitler forbade German nationals from accepting Nobel Prizes in retaliation for the Committee awarding the 1935 Peace Prize to Carl von Ossietzky, an anti-Nazi Jewish pacifist. Thus, Domagk declined the award, but he was able to travel to Stockholm to accept the award (minus the prize money) in 1947.

SEE ALSO Salvarsan (1910), Penicillin (1928), Prontosil (1935), Sulfanilamide (1936).

A photomicrograph of Streptococcus pyogenes *magnified 900x. This spherical Gram-positive bacterium is the cause of many important human diseases ranging from mild skin infections to the life-threatening blood poisoning experienced by Domagk's daughter.*

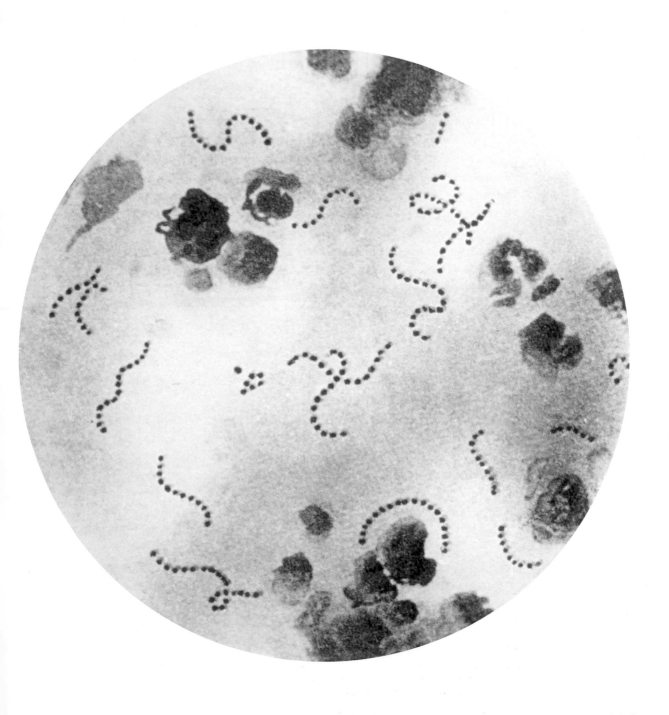

Testosterone

Arnold Adolph Berthold (1803–1861), **Charles-Édouard Brown-Séquard** (1817–1894), **Leopold Ruzicka** (1887–1976), **Adolf Butenandt** (1903–1995)

French printer Henri Estienne (1470–1520) noted, "If youth only knew: if age only could." The eminent French physiologist Charles-Édouard Brown-Séquard was seventy-one years old in 1889. To restore his lost youth, he prepared and injected himself with an extract prepared from the testicles of a dog and guinea pig. It worked, at least on a temporary basis—or so he reported in the prestigious journal *Lancet*. Rather, he demonstrated the power of the placebo, and interest in such "fountain of youth" research evaporated for several decades.

Brown-Séquard's experiment was based on observations going back to prehistoric times and to better-conducted studies by the German physiologist and early endocrinologist Arnold Adolph Berthold. In 1849, Berthold observed that castration of roosters diminished their virility and that after transplantation of testes, they regained their male characteristics.

Reports appeared in 1935 on the isolation of testosterone from the testicles and its synthesis by pharmaceutical company scientists Adolf Butenandt at Organon in the Netherlands and Leopold Ruzicka at Ciba in Switzerland. They were jointly awarded the Nobel Prize in Chemistry in 1939.

Testosterone has two major effects on the body. Its androgenic effects are responsible for the growth and development of the male sex organs, production of sperm, and secondary sex characteristics that make males look like men. In 1951, testosterone's anabolic effects were found to increase muscle mass. Synthetic anabolic steroids, such as **Dianabol**, have increased effects on muscle and, relative to testosterone, reduced androgenic properties. Since their introduction in 1956, these performance enhancers have gained widespread notoriety because of their use by athletes and body builders.

Men with abnormally low testosterone levels, including those with surgical removal of the testes, often have decreases in libido, muscle mass, and energy level. Testosterone replacement therapy (TRT) may reverse these deficiencies. By contrast, TRT has not been shown to reverse the normal changes seen with aging. After the age of thirty, levels of testosterone typically decrease by 1–2 percent per year.

SEE ALSO Dianabol (1956).

Castration of male laboratory animals reduces aggressive behavior, and replacement of testosterone restores their aggressiveness. In humans, by contrast, it is not clear whether testosterone facilitates aggression or encourages social dominance, competitiveness, and impulsiveness.

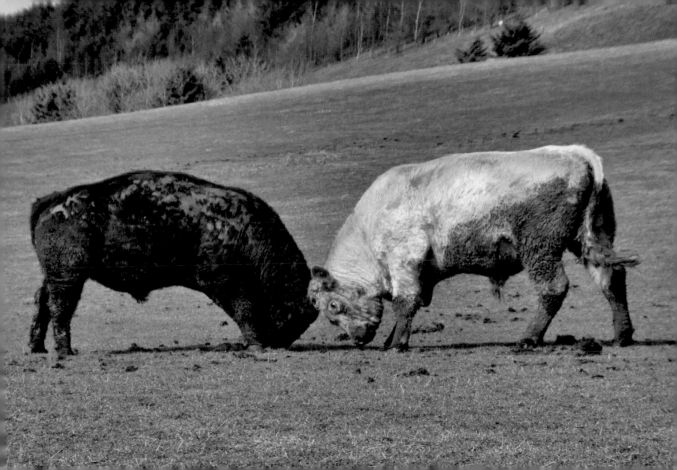

Neostigmine and Pyridostigmine

Thomas Willis (1621–1675), **Mary Walker** (1888–1974)

FROM MYASTHENIA GRAVIS TO GULF WAR SYNDROME. The earliest report of myasthenia gravis (MG) appeared in 1672, when Thomas Willis, famed English anatomist and physician, wrote of a woman "who temporarily lost her power of speech and became 'mute as a fish.'" More common symptoms of this nerve-muscle disorder include drooping eyelids and weakness of the arms and legs, particularly after exercise.

In 1934, **physostigmine** was used as an antidote for **curare** poisoning. Scottish physician Mary Walker thought that because MG symptoms resembled the muscle weakness caused by curare poisoning, a curare-like substance circulating in the blood might cause the disorder. She administered physostigmine to several of her patients. "Then . . . like Lazarus rising from the grave, they rose and walked across the room" (Jane Ellsworth, 1952).

Physostigmine acts by prolonging the effects of acetylcholine (ACh). After being released from nerve endings, the **neurotransmitter** chemical ACh crosses a synapse or gap and activates receptors on muscles, causing them to contract. Physostigmine is an anticholinesterase agent that acts by blocking the enzyme cholinesterase (responsible for the inactivation of ACh), thereby increasing ACh's ability to cause muscle contractions.

In 1935, Walker tested neostigmine, a physostigmine-like drug first synthesized in 1931, and found it far superior. When injected, neostigmine caused more forceful muscle contractions that persisted far longer, with fewer side effects. The next significant advance for treating MG was pyridostigmine (Mestinon), which appeared in 1959. It is taken by mouth, has fewer side effects, and acts for an even longer period—particularly, overnight.

During the Persian Gulf War of 1990–1991, U.S. troops were given pyridostigmine to prevent the toxic effects and mortality associated with exposure to the nerve gas soman. While the conclusions are highly controversial, it has been argued that pyridostigmine, when taken with insect repellents, may have contributed to the Gulf War Syndrome, whose very diverse symptoms include memory problems, fatigue, joint pain, dizziness, and skin and immune system conditions.

SEE ALSO Curare (1850), Physostigmine (1875), Drug Receptors (1905), Neurotransmitters (1920), Tabun and Sarin (1936).

Patients with advanced cases of myasthenia gravis experience profound weakness of the extremities. Mary Walker's first public demonstration that neostigmine could temporarily reverse these symptoms was likened to Lazarus rising from the grave.

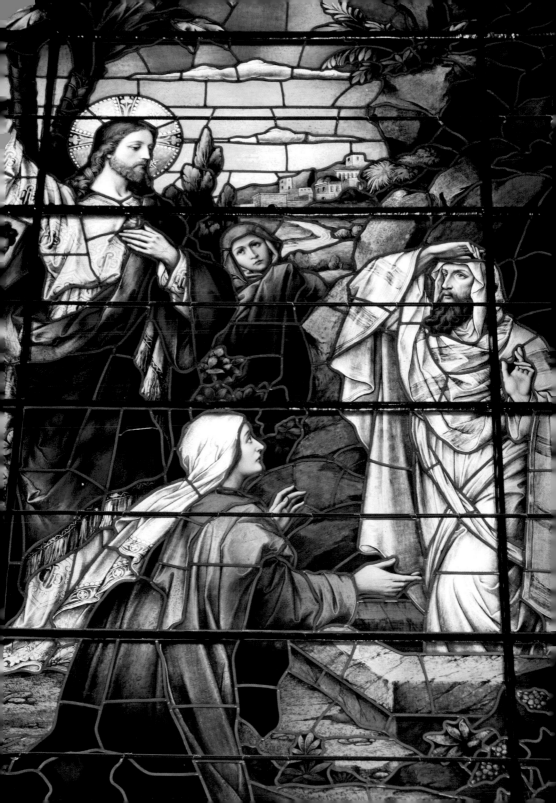

Tabun and Sarin

Gerhard Schrader (1903–1990)

In 1936, the German chemist Gerhard Schrader, working at IG Farben, was seeking to develop an insecticide that would disrupt the function of the insect nervous system. His studies focused upon the *organophosphates*, anticholinesterase chemicals that prevent the breakdown of acetylcholine.

DRUGS OF DEATH. One of these compounds, tabun, proved extremely effective in killing leaf lice, but accidental exposure to a single drop demonstrated dramatically that its toxic effects were not limited to insects. Schrader was overcome with dizziness and had severe difficulty seeing, thinking, and breathing. The focus of Schrader's research was immediately redirected from insect poisons to nerve gases intended for use as chemical-warfare weapons. If used on the battlefield, within minutes after very small amounts are inhaled or one to two hours after being absorbed through the skin, these highly volatile liquids are capable of causing death from respiratory failure.

Schrader, the "father of nerve gas," synthesized tabun (designated GA) in 1936, sarin (GB) in 1939, and soman (GD) in 1944. The German production of nerve gases remained secret until the final months of World War II, but they were never deployed against Allied troops.

The Iraqis were said to have used sarin in their 1980–1988 war against Iran but not during the Persian Gulf War. To protect American combatants against the potential deployment of sarin, the antidote **pyridostigmine** was given. It was thought that American and United Nations troops had been exposed to nerve gases when a chemical depot in Khamisiyah was destroyed in 1991, and many believe that this exposure, in combination with pyridostigmine use, may have contributed to Gulf War Syndrome.

In 1993, the United Nations General Assembly approved the Chemical Warfare Convention that outlaws the production, stockpiling, and use of chemical weapons, including nerve gases, and calls for the destruction of existing stores. This did not end the use of nerve gases, however. In 1995, members of the radical and militant religious organization Aum Shinrikyo released sarin on several Tokyo Metro subway trains, killing twelve and severely injuring more than fifty people, with thousands of others affected.

SEE ALSO Neostigmine and Pyridostigmine (1935), DDT (1939).

Just as early miners brought caged canaries into coal mines to detect gas leaks, rabbits were used to detect leaks at a sarin nerve gas production plant at the Rocky Mountain Arsenal in Commerce City, Colorado.

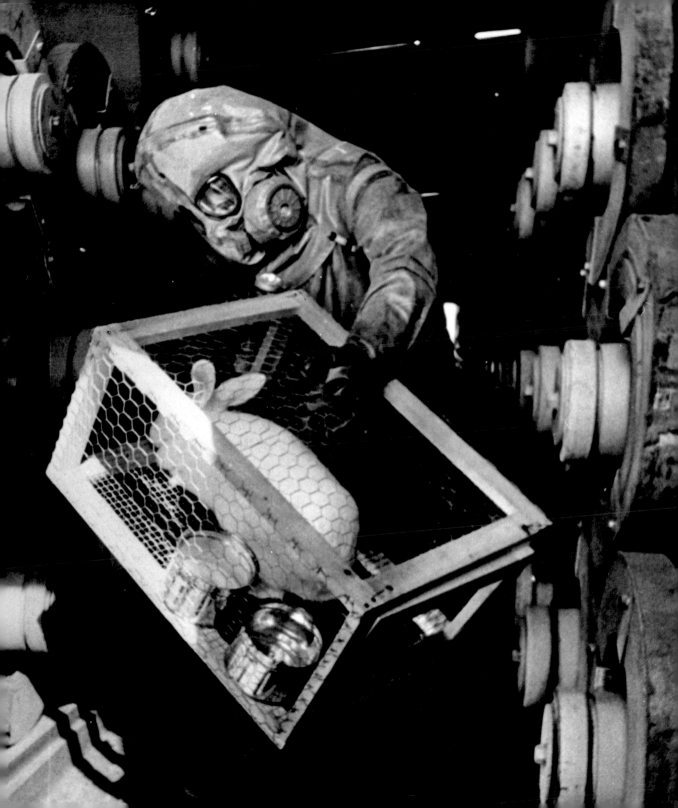

Sulfanilamide

With the discovery in 1935 that the red dye **Prontosil**'s antibacterial effects were attributed to its breakdown product, intense interest focused on sulfanilamide. Unlike Prontosil, it was cheaper, had fewer adverse effects, did not impart a red color to the skin and was not subject to patent restrictions. Sulfanilamide had a simple chemical structure that was highly amenable to being modified into other sulfa (or *sulpha* in British English) drugs that were less toxic and could treat a wider range of infectious diseases. Before the availability of **penicillin** in the first half of the 1940s, sulfas were the best antibacterial drugs available.

SAVING PRIVATE RYAN. Many of these drugs were lifesaving, but not always (see **Federal Food, Drug, and Cosmetic Act**). During World War I, more troops died from combat infections than from enemy bullets and explosives, so in 1941–42 each U.S. soldier's First Aid Packet was equipped with two sulfa drugs to prevent infection from severe wounds. Crystalline sulfanilamide, contained in 5-gram packages, was sprinkled over open wounds—a practice that continued until mid-1944, when it was determined that the powders were more harmful than beneficial. The packet also contained eight sulfadiazine tablets, which were to be taken with water until surgery, if needed. In the film *Saving Private Ryan* (1998), sulfa powder is sprinkled into Medic Wade's multiple abdominal wounds, but to no avail. Former British prime minister Winston Churchill was more fortunate than Medic Wade: Sulfapyridine tablets (M & B 693) effectively treated pneumonia he contracted during a visit to North Africa in December 1943.

With the exception of urinary-tract and respiratory-tract infections, sulfa drugs are now rarely used, having been replaced by penicillin and other antibiotics. The demise of the sulfa drugs was hastened by bacterial resistance, adverse effects on the urinary tract and blood, and hypersensitivity reactions, some of which can be life-threatening.

Sulfa chemicals have been modified to create medicines used for the treatment of leprosy (**Dapsone**), fluid accumulation (**Diuril**), and diabetes (**Orinase**).

SEE ALSO Penicillin (1928), Prontosil (1935), Dapsone (1937), Federal Food, Drug, and Cosmetic Act (1938), Orinase (1957), Diuril (1958).

On the use of a sulfa drug to treat his pneumonia, Churchill said in a 1944 radio broadcast, "This admirable M & B [after M & B, the company that made it] . . . was used at the earliest moment and after a week's fever the intruders were repulsed. I hope that all our battles will be equally well conducted."

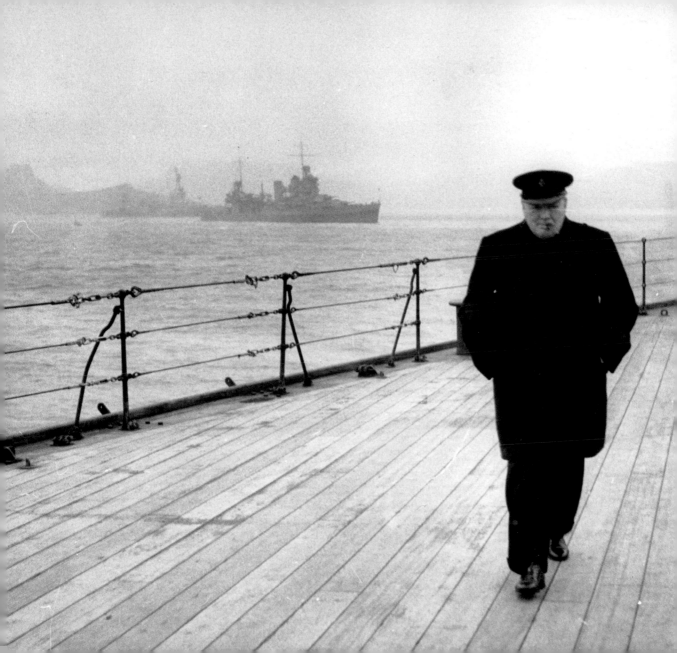

Dapsone

Gerhard Armauer Hansen (1841–1912)

Few disease over the millennia have generated as much terror, superstition, and false beliefs as leprosy, one of the oldest recorded diseases. Scholars believe that the leprosy of the Bible was actually other unrelated benign skin conditions. The leprosy we know was prevalent in Europe between 1000 and 1400, and then it declined. The many works of art from the period support the assumption that it was widespread. Leper houses, estimated to number 19,000 in Europe, were built to house the afflicted, and those not confined were required to wear special garb and to carry a wooden clapper warning the unsuspecting of their approach.

That leprosy was not a Divine punishment, or hereditary, or originating in bad air was established in 1873 by the Norwegian physician Gerhard Armauer Hansen, who discovered the first bacterium found to cause disease in humans: *Mycobacterium leprae*. Leprosy (Hansen's disease) causes disfiguring skin lesions and nerve damage resulting in muscle weakness and a loss of sensation in the skin. Although the afflicted have long been stigmatized, rejected, and excluded from society, this condition is not highly contagious—some 95 percent of people have natural immunity to it—and the symptoms generally appear slowly (three to seven years) after initial infection.

The "modern" era of drug treatment of leprosy has its origins in 1937, when dapsone, a sulfa-related drug, was tested for its antibacterial potential. It proved highly effective but was perceived as too toxic. Dapsone's effectiveness against experimental tuberculosis in animals provided a lead for its use in leprosy, because the two diseases are caused by closely related bacteria.

For more than six decades, dapsone (DDS) has remained the most important drug for leprosy treatment. To reduce the development of bacterial resistance, since the early 1980s dapsone has been given as a key component of multidrug therapy (MDT), in combination with **rifampin** and clofazimine, for at least a two-year treatment period. During the past two decades, this treatment has cured 15 million people worldwide.

SEE ALSO Sulfanilamide (1936), Streptomycin (1944), Rifampin (1967).

Contact with infected armadillos, long used for the testing of anti-leprosy drugs, has been found to be responsible for one-third of the 150–250 leprosy (Hansen's disease) cases that arise in the United States each year.

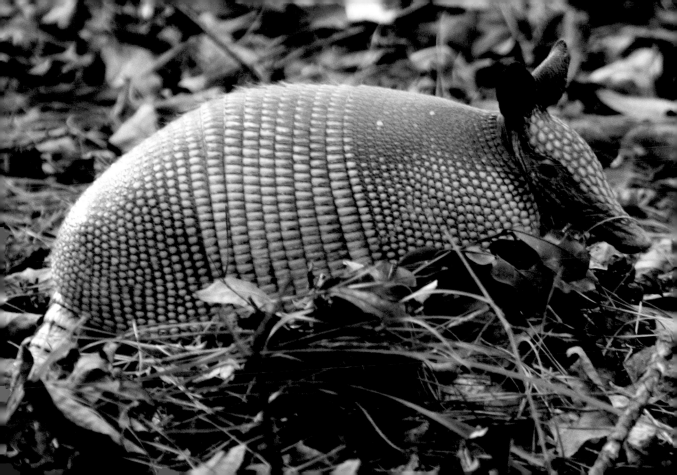

Diethylstilbestrol

Charles Dodds (1899–1973), Charles Huggins (1901–1997)

Estrone and other estrogenic compounds were isolated from human and horse urine during the 1930s and were used to relieve symptoms of menopause. These natural products had limited effectiveness when given orally, however, so they had to be injected. Moreover, their extraction from urine or the laboratory synthesis of such complex molecules was expensive. These problems were solved in 1938 when, in the laboratory of the British biochemist Charles Dodds at Oxford University, diethylstilbestrol (DES, stilbestrol) was synthesized.

DES had a simple nonsteroid chemical structure, was inexpensive to manufacture, and was very active when taken by mouth. Highly effective for the treatment of menopause, it was approved for this use in 1941 and for other estrogen-deficiency disorders in subsequent years. In 1947, its uses were extended to prevent complications of pregnancy—in particular, miscarriages—for which it was widely prescribed.

Later clinical studies failed to support claims of its effectiveness in preventing miscarriages. Moreover, women who used DES during pregnancy had a greater likelihood of developing breast cancer. Far more ominously, a 1971 report provided strong evidence that DES use was associated with vaginal cell cancer in girls and young women whose mothers had taken the drug during pregnancy. That year, the FDA withdrew their approval of DES to prevent miscarriages and emphasized that it should not be given during pregnancy.

Despite its link to breast and vaginal cancers, DES continues to be used for the treatment of prostate cancer. During the late 1930s, Charles Huggins at the University of Chicago noted that castration shrunk prostate tumors in dogs and that DES shut down the production of **testosterone**, producing a chemical castration. From these observations and subsequent studies involving breast cancer, Huggins postulated that certain cancers required hormones to grow and survive—a finding that spearheaded the development of certain classes of anticancer drugs and that earned him the 1966 Nobel Prize in Physiology or Medicine.

SEE ALSO Estrone and Estrogen (1929), Testosterone (1935), Premarin (1941), Tamoxifen (1973), 17P/Progesterone Injections and Gel (2003).

Prostate cancer is the third deadliest cancer in men of all ages and the most common cause of death from cancer in men over seventy-five years of age.

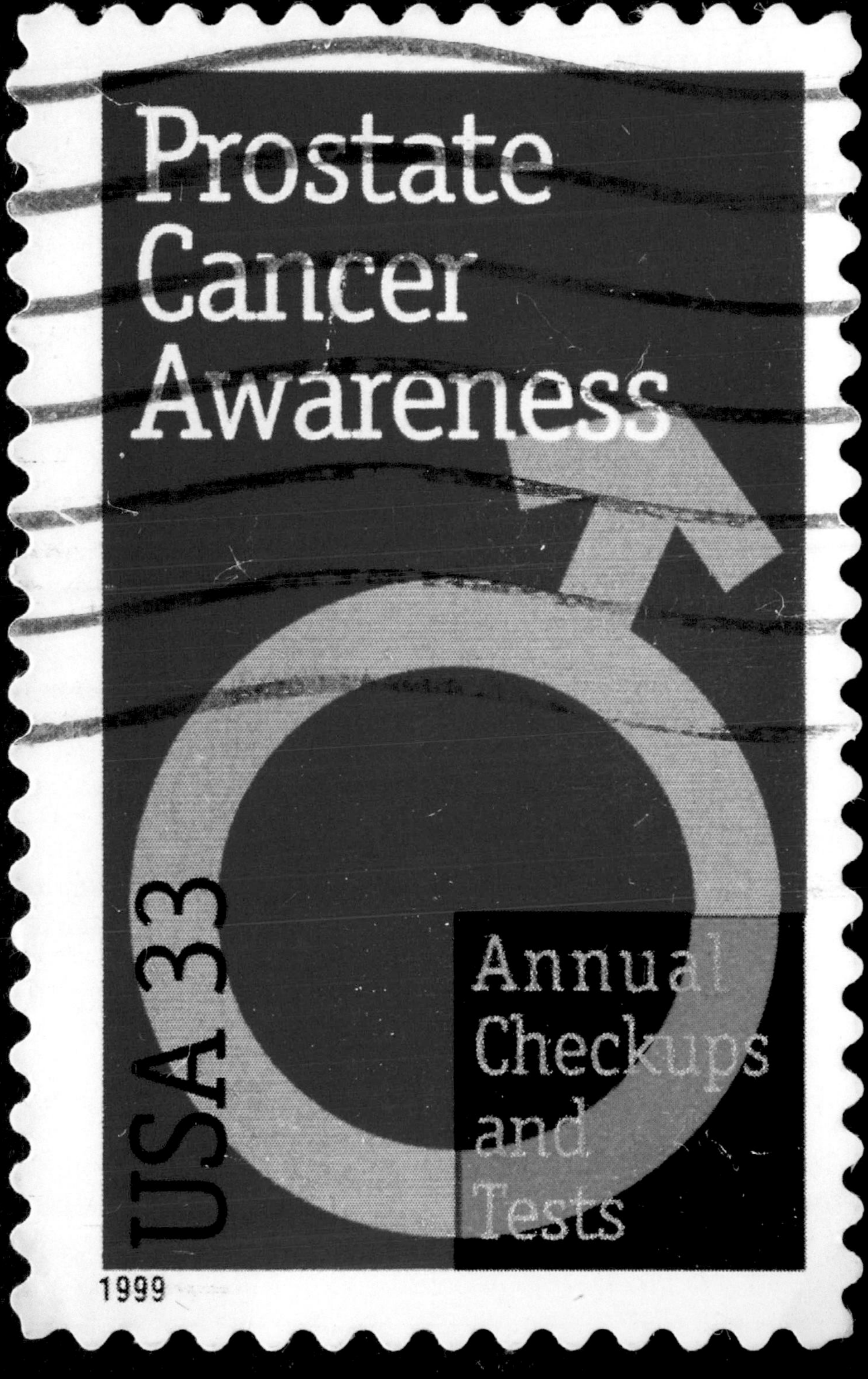

Prostate Cancer Awareness

USA 33

1999

Annual Checkups and Tests

Dilantin

Heinrich Biltz (1865–1943), Tracy J. Putnam (1894–1975), H. Houston Merritt (1902–1979)

The antiepileptic effects of the **bromides** and **phenobarbital** were discovered quite by accident. Not so for Dilantin. These earlier drugs controlled seizures but caused considerable drowsiness. Dilantin (phenytoin) demonstrated for the first time that sedation was not essential to controlling seizures.

Evaluation of potential antiseizure drugs required a device that could measure brain waves in humans. During the mid-1930s, Tracy J. Putnam and H. Houston Merritt, at Boston City Hospital—then the leading hospital in the United States in neurology— established the world's first electroencephalographic (EEG) laboratory to study brain waves in patients, including the characteristic violent EEG activity associated with epileptic seizures. An analogous recorder was devised to test potential drugs in animals.

One of the compounds tested was phenytoin, synthesized in 1908 by Heinrich Biltz, a professor of chemistry at the University of Kiel in Germany. Biltz sold the compound to the Detroit pharmaceutical company Parke-Davis, which shelved it for almost three decades until 1937, when positive antiseizure test results in animals were subsequently confirmed in human subjects. Phenytoin rivaled phenobarbital in preventing seizures but caused less sedation. Phenytoin (previously named diphenylhydantoin), marketed in 1938 as Dilantin, was effective against almost all seizure types, including the classic tonic-clonic (grand mal) seizures in which the patient experiences a loss of consciousness, convulsions, and severe muscle spasms throughout the body.

Some 50 million persons worldwide have epilepsy, a condition controlled but not cured with drugs. Sometimes several drugs are required to render 50 percent of patients seizure-free, while another 25 percent of sufferers derive significant benefit from them. Among the famous epileptics was the Russian writer Fyodor Dostoyevsky (1821–1881), as were his memorable characters Prince Myshkin in *The Idiot* and Smerdyakov in *The Brothers Karamazov*. Dilantin was administered as an anticonvulsant and used to control inmates, as depicted in Ken Kesey's 1962 novel *One Flew Over the Cuckoo's Nest*.

SEE ALSO Bromides (1857), Phenobarbital (1912), Valproic Acid (1967).

Dilantin was the first drug found to control epileptic seizures without causing excessive drowsiness. Electroencephalographic (EEG) recordings measure brain waves, which are used to distinguish among epileptic seizure types, so that the most appropriate antiepileptic drug may be selected.

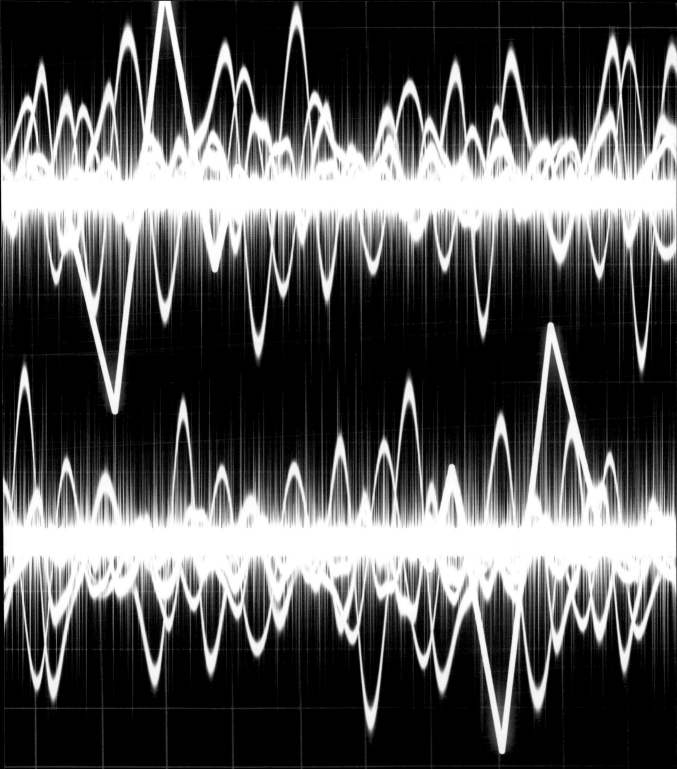

Federal Food, Drug, and Cosmetic Act

The newly introduced **sulfanilamide** tablets had been found safe and effective for the treatment of streptococcal infections, and there was a call for a liquid. After trying a number of solvents, Harold Cole Watkins, chief chemist and pharmacist at S.E. Massengill Co., Bristol, Tennessee, found that he could dissolve the drug in diethylene glycol. Elixir Sulfanilamide, as it was called, looked good, and its raspberry flavor tasted fine. Shipped out countrywide in September 1937, it had never been tested for toxicity, which was not required by law.

Within weeks, the first deaths were reported, and before the drug shipments were recovered, 105 of 353 patients who had consumed it in fifteen states had died—many of them children treated for sore throats. The solvent diethylene glycol, used as antifreeze, was responsible for fatal kidney failure. The **Food and Drug Administration** seized some of the drug because it had been misbranded as an "elixir" (an alcoholic solution) when it did not contain **alcohol**.

Three consequences arose directly from this disaster: Massengill paid out $500,000 in injury claims; chemist Watkins died of a self-inflicted gunshot wound to his heart in January 1939; and, most significantly, the 1906 **Pure Food and Drug Act**, which had only prohibited the adulteration or misbranding of drugs, was thoroughly revised. With the sulfanilamide disaster fresh in mind, Congress enacted the 1938 Federal Food, Drug, and Cosmetic Act, which required that new drugs be tested for toxicity and approved by the Food and Drug Administration *before* they were marketed. (This protected the American public against the marketing of **thalidomide** in 1960.) Other provisions of the law required that drug containers provide adequate directions for use of the drug and differentiated between prescription drugs and those that could be sold over the counter. Laws now mandated that drugs be pure and safe, but proof of their effectiveness had to wait until 1962.

SEE ALSO Alcohol (c. 10,000 BCE), Pure Food and Drug Act (1906), Food and Drug Administration (1906), Sulfanilamide (1936), Thalidomide (1957), Kefauver-Harris Amendment (1962).

In the aftermath of the devastating Hurricane Katrina in October 2005, barrels of antifreeze (diethylene glycol) and synthetic oil were scattered over lawns and roadways in Venice, Louisiana. This same diethylene glycol was used in "Elixir Sulfanilamide."

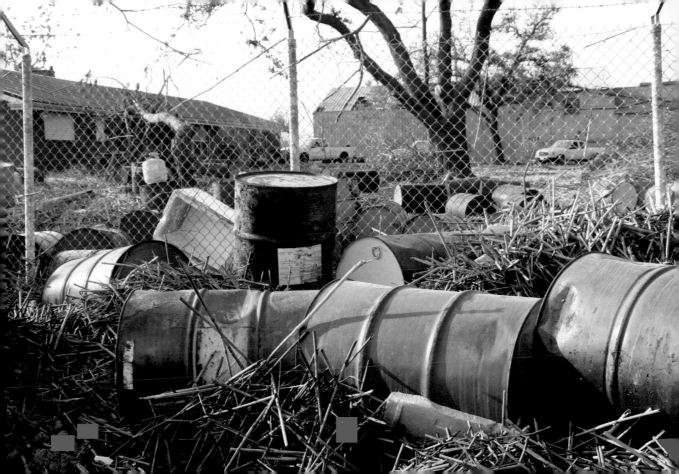

DDT

Paul Müller (1899–1965), **Rachel Carson** (1907–1964)

Typhus epidemics have accompanied us throughout history, generally during wars and famine. The disease was responsible for three million deaths during World War I and hundreds of thousands of deaths among Nazi concentration camp prisoners during World War II. DDT's application to the clothing of more than one million persons during the winter of 1943–1944 averted a major typhus epidemic in Naples by killing the lice responsible for carrying the bacterium causing typhus.

DDT (*dichlorodiphenyltrichloroethane* or chlorophenothane) was synthesized in 1874, but it was not until 1939 that Swiss chemist Paul Müller, at J. R. Geigy in Basel, Switzerland, discovered its insecticidal properties. In particular, he found that DDT readily crossed the insect exoskeleton (cuticle) and fatally disrupted its nervous-system function. In 1948, Müller received the 1948 Nobel Prize in Physiology or Medicine.

DDT's popularity stemmed from its effectiveness, very low cost, persistency after application to plants, and relatively low toxicity to mammals. Malaria, the most common human disease, affects some 250 million people worldwide and causes almost one million deaths annually. The World Health Organization initiated an international program in 1955 utilizing DDT to eradicate the mosquito vector of malaria.

HEALTH MIRACLE OR ENVIRONMENTAL DISASTER? DDT's accolades were not to endure! Poor management of the malaria-eradication program, inadequate funding, and indiscriminate DDT use led to insect resistance and loss of effectiveness. Of far greater impact in DDT's demise was Rachel Carson's book *Silent Spring* (1962), which documented the disastrous effects the indiscriminate use of pesticides, such as DDT, were having on the environment. Its use was linked to extensive fish kills and a thinning of eggshells, most famously for the bald eagle.

Silent Spring not unexpectedly generated vituperative criticism from the pesticide manufacturers and others emphasizing DDT's benefits to public health, although the book received overwhelming support from the scientific community and public and was instrumental in mobilizing a global environmental movement. The use of DDT was banned in the United States in 1972 and most developed countries by the 1980s.

SEE ALSO Quinine (1820), Chloroquine (1947), Malathion (1951), Artemisinin (1972).

The human body louse is the primary carrier of rickettsiae, the microbe responsible for causing epidemic typhus, one of history's most significant human diseases. When applied to the skin as a powder, DDT very effectively kills body lice and persists on the skin long enough to kill young lice as they emerge from their eggs.

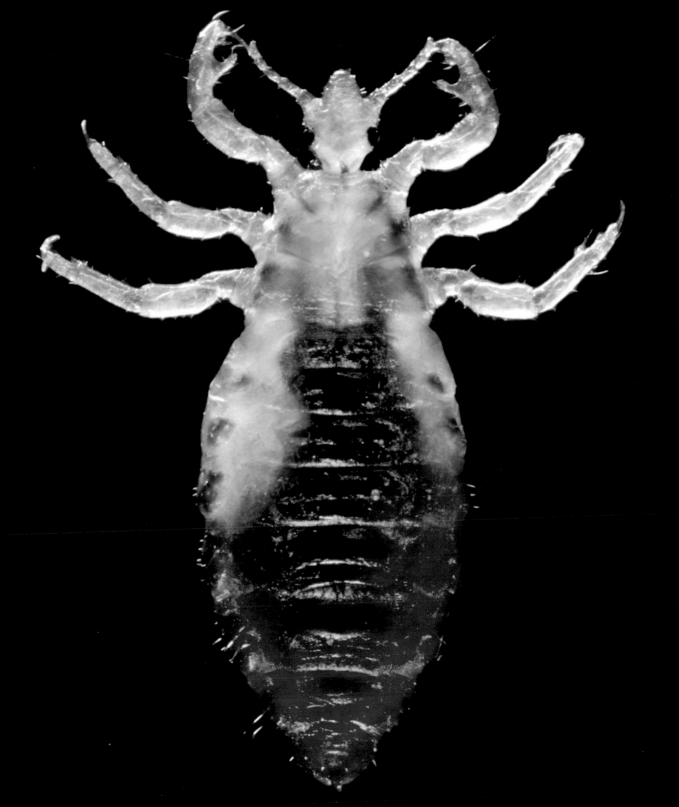

Percorten

Tadeus Reichstein (1897–1996)

Almost forty years after President John F. Kennedy's death in 1963, his medical records were publicly disclosed. Although his outward image exuded vigor and athleticism, throughout much of his adult life he was plagued with a variety of medical conditions and experienced constant and unremitting severe back pain. During his presidency, he reportedly took ten to twelve medicines a day. In 1947, at the age of thirty, he was officially diagnosed with Addison's disease, a life-threatening condition characterized by a deficiency of adrenal gland hormones, the replacement of which he required for the remainder of his life.

The adrenal glands sit atop each kidney and contain two parts. The inner medulla secretes hormones, such as **epinephrine/adrenaline**, which play an important role in the control of blood pressure and heart rate. The outer cortex secretes several types of essential hormones, including the glucocorticoids and mineralocorticoids. A deficiency of glucocorticoidal hormones, including **cortisone**-related compounds, leads to difficulties in controlling blood glucose (sugar) levels and the body's response to stress. Inadequate supply of the primary mineralocorticoid, aldosterone, causes salt imbalances and excessive water loss in urine, potentially leading to dehydration and shock.

During the 1920s and 1930s, study of the adrenal cortex became an active area of research interest, and gland extracts were used to treat Addison's patients. In 1938, Tadeus Reichstein, a Polish-born Swiss chemist at the University of Basel, isolated desoxycorticosterone from an extract of the adrenal cortex, and Ciba marketed it as Percorten the following year. This first corticosteroid to be synthesized and used for Addison's corrected the salt and water imbalances. Percorten is no longer used to treat Addison's in humans, but it continues to be prescribed for dogs.

Although Reichstein is best known for his studies on adrenal cortex hormones—including the isolation of cortisone (for which he was a co-recipient of the 1950 Nobel Prize for Physiology or Medicine)—his early research dealt with the chemicals contributing to the aroma of **coffee**.

SEE ALSO Coffee (c. 800), Epinephrine/Adrenaline (1901), Cortisone (1949).

An August 1963 photograph of brothers Robert, Edward "Ted," and President John F. Kennedy outside the Oval Office. JFK suffered from Addison's disease, a debilitating condition formerly treated with the use of the corticosteroid Percorten.

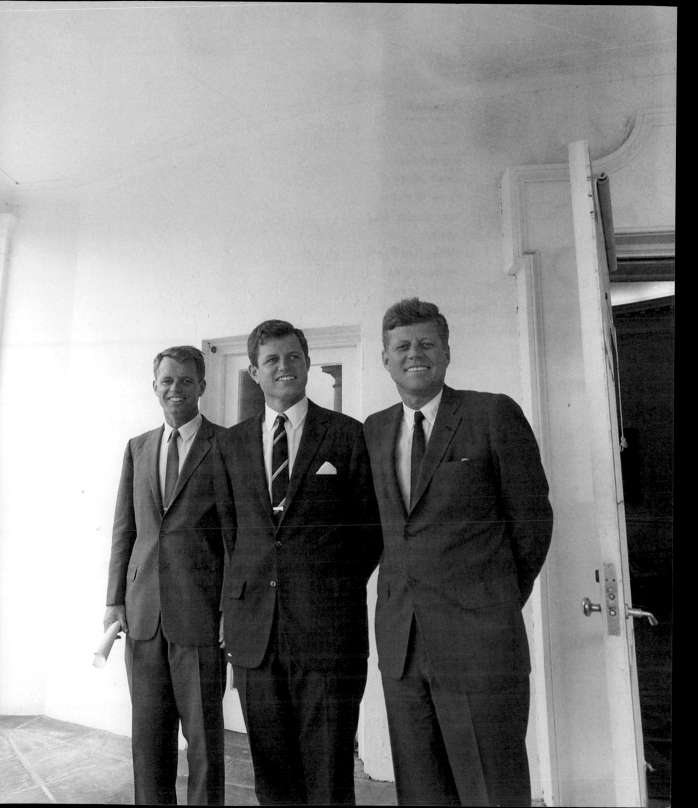

Warfarin

Frank W. Schofield (1889–1970), Karl Paul Link (1901–1978)

During the winter of 1921–1922, veterinarians in Alberta Province, Canada, and North Dakota were faced with a new disorder in cattle. The animals bled excessively and sometimes fatally after experiencing mild injury or minor surgery such as dehorning or castration. Frank W. Schofield, a Canadian veterinary pathologist, identified the cause of "sweet clover disease" to be a clotting defect resulting from ingesting a substance in the spoiled clover.

In the 1930s, Karl Paul Link, a biochemist at the University of Wisconsin–Madison, had set out to identify the anticoagulant (blood thinner), which he then isolated in 1940 in pure form from the clover, calling it dicoumarol. A longer-acting and more powerful synthetic derivative of dicoumarol, warfarin, was named after the Wisconsin Alumni Research Foundation. WARF funded Link's research and was the beneficiary of the royalties from warfarin sales as Coumadin and other trade-named products. Warfarin's first market in 1948 was as a rodenticide, and for many years it proved very popular worldwide. Because of its toxicity in animals, there was initial reluctance to using warfarin as a medicine. This obstacle was overcome in 1951 after a U.S. Army service member attempted suicide by ingesting a very large dose of a warfarin-containing rodenticide and survived. Warfarin was subsequently approved for medical use in 1954.

Warfarin, taken orally, prevents the synthesis of clotting factors, the formation of clots, and the dislodgement of such clots in veins, which block blood flow to vital organs. It is commonly used to prevent clotting in patients with artificial heart valves and atrial fibrillation, an abnormal heart rhythm. One of the earliest notable patients was President Dwight D. Eisenhower, who took warfarin in 1955 after a heart attack.

One of the great challenges associated with the use of warfarin is adjustment of its dose to achieve an ideal, personalized blood level: If too high, bleeding results; if too low, clots form. Moreover, warfarin interacts with a great number of drugs that can increase or decrease its blood levels.

SEE ALSO Aspirin (1899), Heparin (1916), Plavix (1997), Pradaxa (2010).

Mamie and Second Lieutenant Dwight D. Eisenhower in 1916, the year of their marriage, and one year after his graduation from the U.S. Military Academy at West Point. Nearly forty years later, Eisenhower began using warfarin, following a heart attack.

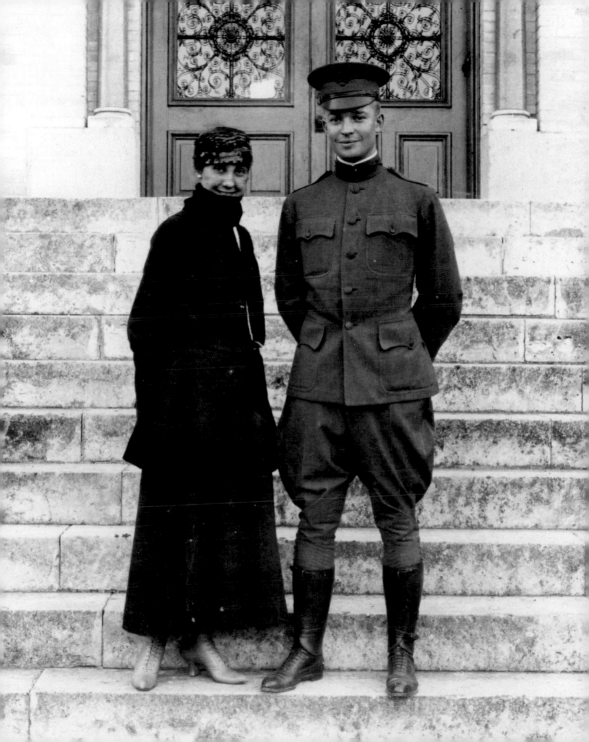

Premarin

Before 2002, hormones were routinely prescribed to women experiencing menopausal symptoms. Not only did **estrogen** (Premarin) or estrogen-**progestin** combination (Prempro) effectively treat the hot flashes, night sweats, and discomforting vaginal symptoms; women reported feeling great.

In 1941, the Canadian company Ayerst, McKenna & Harrison, Ltd., released a product obtained from *preg*nant *mares'* ur*ine*—Premarin—that contained a mixture of some ten estrogens. Approved for treating menopausal symptoms in the United States in 1942, it was natural, meaning "safe," to many. Between the late 1950s and early 1970s, a series of medical papers and popular books portrayed menopause as a *disease* of estrogen deficiency and extolled the long-term use of Premarin (hormone replacement therapy, HRT) to combat it, to prevent osteoporosis, and to protect the heart in menopausal and postmenopausal women. Sales increased significantly.

Scientific reports in 1975 established that estrogen therapy increased the risk of endometrial (uterine) cancer, and sales dropped precipitously by 1980. Yet, thanks to aggressive promotion to doctors and direct-to-consumer ads, from 1992 to 2000 Premarin became one of the two most popular drugs in America. The addition of a progestin to estrogen in 1995 reduced the danger of endometrial cancer.

The Women's Health Initiative (WHI) initiated two extensive, long-term clinical trials in the early 1990s to scientifically establish the beneficial effects of Prempro and Premarin in postmenopausal women. The Prempro study ended early in 2002 and unexpectedly concluded that Prempro users had a higher incidence of heart attacks, strokes, blood clots in the lungs, and breast cancer than **placebo** users; conversely, there were fewer cases of colorectal cancer and bone fractures. In the Premarin study, drug users had greater risks of strokes, blood clots, breast cancer, and possibly heart disease and dementia. Understandably, sales of Prempro and Premarin plunged!

Some of WHI results have been challenged and are being reevaluated for subsets of postmenopausal women. While HRT is highly effective in relieving menopause symptoms, women should critically weigh the risks. If drugs are used, it should be at the lowest doses for the shortest time (one to two years).

SEE ALSO Estrone and Estrogen (1929), Progesterone and Progestin (1933), Diethylstilbestrol (1938), Placebos (1955).

Menopause has been a source of humor but not for those experiencing its sometimes highly distressing symptoms. Premarin's and Prempro's ability to relieve these symptoms is well accepted, but do their benefits outweigh potential long-term risks?

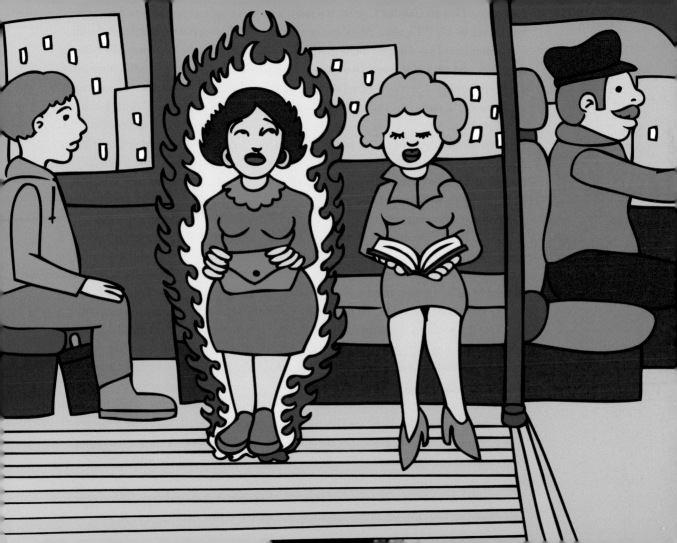

Nitrogen Mustard

Louis Goodman (1906–2000), **Alfred Gilman** (1908–1984)

FROM WAR GAS TO CANCER CHEMOTHERAPY. The backstory for cancer chemotherapy began on July 12, 1917, when Allied troops near Ypres in Flanders were bombarded with German mustard gas–charged shells. Early attention focused on the blistering effects on the skin, eyes, and respiratory tract. Two years later, the ability of mustard gas (sulfur mustard) to decrease the number of white blood cells and to break down lymph tissue was recognized.

The story continued during World War II. In 1942, Yale pharmacologists Louis Goodman and Alfred Gilman conducted wartime secret studies with a series of nitrogen mustard derivatives for potential use as war gases. In 1943, Bari, a major Italian seaport for supplying Allied troops, was subject to a German air raid. Seventeen ships, including the Liberty ship USS *John Harvey* and its secret cargo of nitrogen mustard, were lost along with some 1,000 servicemen. Survivors exposed to nitrogen mustard experienced a dramatic decrease in white blood cells. At the war's conclusion in 1946, the results of Goodman and Gilman's studies were published. The nitrogen mustards caused shrinkage of tumors of lymphoid cells, pointing to their potential use for treating lymphoma, Hodgkin's disease in particular. Cancer treatment options were no longer limited to radiation and surgery.

From these studies came the first cancer chemotherapeutic drugs, which prevent the cancer cell from dividing and growing. The first of these nitrogen mustard alkylating agents was HN2 or nitrogen mustard (Mustargen), given intravenously. Over the next decade, others included chlorambucil (Leukeran), busulfan (Myleran), and cyclophosphamide (Cytoxan)—all orally active drugs that are most effective against slow-growing tumors.

Although effective against many cancers and potentially lifesaving, alkylating agents are far from innocuous. They are also toxic to noncancerous cells that grow rapidly. These effects include depression of bone marrow, in which blood cells are produced (the most serious side effect that limits the dose of drug); hair follicle injury causing hair loss; and severe nausea and vomiting.

Goodman and Gilman's greatest legacy is their authorship and then editorship of *The Pharmacological Basis of Therapeutics*, a classic text first published in 1941, and its eleventh edition, in 2006.

SEE ALSO Amethopterin and Methotrexate (1947), Mercaptopurine (1953).

After being exposed to mustard gas during World War I, Allied troops (and their military dogs and horses) stationed on the Western front were issued gas masks. A gas mask covers and protects the mouth, nose, and face and is equipped with a filter canister that absorbs the toxic gas.

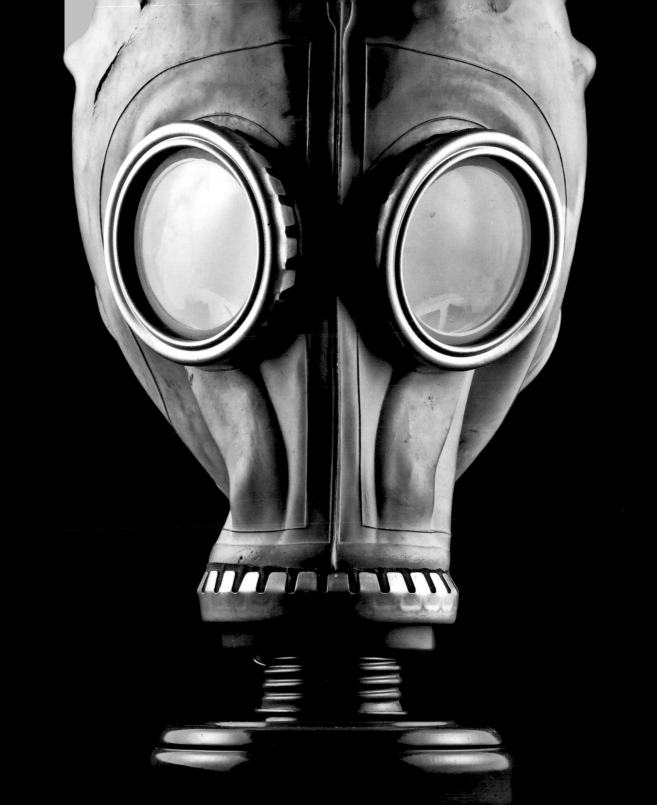

LSD

Albert Hofmann (1906–2008)

On Friday, April 16, 1943, Swiss chemist Albert Hofmann felt ill and left his Sandoz laboratory mid-afternoon. Lying down at home, he reported that "there surged in upon me an uninterrupted stream of fantastic images of extraordinary vividness and accompanied by intense, kaleidoscope-like play of colors." Suspecting a link between these effects and a chemical on which he had been working—initially synthesized in 1938 and then put aside—the following Monday he ingested an extremely small amount of the chemical: 250 micrograms (0.25 mg). Forty minutes later, during his "bicycle day" ride home and for the next six hours, disordered and multicolored images ran through his head.

Hofmann's seemingly minute dose of lysergic acid diethylamine (LSD-25, lysergide) was actually five to ten times higher than a normal dose. (LSD is the most potent hallucinogenic substance known, acting in the brain at seemingly infinitesimal doses). His 1947 scientific report captured the attention of a widely diverse range of readers, including scientists, psychiatrists, the CIA, the army, and recreational users.

In the 1950s, when the biomedical community was focused on the brain and mental disorders, LSD was utilized to better understand the brain and to study the cause and treatment of schizophrenia. It was given to enhance psychotherapy sessions and to combat alcoholism.

The CIA and army conducted experiments with more than 1,000 soldiers and civilians, testing LSD's potential to behaviorally disrupt the enemy and to elicit obedience in prisoners and spies. In the mid-1970s, when these army-sponsored 1950s-era studies were disclosed, it was obvious that ethical codes of human experimentation had been violated. Many of the subjects were not willing volunteers, neither were they informed about the nature and risks of the studies.

SEEING SOUNDS IN LIVING COLOR. Inspiring the emergence of psychedelic rock in the 1960s and 1970s, LSD has long attracted the interest of artists, writers, and musicians, who used LSD to expand their consciousness, creativity, and insights. Although experts have not found concrete evidence for such mind-altering effects, LSD can cause synesthesia (a mixing of the senses) in which sounds are seen. Research continues into possible beneficial effects of LSD for alcoholics, terminally ill patients, and others.

SEE ALSO Clinical Testing of Drugs (1753), Mescaline (1897), Ergotamine and Ergonovine (1925).

Psychedelic art is work inspired by hallucinogenic experiences from LSD, mescaline, or psilocybin. Surrealistic subject matter, kaleidoscopic patterns, bright colors, details, and the morphing of objects or themes characterize this genre.

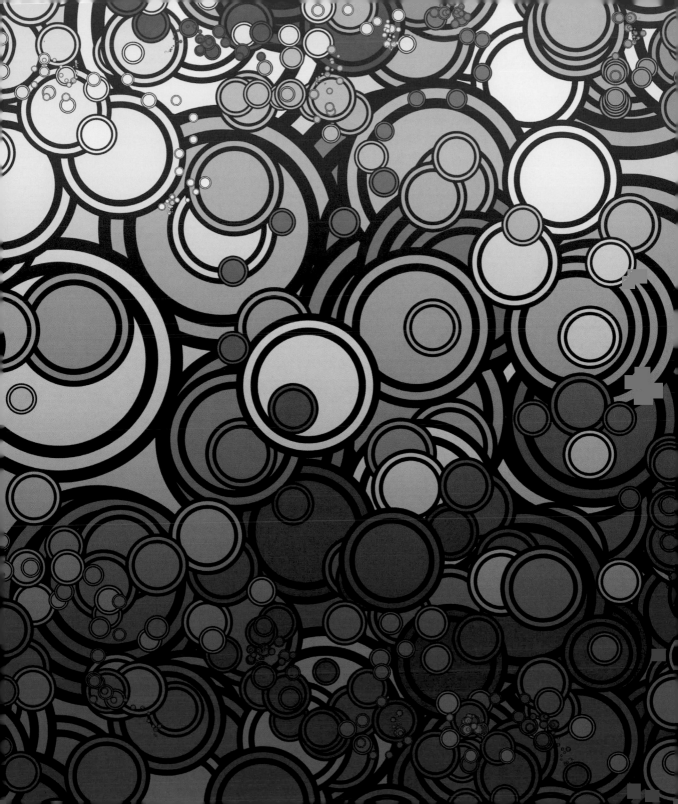

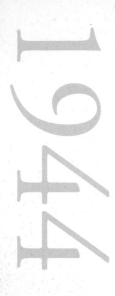

Streptomycin

Selman Waksman (1888–1973), **Albert Schatz** (1922–2005)

OVERCOMING THE WHITE PLAGUE. Evidence of tuberculosis (TB) dates back 6,000 years. During the nineteenth century, one in four deaths in Europe was caused by consumption or White Plague, as TB was then known. The disease was even romanticized in the deaths of heroines in *La Bohème*, *Les Misérables*, and *La Traviata*. Since 1877, it was known that certain soil-dwelling bacteria and fungi were able to kill or interfere with the growth of disease-causing microbes (termed *antibiosis*), including the *tubercle bacillus*, the bug responsible for TB.

Selman Waksman was born in a peasant village near Kiev, now in Ukraine. He came to the United States in 1910 and, after completing his education, became a faculty member in biochemistry and microbiology at Rutgers University. Over four decades, he and his associates discovered more than twenty antibiotics (Waksman coined the word), including neomycin and streptomycin. From among the 10,000 soil samples he tested was streptomycin, the first effective anti-TB drug. Discovered in 1944, it was the first choice for TB treatment for many years, but the rapid development of bacterial resistance and toxicity interfered with its effectiveness, and the injectable drug was displaced by less toxic drugs that could be given by mouth (e.g., **isoniazid**, **rifampin**).

Streptomycin was also effective in treating infections resistant to **penicillin**, the first antibiotic. Among these were high-mortality tularemia (rabbit fever) and meningitis, as well as urinary-tract infections. Streptomycin fathered a new family of antibiotics: the aminoglycosides, which include **gentamicin**.

Scientific acclaim and financial rewards were showered upon Waksman. Neglected was his graduate student, Albert Schatz, who claimed to have been a co-discoverer of streptomycin, the subject of his doctoral dissertation. Schatz was the first author on the scientific paper announcing its discovery and was listed second on its patent. Although a 1950 out-of-court settlement, with undisclosed terms, granted Schatz both recognition as a co-discoverer and a fraction of the royalties, only Waksman received the 1952 Nobel Prize in Physiology or Medicine. In Waksman's acceptance speech, Schatz was inconspicuously mentioned as only one of eighteen students and associates.

SEE ALSO Penicillin (1928), Isoniazid (1951), Gentamicin (1963), Rifampin (1967).

This 1953 photograph shows Selman Waksman in his laboratory at Rutgers University in New Jersey.

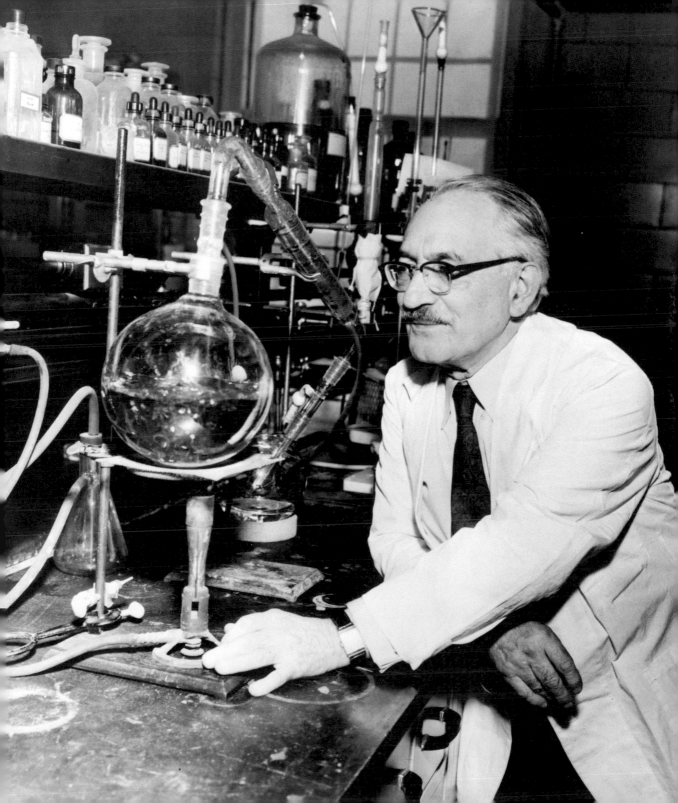

Neo-Antergan

Henry Hallett Dale (1875–1968), **Daniel Bovet** (1907–1992)

During the first three decades of the twentieth century, histamine was isolated from **ergot**, a fungus, and then from animal tissues. It was also found to have profound effects that resembled anaphylactic shock and shown to play a role in allergies. Many of these discoveries were the product of work by Henry Hallett Dale and his laboratory colleagues at the Wellcome Research Laboratory and National Institute for Medical Research, both in London.

THE FIRST ANTIHISTAMINE. If we consider that some 10–15 percent of the population suffers from allergies, the commercial impetus to develop a drug that could antagonize histamine was indeed compelling. In 1937, the Swiss-born Italian pharmacologist Daniel Bovet, working at the famed Pasteur Institute in Paris, began systematically testing a series of potential antihistaminic compounds on guinea pigs. Compound 929F effectively protected guinea pigs exposed to histamine but was too toxic. In 1944, Bovet's efforts were rewarded with the discovery of Neo-Antergan (mepyramine, pyrilamine), among the first marketed antihistamines. In 1957, Bovet was awarded the Nobel Prize in Physiology or Medicine for his work on antihistamines and **curare**-like drugs.

The marketplace response to Neo-Antergan, **Benadryl**, and other antihistamines was overwhelmingly positive and led to the introduction of dozens of comparable products. Some were also marketed for the treatment of motion sickness and the common cold, while others, including mepyramine, were applied to the skin to relieve itching. Antihistamines caused varying levels of drowsiness. For many years, mepyramine was used in nonprescription sleep aids but has since been replaced by Benadryl (diphenhydramine).

Likely not enamored of antihistamines, Goodman and Gilman, authors of the leading textbook of pharmacology, noted in 1955, "Perhaps in no other class of therapeutic agents does the physician enjoy a wider choice of preparation; but in no other group of drugs does a discerning choice offer less reward." All this changed in the 1990s, with the introduction of **Claritin** and other non-sedating antihistamines.

SEE ALSO Ergot (1670), Curare (1850), Ergotamine and Ergonovine (1925), Tubocurarine (1935), Benadryl (1946), Claritin (1993).

Guinea pigs were commonly used as test animals for biological research in the nineteenth and twentieth centuries; hence, test subjects are often referred to as guinea pigs. These cute animals are particularly sensitive to the effects of histamine and were extensively used to evaluate antihistamines, such as Neo-Antergan.

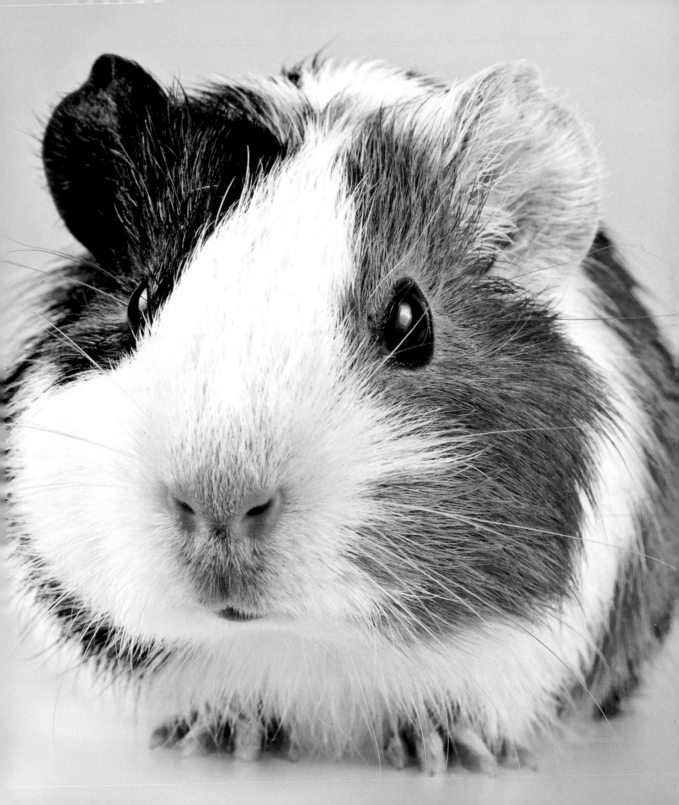

Methamphetamine

First approved in the United States for the treatment of depression, alcoholism, and narcolepsy in 1944, methamphetamine is among the most powerful brain stimulants. Its effects are very similar to **amphetamine**, as are its current medical uses for the treatment of attention deficit hyperactivity disorder and weight reduction. However, these medical uses have been totally overshadowed by its abuse.

During World War II, methamphetamine was taken by both the Allied and Axis combatants to enhance their physical and mental effectiveness; in Japan, it maintained the motivation and improved the efficiency of factory workers. After the war, the huge military stockpile was made available to the Japanese civilian market, leading to its widespread abuse.

During the 1960s, increased amphetamine abuse lead to increased restrictions on physicians prescribing it and on its legal manufacture in the United States. The illicit market responded by setting up clandestine home meth (crank) laboratories throughout the rural South and Midwest. Pseudoephedrine and ephedrine, legal ingredients in nonprescription cold and allergy products, were used as starting materials. Notwithstanding federal restrictions on the sale of products containing these ingredients since the 1980s, as well as the potential dangers for the "stovetop chemist" exposed to toxic chemicals and fumes, meth is relatively easy to prepare. The market is extensive, and the profits are high. In recent years, most of the meth in the United States has been prepared in Mexico. Since 1999, meth usage has steadily decreased.

Meth is most commonly injected intravenously by "shooting up" or "mainlining," smoked by vaporizing "crystal meth" or "ice" and inhaling the fumes, or snorted by inhaling the finely crushed powder.

Methamphetamine has more pronounced behavioral effects than amphetamine, producing intense euphoria, hallucinations, psychotic behavior, as well as increased physical and mental activity, self-confidence, and sex drive. Abrupt discontinuation after long-term use leads to withdrawal effects characterized by fatigue and depression. Meth possesses very strong addiction potential that is extremely difficult to treat. Long-term users are often depressed and suicidal, and they may develop a schizophrenia-like psychosis. Other health risks include loss of teeth (meth mouth) and HIV in gay and bisexual men via higher rates of unprotected sex.

SEE ALSO Amphetamine (1932), MDMA/Ecstasy (1976), Crack Cocaine (1986).

After being injected or smoked using a glass pipe, crystal methamphetamine produces longer-lasting and more intense stimulation than its powdered form. It can also be snorted, swallowed, or inserted into the anus or urethra, with euphoric effects lasting up to twelve hours.

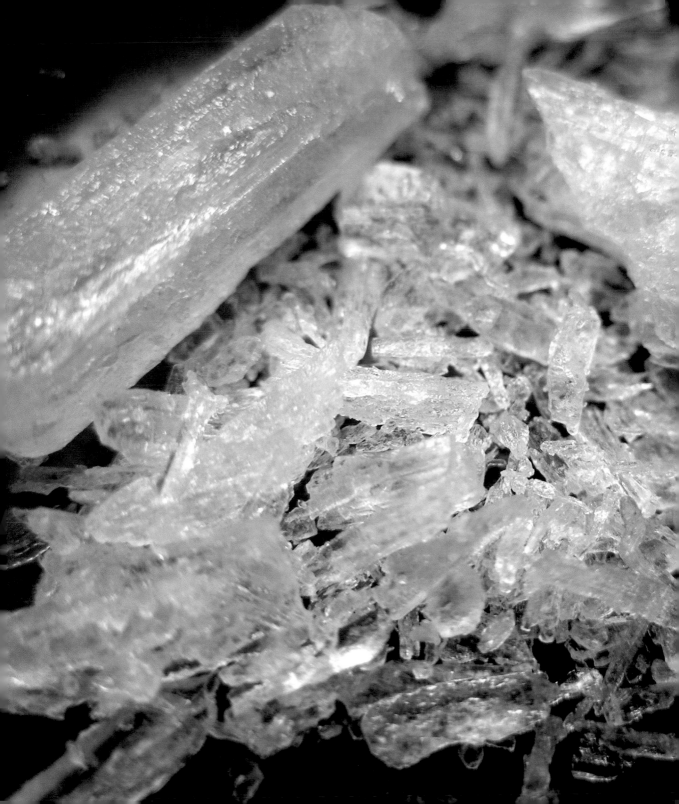

Fluorides

Which public-health accomplishments in the United States during the twentieth century have had the greatest impact on death, disease, and disability? If we limit our tabulation to those in which drugs have played a major role, we can readily include: eradication or prevention of infectious diseases with vaccines; treatment and cure of infectious diseases with antibiotics and other chemotherapeutic agents; reduction of deaths caused by coronary heart disease and stroke; and family planning with hormonal contraceptives.

A far less obvious inclusion on this list, compiled by the U.S. Centers for Disease Control and Prevention (CDC), is the prevention of tooth decay by the addition of fluorides to drinking water and toothpastes. Since 1945, this measure has safely and very inexpensively reduced tooth decay by 40–70 percent in children and 25–30 percent in adults. Additionally, tooth loss in adults has declined by 40–60 percent. For every dollar spent on fluoridation, an estimated $38 is saved on dental treatment. Fluoridation of drinking water has been most commonly adopted in the United States, Canada, the United Kingdom, and Australia, while fluoridated salt is widely utilized in continental Europe.

When ingested, fluoride is incorporated into the structure of developing teeth and acts on the surface of teeth. It both prevents the acid in plaque from demineralizing tooth enamel and enhances the rate at which teeth repair themselves by remineralization. Fluoride levels of 0.5–1.0 parts per million (ppm) in drinking water generally provide optimal benefits. International medical and dental experts agree that there is only one adverse effect associated with excessive exposure to fluorides. When teeth are developing before the age of eight, dental fluorosis—a discoloration or mottling of permanent teeth—may occur.

PROMOTING PUBLIC HEALTH OR UNDERMINING INDIVIDUAL FREEDOM?

Opponents of fluoridation of community drinking water argue that it causes major adverse health problems or that its expense outweighs its benefits. By imposing compulsory mass medication, it violates the individual's right to choose. As depicted in Stanley Kubrick's 1964 classic film *Dr. Strangelove*, during the post-World War II Cold War period, conspiracy theorists argued that it was a Communist plot designed to undermine the public health of Americans.

Noted sociologist and photographer Lewis Hine took this picture of a dentist at work at the Hood Rubber Company Hospital in Cambridge, Massachusetts, in 1917.

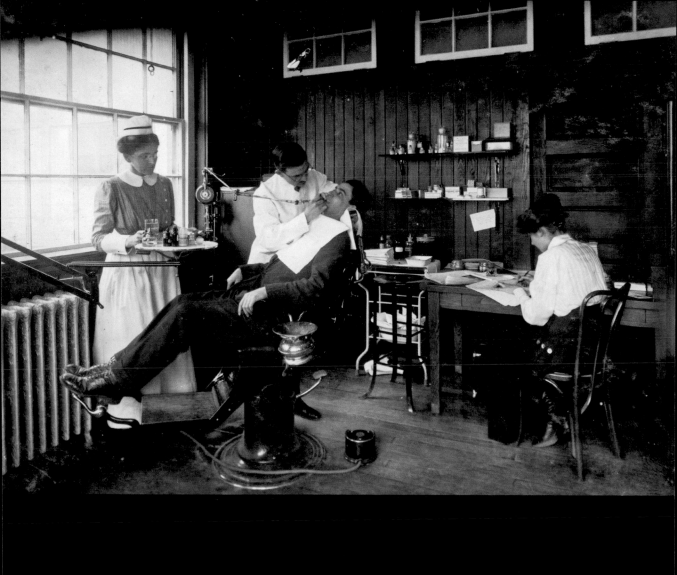

Benadryl

George Rieveschl (1916–2007)

During the course of attempting to find a muscle relaxant in the early 1940s, George Rieveschl, chemistry professor at the University of Cincinnati, synthesized diphenhydramine. In 1943, he took himself and his new compound to Parke-Davis, then the oldest and largest pharmaceutical company in the United States, who marketed it as Benadryl in 1946. Sensing an extremely lucrative potential market for antihistamines, Benadryl was joined in the marketplace by tripelennamine (Pyribenzamine), methapyrilene (Histadyl), and chlorpheniramine (Chlor-Trimeton), among others, by 1950.

As a class of drugs, antihistamines proved to be highly effective for the treatment of allergic disorders and hives. In short order, many of these drugs were promoted for motion sickness, morning sickness, and itching when applied to the skin. But more exciting news poured in. According to a 1949 article in *Reader's Digest*, the "best health news of the year" was the dramatic announcement that antihistamines could *prevent and cure* the common cold. The public response to the ensuing multidimensional promotional campaign was enthusiastic, and individuals with vested financial and scientific interests tended to overlook the shortcomings of the studies leading to these conclusions. More critical tests and analysis of the older results revealed that antihistamines were no more effective than **placebos** and, at best, only provided symptomatic relief of runny noses. Nevertheless, most products intended to treat symptoms of the common cold contain an antihistamine ingredient.

Benadryl is a highly effective drug for treating allergies and is still used for that purpose, but relief is accompanied by a considerable degree of drowsiness. This downside has transformed diphenhydramine into the most widely used nonprescription sleep-aid drug. However, not all allergy sufferers have insomnia; the appearance of **Claritin** in 1993 addressed this consideration.

SEE ALSO Neo-Antergan (1944), Placebos (1955), Claritin (1993).

The most common pollen allergy is allergic rhinitis (hay fever), which occurs when pollen spores are inhaled, causing the release of histamine and other chemicals in susceptible individuals. Antihistamines, such as Benadryl, block the effects of histamine.

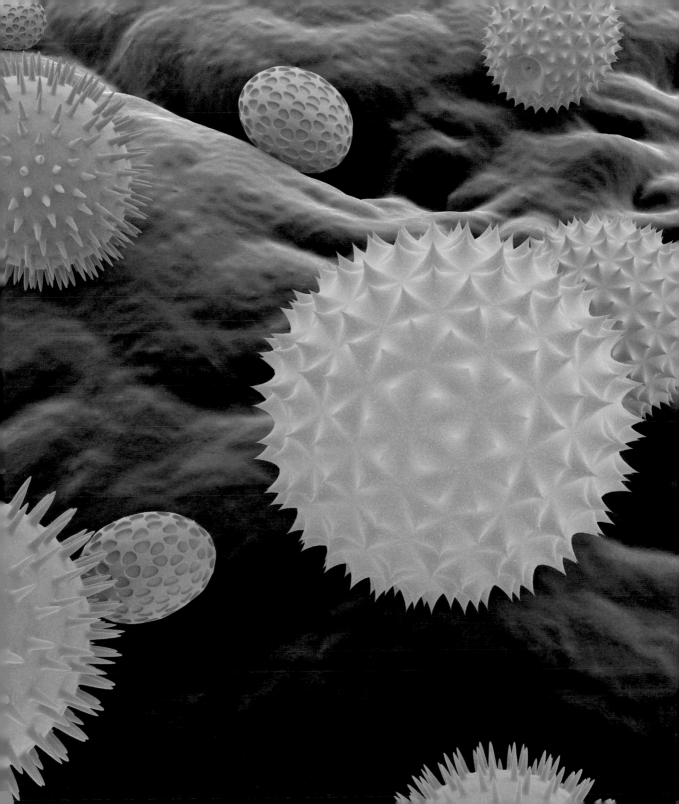

Radioiodine

Pierre Curie (1859–1906), **Marie Sklodowska-Curie** (1867–1934)

THE CURIE LEGACY. In 1898, Marie and Pierre Curie discovered radium, which in 1901 was the first radioisotope used in medicine, initially for the treatment of skin disorders. However, it wasn't until 1946, when artificially produced radioisotopes became available in large quantities, that their medical applications really took off. Currently, there are some thirty radioisotopes used for medical purposes, with more than fifty applications; 95 percent of these radiopharmaceuticals are used for the diagnosis of diseases, with the remainder used for disease treatment. Radioactive iodine (iodine-131), commonly called radioiodine, was among the earliest radiopharmaceuticals and is used to both treat and diagnose disorders of the thyroid gland.

Hormones from the thyroid gland have major effects in adults, such as mediating the rate of metabolism of most cells and the rate and force with which the heart contracts. Synthesis of thyroid hormones is dependent on the availability of iodine in the diet. The thyroid gland very actively and effectively concentrates the body's stores of iodine and radioiodide, capturing levels twenty to fifty times the concentration found in plasma.

In Graves' disease, the most common cause of hyperthyroidism, the individual has an enlarged thyroid gland (goiter) and typically a rapid and abnormal heartbeat, as well as nervousness and an elevated metabolic rate, which increases body temperature and weight loss.

Graves' disease can be treated by surgically removing the thyroid gland or by administration of radioiodine to partially destroy the gland, which spares the patient the risks and expense of surgery. The properties of beta particles emitted from this isotope are such that they don't travel outside the thyroid gland, thus producing minimal damage to surrounding tissues. However, following surgery or administration of radioiodine, the patient must take thyroid hormone pills for a lifetime. Unlike surgery, the full benefits of radioiodine may not be apparent for months.

Radioiodine is also used to diagnose a range of thyroid disorders. After the oral administration of radioiodide, the thyroid gland is scanned for radioactivity. The amount and extent to which the gland takes up the radioisotope serves as a measure of thyroid activity.

SEE ALSO Thyroxine (1914), Synthroid (1997).

Pierre and Marie Curie are shown in their laboratory, with Pierre holding a vial of radium.

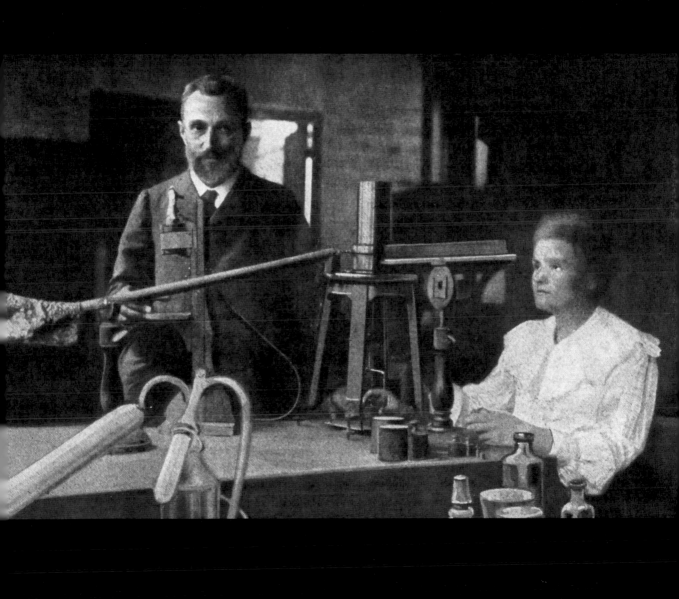

Methadone

Vincent Dole (1913–2006), **Marie Nyswander** (1919–1986)

Among the substitutes for **morphine** synthesized by German scientists before and during World War II was methadone. After the war, all German patents were expropriated by the Allies and confiscated by the U.S. Department of State. Eli Lilly acquired the rights to methadone in 1947 and marketed it as an analgesic (painkiller) and cough suppressant under the trade name Dolophine. Two decades later, it was the most widely used drug for the treatment of **heroin** addiction—a use that has been derided by some.

Methadone does not resemble morphine chemically but produces many of the same effects, including addiction. However, unlike morphine, it is very effective when taken by mouth and acts for extended periods. In the mid-1960s, Vincent Dole and his wife Marie Nyswander, working at the Rockefeller Institute (now Rockefeller University), introduced methadone for the treatment of heroin addiction.

Daily doses of methadone reduce the craving addicts have for heroin and prevent the withdrawal symptoms in physically dependent individuals. Those who quit using heroin and remain in the methadone maintenance treatment (MMT) program engage in fewer criminal activities (as they are obtaining methadone legally) and are more likely to assume family responsibilities and gainful employment. Moreover, because methadone is taken by mouth, the transmission of hepatitis and HIV by contaminated needles is reduced.

SUBSTITUTE ADDICTION: GOOD OR BAD? MMT is not without detractors or problems. Because methadone is often used for extended periods—for some, a lifetime—methadone addiction often replaces heroin addiction. Loose control of methadone distribution at some clinics has led to accidental overdoses and deaths. In addition, numerous private methadone clinics in the United States may charge clients $50–300/week. Without insurance, methadone is, thus, unaffordable for many users, and even well-motivated addicts may face long waits before entering programs. Although methadone offers hope for the heroin addict, it is not the final solution to this intractable societal problem.

SEE ALSO Morphine (1806), Heroin (1898), Opioids (1973), OxyContin (1996).

For those unable or unwilling to go "cold turkey," methadone provides a weapon to break the shackles of heroin addiction. Not infrequently, individuals may need the persuasion of a significant other to enroll in a methadone maintenance program; in other instances, courts may offer an addict the option of either incarceration for heroin-related offenses or successful participation in a methadone program.

DRUG

30s

FIGHT

ABUSE

40s

PILIPINAS

Drug Metabolism

Richard Tecwyn Williams (1909–1979)

What happens to a drug after it has entered your blood and acted for some finite period? Is it doomed to sail eternally around your body like the legendary ship *The Flying Dutchman*? Drug metabolism prevents our bodies from becoming junkyards for all the drugs we have ever taken. The drug-clearing process of metabolism (or biotransformation) chemically converts drugs into products called metabolites that can be more readily excreted from the body by the kidney, the major organ of drug elimination. These chemical changes require the presence of biological catalysts called enzymes, primarily located in the liver, which permit animals to eliminate foreign toxic chemicals. In his classic 1947 work, *Detoxification Mechanisms*, R. T. Williams defined these reactions and laid the foundation for the study of drug metabolism.

The speed at which drugs are metabolized determines the intensity and length of their effects. If the rate of metabolism is slowed by reducing the activity of these drug-metabolizing enzymes, the drug will act with greater force for a longer than normal period, increasing the risk of toxicity. Conversely, speeding up the rate of metabolism (enzyme induction) by smoking cigarettes, for example, can reduce the intensity and effectiveness of the drug and shorten the time it continues to act.

Metabolism explains, in part, why some individuals or groups of individuals are highly sensitive to drugs, while others are more resistant. Some differences can be attributed to other drugs taken concurrently that have the potential to stimulate or inhibit the activity of drug-metabolizing enzymes. Other factors that modify the rate of metabolism include the age of the patient (low enzyme activity in infants, young children, and the elderly) and genetic factors. Members of certain Asian groups (Chinese, Japanese, Koreans) are more sensitive to the effects of alcohol than Caucasians—a difference attributed to a deficiency of the enzyme aldehyde dehydrogenase.

In the past, metabolism was thought to transform chemical compounds into metabolites that had less biological activity than their parent drug. Usually this is true, but not always. Levodopa is inactive, but when it enters the brain it is metabolized to dopamine, which is effective for the treatment of Parkinson's disease.

SEE ALSO Chloramphenicol (1949), Succinylcholine (1951), Isoniazid (1951), Malathion (1951).

Certain ethnic groups, or individuals within a given ethnic group, may differ from the general population in their ability to metabolize drugs. New drugs are increasingly being tailored to treat those few individuals whose unusual response to them is based on a genetically associated, atypical drug metabolism.

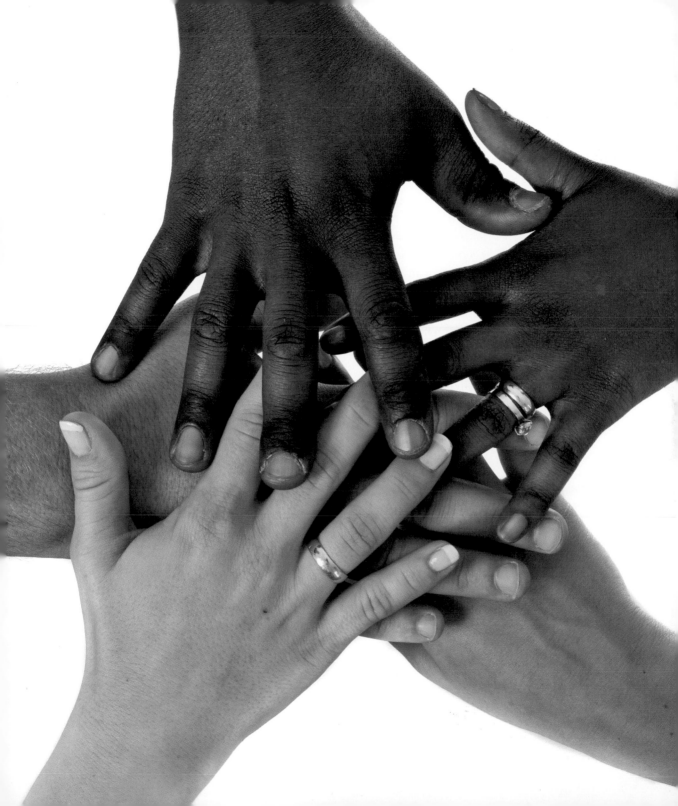

Chloroquine

Hans Andersag (1902–1955)

Malaria is one of the major causes of death worldwide and the most critical health problem in more than ninety countries, home to 40 percent of the world's population. There are four different strains of *Plasmodium*, the malaria-causing protozoan parasite, and these are transmitted by a bite of the female *Anopheles* mosquito. The two most common forms of malaria are caused by *P. vivax* and *P. falciparum*, which are responsible for the characteristic high fever, chills, and profuse sweating. Unlike *P. vivax*, which is common outside of Africa and relatively mild, *P. falciparum* is responsible for some 90 percent of all human infections (200–300 million cases annually)—98 percent of which are in Africa—and 90 percent of all malaria deaths.

When supplies of **quinine** were cut off by the Japanese during World War II, an all-out effort was initiated in the United States to discover quinine substitutes to treat malaria. Of the 14,000 compounds screened, chloroquine proved to be the most effective. In retrospect, it was determined that chloroquine was first synthesized at the Elberfeld laboratories of IG Farben in Germany in 1934 by Hans Andersag and named Resochin but not used because of its perceived toxicity.

More powerful and less toxic than quinine, chloroquine (Aralen) has been the drug of choice for the prevention and treatment of malarial infections since the mid-1940s. Its many advantages include its effectiveness, quick action, long-lasting effects, few adverse reactions, safety during pregnancy, and very low cost. In the late 1950s, early signs of resistance began to appear. By the 1980s, chloroquine-resistant strains of *P. falciparum* became widespread throughout much of the world, with the exception of the Caribbean islands, parts of Central America, North Africa, and the Middle East, where chloroquine remains highly effective. Hints are emerging that it may be regaining its effectiveness in Africa.

SEE ALSO Quinine (1820), Artemisinin (1972).

Charles Alphonse Laveran (1845–1922) made this drawing of malaria parasites. A French physician who discovered in 1880 that protozoa caused malaria, he was the first person to identify protozoa as diseasing-causing agents, and for which he was awarded the 1907 Nobel Prize in Physiology or Medicine.

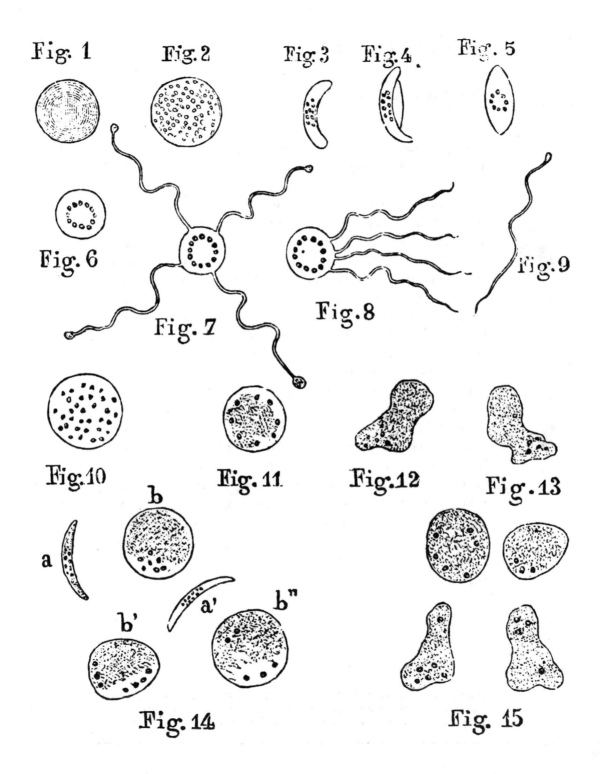

Fig. 1   Fig. 2   Fig. 3   Fig. 4.   Fig. 5

Fig. 6

Fig. 7

Fig. 8

Fig. 9

Fig. 10   Fig. 11   Fig. 12   Fig. 13

a   b

b'   a'   b"

Fig. 14

Fig. 15

Amethopterin and Methotrexate

Sidney Farber (1903–1973)

Methotrexate and the very closely related drug aminopterin occupy a significant place in the history of cancer chemotherapy: They were the first drugs found to cause a remission in leukemia and cure a solid tumor. During the 1930s and early 1940s, scientists observed that folic acid–rich foods stimulated the growth and development of bone marrow, the site of blood-cell production. This benefited anemia patients but worsened leukemia in children. For these children, their prognosis was the same in 1940 as it was when the disease was first identified in 1845: Once diagnosed with leukemia, their life expectancy was measured in weeks.

FIRST HOPES IN CHILDHOOD CANCER TREATMENT. Sidney Farber was a Harvard Medical School pediatric pathologist. He hypothesized that if folic acid stimulated the bone marrow, administering a drug that blocked folic acid would depress the bone marrow and shut down excessive production of white blood cells in leukemia. Farber contacted Lederle Laboratories, a company then interested in folic acid, and requested that they develop a chemical that could antagonize folic acid. In 1947, Farber found that the first of these anti-folate compounds, aminopterin, completely— but only temporarily—improved the condition of ten of sixteen children with acute lymphoblastic leukemia. Amethopterin was the first drug effective against non-solid tumors—cancers that are widespread in the body and that cannot be removed surgically.

Methotrexate, a far safer, close chemical derivative of aminopterin, is currently in use. In 1958, methotrexate was shown to cure choriocarcinoma, a malignant solid tumor of the uterus. It is also used for a wide range of rapidly growing cancers, as well as psoriasis and rheumatoid arthritis as a disease-modifying anti-rheumatic drug (DMARD).

Farber was advised early on that children with leukemia should be left to die in peace. His hunches about anti-folate compounds were vindicated, and he is now regarded as the "father of modern cancer chemotherapy."

SEE ALSO Enbrel, Remicade, and Humira (1998), Gleevic/Glivec (2001).

Sidney Farber, "the father of modern cancer chemotherapy," founded the Children's Hospital Center Research Foundation, which expanded the scope of its patient population and became the Dana-Farber Cancer Institute in 1947, a renowned comprehensive cancer treatment and research center.

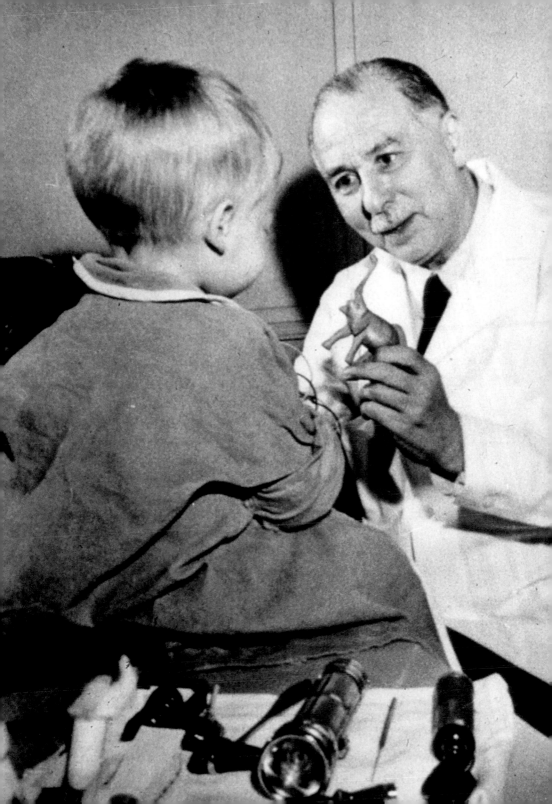

Tetracyclines

Benjamin Minge Duggar (1872–1956), Lloyd Conover (b. 1922)

In 1948, Benjamin Minge Duggar, a seventy-six-year-old retired professor of botany working as a consultant for Lederle Laboratories, made the discovery that immortalized him. He found chlortetracycline (Aureomycin), which was produced by a golden-colored bacterium of the *Streptomycetes* genus. Chlortetracycline was active in combating a very wide range of bacteria, plus a variety of microbes that had failed to be curbed by any of the existing drugs. Two years later, a team of scientists at Pfizer found oxytetracycline (Terramycin). In 1952, Lloyd Conover, also at Pfizer, synthesized tetracycline, the first antibiotic made in the lab from a natural drug. Within three years, tetracycline, the most illustrious and financially successful of the triumvirate, became the most widely prescribed broad-spectrum antibiotic in the United States.

The 1950s witnessed highly contentious patent-infringement suits involving rival manufacturers of tetracycline with dueling trade names that included Achromycin, Tetracyn, Panmycin, and Sumycin. These suits remained unresolved until 1982. In addition, the Federal Trade Commission raised illegal price-fixing charges against five companies, alleging that they had colluded to keep the price of tetracycline artificially high.

Over the years, the tetracyclines were widely popular but indiscriminately prescribed for minor disorders. This led to the development of resistance by bacteria that had readily succumbed to the effects of tetracyclines in the past. Now, decades later, these drugs have lost their initial luster and are recommended for treating only a very limited number of microbial diseases.

The tetracycline antibiotics gain access to tissues and fluids throughout the body, including the bones and teeth, where they are stored. If taken between the ages of two months and five years, when permanent teeth are being calcified, they can cause brown discoloration of teeth. Similarly, when the tetracyclines are given to pregnant women, particularly during the second and third trimesters of pregnancy, discoloration of their offspring's teeth may occur.

SEE ALSO Streptomycin (1944), Chloramphenicol (1949), Ampicillin (1961).

The test in this Petri dish is to determine the sensitivity of a bacterial culture to tetracycline and three other antibiotics. The large dark circle in the upper left shows a powerful antibiotic response to bacterial growth. The circle in the lower left shows a weak response. These kinds of results are used when selecting the most effective antibiotic to treat a bacterial infection.

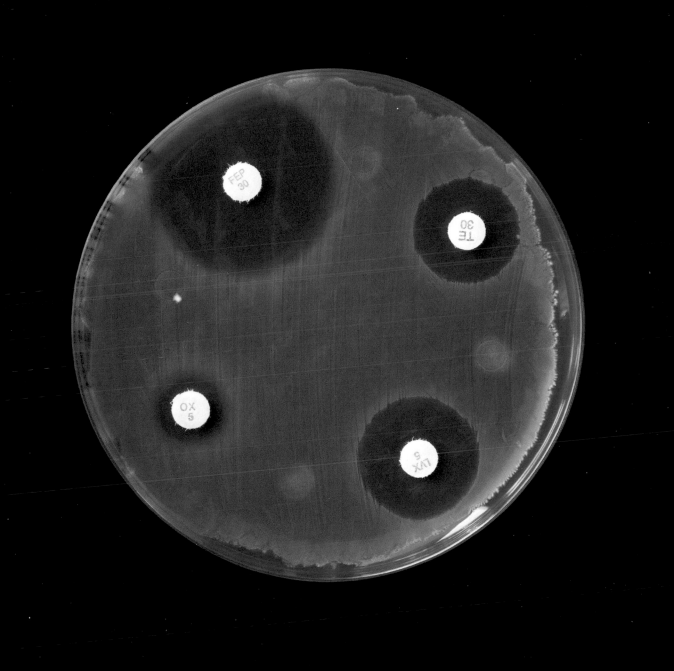

Xylocaine

Hans von Euler-Chelpin (1873–1964), **Nils Löfgren** (1913–1967)

For almost five decades, procaine was the standard against which all local anesthetics were compared. In 1948, when Xylocaine (lidocaine) was first marketed, it rapidly displaced **Novocain** (procaine) because of its effectiveness and numerous applications.

Lidocaine's backstory begins in the laboratory of Hans von Euler-Chelpin, a German-born Swedish biochemist, who was co-recipient of the 1929 Nobel Prize in Chemistry in recognition of his studies on the role of enzymes in the fermentation of sugars. (In 1970, his son Ulf von Euler was awarded the Nobel Prize in Physiology or Medicine.) During the course of his plant chemistry studies at the University of Stockholm in 1935, Euler-Chelpin discovered a chemical that numbed his tongue. Over the next seven years, members of his laboratory prepared almost five dozen chemicals, searching for a local anesthetic that was not irritating to the skin.

That search culminated in 1943 with the discovery of lidocaine by Bengt Lundqvist and Nils Löfgren (the subject of the latter's doctoral dissertation). In 1948, after years of biological testing, it was sold to Astra, then a small Swedish pharmaceutical company, which marketed it as Xylocaine.

A Local Anesthetic for All Seasons. Lidocaine produces faster, more intense, and longer-lasting pain relief than procaine and can be used as a substitute in persons who are allergic to procaine and chemically related local anesthetics. Whereas procaine is only effective when injected, lidocaine can be injected for virtually all types of local anesthetic needs and can be applied to the skin and mucous membranes in gels, ointments, and creams. Lidocaine nasal spray and drops are available for short-term relief of migraine headaches, as is a skin patch to relieve shingles pain.

In 1950, intravenously injected lidocaine was found to be highly effective for controlling abnormal heart rhythms of the ventricles (the lower chambers of the heart) associated with heart attacks and is the preferred drug for these conditions. Astra's profits from the sales of Xylocaine were instrumental in funding the research and development of other new drugs and propelling the growth of the company, now called Astra-Zenica, into one of the world's largest pharmaceutical companies.

SEE ALSO Cocaine (1884), Novocain (1905).

Xylocaine and related drugs are the preferred local anesthetics because they act faster and longer than procaine (Novocain) and produce a greater degree of pain relief.

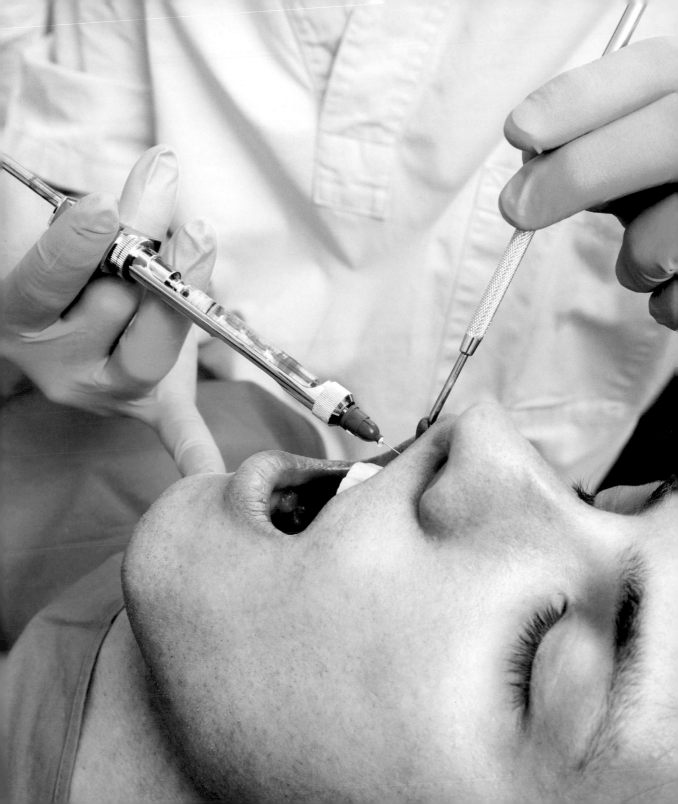

Lithium

John Cade (1912–1980), Morgens Schou (1918–2005)

As the old spiritual song aptly tells us, "I'm sometimes up and I'm sometimes down." Fluctuations in mood are a very normal pattern in life, but it's not considered normal when the ups are too high and the downs are too low. Disorders of mood—so-called "affective disorders"—can be incapacitating to the patient and family members. Luckily, mood stabilizers such as lithium can bring relief.

Several decades after its discovery and isolation as a metal, lithium was used in the 1840s for the treatment of bladder stones and gout, and during the last three decades of the nineteenth century, it was used to treat mood disorders. Lithium chloride reappeared in the 1940s as a substitute for table salt (sodium chloride), when salt-free diets were shown to be beneficial in the management of patients with heart disease and high blood pressure. This seemed reasonable, since lithium resembles sodium chemically, pharmacologically, and in taste. In practice, however, it was responsible for kidney toxicity and a number of deaths in 1949. All lithium-containing products were withdrawn from the market.

That same year, after the Australian psychiatrist John Cade observed that injections of lithium urate caused guinea pigs to become sedated rather than excited. He observed that lithium carbonate calmed ten manic patients but was without effect in schizophrenics. During the 1950s and 1960s, the Danish psychiatrist Morgens Schou, following up on Cade's results, conducted large-scale clinical studies demonstrating lithium's effectiveness in preventing mania. Concerned about the toxicity of lithium, the **Food and Drug Administration** delayed approval of it in the United States until 1970, years after it was marketed in Europe. Lithium is now used to treat episodes of mania and to prevent reoccurrences of the wild mood swings seen in bipolar (manic-depressive) disorders.

Lithium is an unusual drug for the treatment of mental disorders, because, unlike related drugs such as **Haldol**, it has no effects on behavior in (behaviorally) normal individuals. It merely normalizes extreme mood and permits the manic patient to "come down" without feeling drugged or tranquilized.

SEE ALSO Haldol (1958).

The exact nature of Vincent van Gogh's medical conditions remains a subject of active inquiry. His feverish outpouring of art during his final years suggest that he suffered from mania or bipolar disorder (manic-depression), a mood disorder now commonly treated with the use of lithium and other mood stabilizers. This self-portrait was painted in 1888.

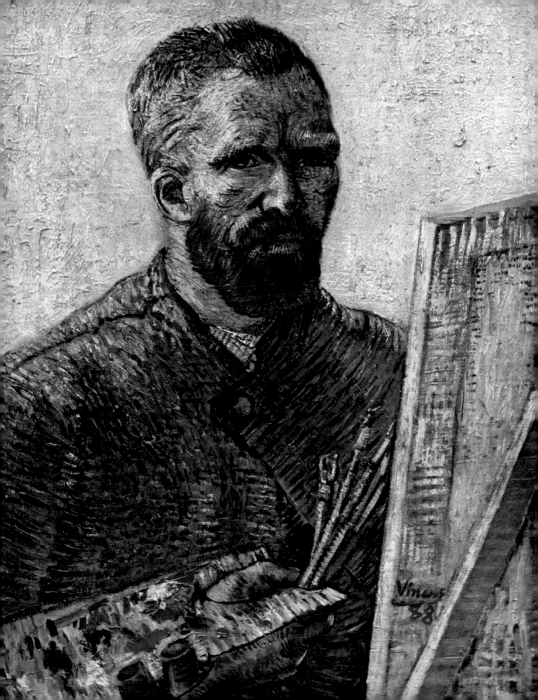

Chloramphenicol

Streptomyces is a genus of soil bacteria that is a virtual biological drug-making factory. It produces a wide range of drugs used to combat infections caused by bacteria (**tetracycline**, **streptomycin**, vancomycin, neomycin), fungi (**nystatin**, **amphotericin B**), and parasites (ivermectin), as well as anticancer drugs (bleomycin). Chloramphenicol is an antibacterial antibiotic that was isolated from one of the more than 550 *Streptomyces* species—this one from a soil sample in Venezuela.

When chloramphenicol (Choromycetin) hit the market in 1949, Parke-Davis appeared to have a blockbuster drug. Along with the tetracyclines, it was one of the first broad-spectrum antibiotics that were effective against a wide range of microbes. Moreover, chloramphenicol's long reach to fluids and tissues throughout the body prevented disease-causing microbes from evading it.

FATAL FLAWS IN A LIFESAVING DRUG. However, its potentially life-threatening effects on the bone marrow—the site of blood cell manufacture in adults—prevented chloramphenicol from achieving its potential in medicine. The most serious effects are pancytopenia (a decrease in red and white blood cells and platelets) and aplastic anemia, in which the bone marrow fails to make enough blood cells—in particular, red cells.

In addition, non-blood-related problems were seen in the very young. Infants, especially premature infants, do not metabolize drugs as effectively as older children and adults. This lesson was tragically learned with chloramphenicol. In the late 1950s, what appeared to be "reasonable" doses were given to premies, after which their bodies became limp, their skin assumed ashen-gray coloration, their blood pressure dropped, and they became cyanotic; 40 percent died within days. This "gray baby syndrome" was found to result from the very low activity of UDP-glucuronyl transferase enzymes. Current uses of chloramphenicol are limited to serious infections when safer drugs are not effective. These include bacterial meningitis, typhoid fever, Rocky Mountain spotted fever, and related infections caused by the *Rickettsia* genus.

SEE ALSO Drug Metabolism (1947), Streptomycin (1944), Tetracyclines (1948), Nystatin (1954), Amphotericin B (1956).

The female American dog tick or wood tick is the primary carrier of the rickettsia that causes Rocky Mountain spotted fever. In humans, RMSF has a mortality rate of 20–25 percent if untreated and 5 percent if treated with chloramphenicol.

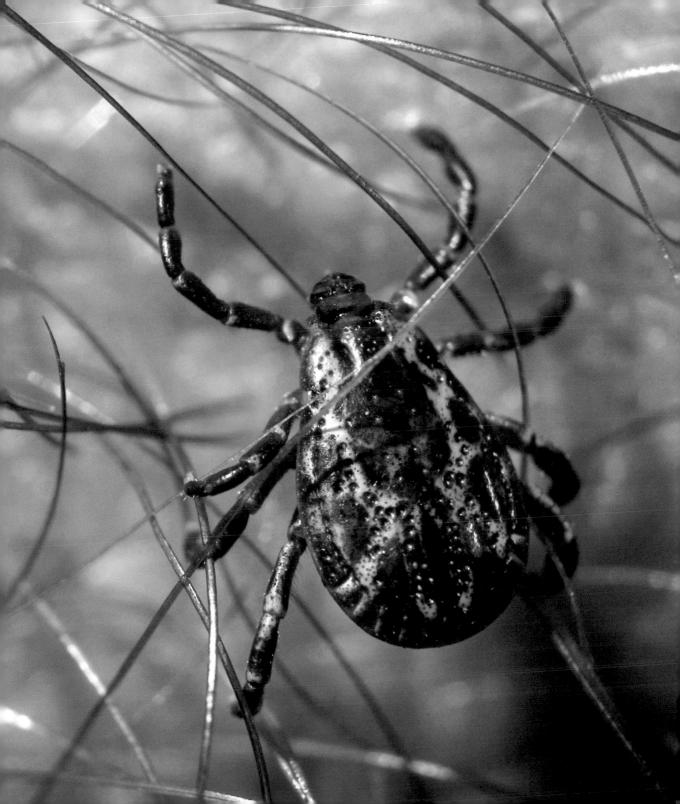

Cortisone

Edward C. Kendall (1886–1972), **Phillip S. Hench** (1896–1965), **Tadeus Reichstein** (1897–1996), **Lewis H. Sarett** (1917–1999)

In 1941, rumors surfaced that *Luftwaffe* pilots were receiving injections of steroid hormones from the adrenal cortex, enabling them to withstand high-altitude stress. Among the chemists the American military contacted to deal with this one-upmanship was Edward C. Kendall, a research biochemist at the Mayo Foundation in Rochester, Minnesota, who had previously conducted research on adrenal-gland chemistry. Although the rumor proved false, Kendall, collaborating with Merck chemist Lewis H. Sarett, began producing large quantities of "Kendall's Compound E." This was to become one of the most important drugs ever discovered.

At about the same, Phillip Hench at the Mayo Clinic observed that women with rheumatoid arthritis experienced fewer arthritic symptoms while pregnant. Hench speculated that their temporary pain relief resulted from release of an antistress hormone during pregnancy. In 1948, Hench tested "Kendall's Compound E" in a severely arthritic woman, and after several injections, she was free of pain and was able to walk. These dramatic early results were replicated in additional patients in 1949, but relief continued only as long as the drug, now named cortisone, was taken.

Within a few years, cortisone and related drugs were found to provide major benefits in scores of medical conditions, including allergies, asthma, cancers, and conditions affecting the skin, eyes, blood, and bowels. However, the price of cortisone's sometimes lifesaving benefits was considerable. Cortisone caused major aberrations in the body's metabolism, behavioral alterations, stomach ulcers, and major imbalances in salt and water, which impaired heart function.

Merck's cortisone was almost immediately followed on the market by hydrocortisone (cortisol), the active form of cortisone in the body. Thereafter, numerous modifications made in their steroid chemistry produced drugs that are far more active at lower doses and that, more important, do not cause the retention of salt and water by the body. Still other steroids have been formulated for application to the skin and to be inhaled for the treatment of asthma. The 1950 Nobel Prize in Physiology or Medicine was awarded to Kendall, Hench, and Swiss collaborator/chemist Tadeus Reichstein.

SEE ALSO Aspirin (1899), Percorten (1939), Albuterol/Salbutamol (1968), Beclovent (1976), Endrel, Remicide, and Humira (1998).

Pierre-Auguste Renoir (1841–1919) suffered from severe rheumatoid arthritis. During his last years, his hands were completely deformed, and he had to wedge a paintbrush between his fingers to paint this 1910 self-portrait.

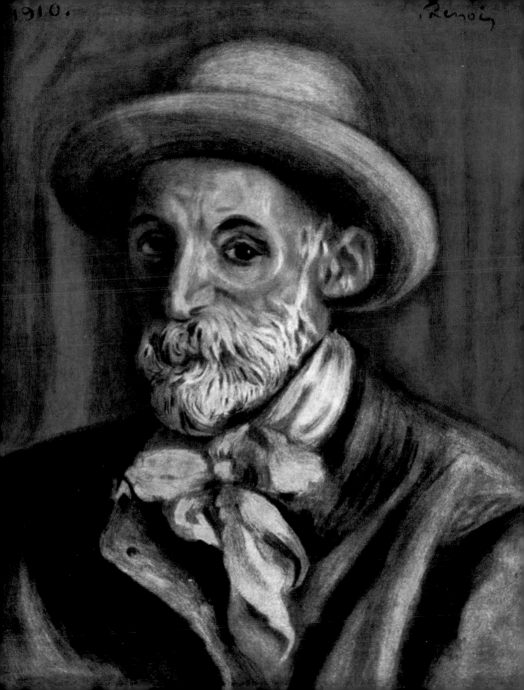

1910.

Renoir

Succinylcholine

Werner Kalow (1917–2008)

Succinylcholine is an excellent choice of poisons, because it breaks down rapidly in the body and leaves few traces. In the 1960s, Carl Coppolino, a New Jersey anesthesiologist, was accused but acquitted of using succinylcholine to murder his lover's husband. He was subsequently convicted of using the same drug to fatally poison his wife.

During surgery—particularly surgery involving the abdomen—drugs are used to relax muscles. Voluntary muscles become flaccid, causing whole-body paralysis. Breathing muscles are also paralyzed, and breathing must be maintained artificially using a mechanical respirator. **Tubocurarine**-like drugs are used to produce muscle relaxation over periods that often exceed thirty minutes, but sometimes it is only necessary to relax muscles for several minutes. Common procedures that require short-term paralysis include preventing the gag reflex when a breathing tube is inserted into the trachea. Brief muscle relaxation also prevents convulsions and possible fractures of the spine during electroconvulsive shock therapy used to treat severe depression.

Succinylcholine (suxamethonium, Anectine) produces muscle relaxation within one minute of an injection, and its effects on breathing and muscle paralysis *usually* persist for only three to five minutes. Usually, but not always. Normally, succinylcholine is very rapidly broken down and inactivated by pseudocholinesterase, an enzyme present in the plasma. However, about one in 3,000 individuals has a genetic abnormality involving a defective form of pseudocholinesterase. For those people, succinylcholine produces paralysis and an inability to breathe unassisted for two hours or longer. The study of the genetic basis for our different responses to drugs, pharmacogenetics, is now one of the hottest areas of drug research. A pioneer in this field was Werner Kalow. Kalow served in the German navy during World War II, was a prisoner of war in Arizona, and in 1951 became professor of pharmacology at the University of Toronto. There he studied, in detail, the pharmacogenetics of succinylcholine, inspired by a patient's death from this drug.

SEE ALSO Tubocurarine (1935), Drug Metabolism (1947), Isoniazid (1951).

Succinylcholine is a very short-acting muscle relaxant used primarily for insertion of breathing tubes and laryngoscopes.

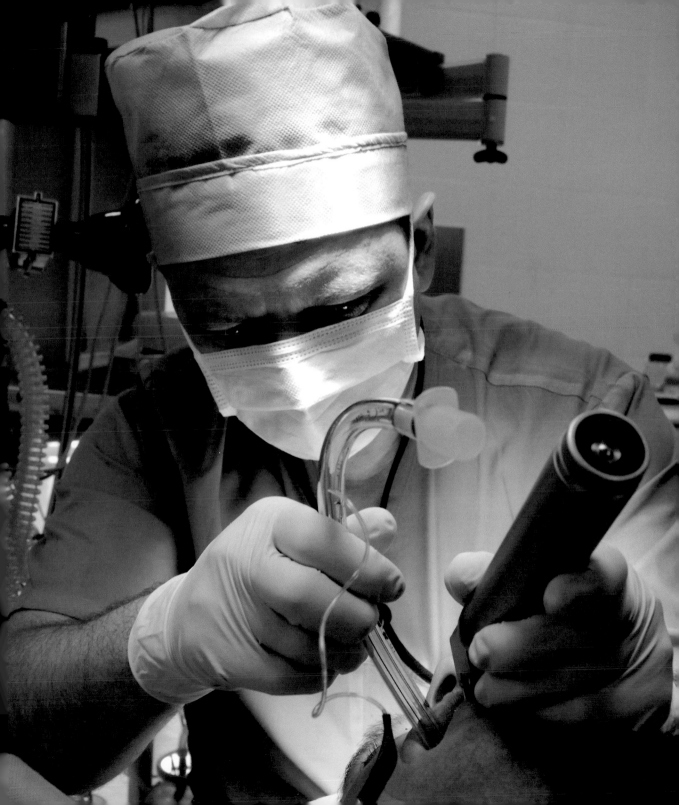

Isoniazid

Isoniazid was first synthesized in 1912 at the German University of Prague by Hans Meyer and Josef Malley, and then it languished on chemistry shelves for four decades. In 1951, its effectiveness against tuberculosis (TB) was recognized, and it appeared in clinics the following year. Early results were highly promising, and it very rapidly assumed a preeminent place in TB treatment, displacing **streptomycin**. The lay public and members of the medical community predicted that TB would soon become a disease only found in medical history books.

TB did not become extinct. The tubercle bacillus, the microbe responsible for TB, rapidly became resistant to isoniazid (Nydrazid, Laniazid). Nevertheless, because of its high degree of effectiveness by mouth, relatively low toxicity, and affordability, it has remained the primary anti-TB drug worldwide, always used in combination with other drugs, such as **rifampin**, to delay the development of bacterial resistance. Susceptible individuals and those in close contact with TB patients also use isoniazid alone to prevent TB contagion.

Most drugs, including isoniazid, must be chemically changed (metabolized or biotransformed) before they can be eliminated from the body. The liver is the major organ responsible for **drug metabolism**. After a given dose, the blood levels of most drugs follow a normal or Gaussian distribution, such as the variation seen in IQ scores. Some levels are high, some low, but most fall in an intermediate range. This was not the case for isoniazid!

Half the Caucasian and African-American people in the United States rapidly metabolize isoniazid (and thus have low blood levels), while the other half are slow metabolizers (have high blood levels) and are more likely to experience drug toxicity. The proportion of slow metabolizers is markedly different for other ethnic groups: Native Americans, 21 percent; Japanese, 13 percent; and Eskimos, 5 percent. Slow metabolism has been attributed to an inherited recessive trait that reduces the amount of the enzyme acetyltransferase. Isoniazid serves as a classic example of pharmacogenetics: the influence of genetic factors on drug response.

SEE ALSO Streptomycin (1944), Drug Metabolism (1947), Iproniazid (1951), Rifampin (1967).

Photomicrograph of sputum containing Mycobacterium tuberculosis, *the bacterial cause of tuberculosis. TB is spread when the infected individual coughs or sneezes, and the bacteria, contained in microdroplets, are inhaled.*

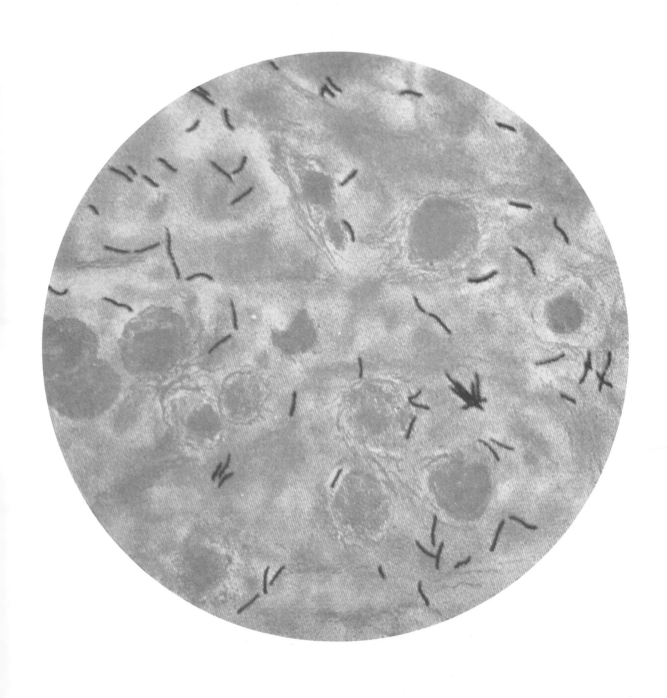

Malathion

When using an antibiotic to treat an infection caused by a microbe, the drug must be more toxic to the microbe than to the patient. This basic concept, referred to as selective toxicity, is predicated on exploiting an important biological difference between the microbe and the patient. For example, many bacteria require an intact cell wall to survive. **Penicillin** kills susceptible bacteria by interfering with their ability to manufacture cell walls, but it does not adversely affect mammalian cells, which lack this structure.

Selective toxicity also applies to insecticides: the chemical should effectively kill the insect without harming humans or animals. Parathion, an insecticide that appeared in the 1940s and now banned in many countries, is toxic to insects but also injurious to humans and wildlife. By contrast, malathion, developed in 1951, is far more toxic to insects than to mammals. The basis for this selective toxicity occurs because of relative differences in their enzyme activity. Malathion is inactive in mammals and insects and chemically transformed in the body to the toxic malaoxon. Further, both malathion and malaoxon are inactivated by the enzyme carboxyesterase. So, how does our body's response differ from that of insects?

Mammals have high carboxyesterase activity and very rapidly convert malathion to an inactive product *before* it can be converted to malaoxon. Insects are less fortunate because they have low carboxyesterase activity, and, thus, are poisoned by the buildup of malaoxon. Cases of insect resistance to malathion have been attributed to increases in the carboxyesterase enzyme.

Malathion is widely used as an insecticide on agricultural crops, in home gardens, and to kill mosquitoes and Mediterranean fruit flies in large outdoor areas. It is also used to kill fleas on household pets and as a lotion to treat head lice and their eggs in humans.

SEE ALSO Penicillin (1928), DDT (1939), Drug Metabolism (1947).

Crop dusters have been used to apply malathion in agricultural settings to eliminate Mediterranean fruit flies and protect cotton fields against boll weevils. In such urban centers as New York City and Winnipeg, aerial sprays have been used to eradicate mosquitoes and, by extension, the West Nile virus.

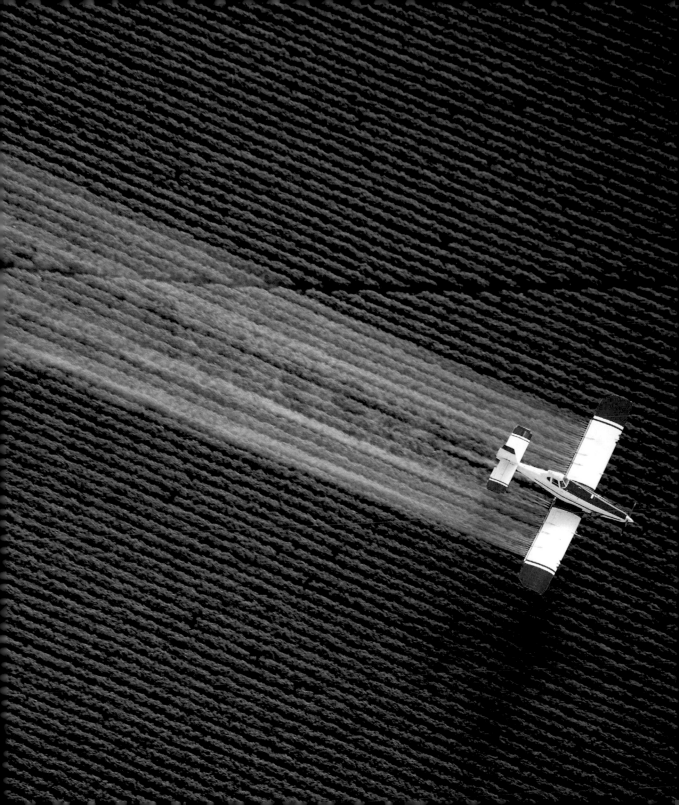

Phenergan

During the 1940s, interest focused on a new class of drugs that could antagonize histamine and be used for the treatment of allergic disorders. The French company Rhône-Poulenc focused their attention on drugs of the phenothiazine class. The two most important products to emerge from this research were the antischizophrenic drug **chlorpromazine** (Thorazine, Lacgactil) and the antihistamine promethazine (Phenergan), the latter appearing in 1951.

In addition to its antihistaminic properties, Phenergan, like many phenothiazines and other "first-generation" antihistamines, has strong sedative properties. It is available as a nonprescription sleep aid in some countries, including Australia, Canada, and the United Kingdom. Since 1955, it has also been used, by injection, for motion sickness and to control severe nausea and vomiting.

In 2009, Phenergan was the focus of a U.S. Supreme Court decision that has far-reaching ramifications. In the case of *Wyeth v. Levine*, Vermont bass player Diana Levine received an injection of Phenergan for the treatment of nausea resulting from a severe headache. The drug was inadvertently injected into an artery instead of its intended vein, resulting in tissue damage, gangrene, and the amputation of her lower arm. Because of this potential danger, the Food and Drug Administration and Wyeth, the drug manufacturer, warned against but did not prohibit this "IV push" method of injection. The company argued that since the FDA had approved the drug and the wording on the label regarding its use, Ms. Levine should not be permitted to sue for damages in state court—a legal theory known as FDA Preemption.

Is FDA Approval a Liability Shield? In a 6-3 decision, the high court ruled that FDA approval of a medication (including the labeling of that medication) does *not* shield the manufacturer from liability for any injuries caused by the medication. Understandably, consumer groups and plaintiff attorneys applauded this decision, but pharmaceutical manufacturers derided it.

The prescription cough syrup promethazine + **codeine**, called "purple drank" and "syrup," is a recreational drug in the southern United States. Rap stars such as Lil' Wayne have popularized it in hip-hop song lyrics.

SEE ALSO Codeine (1832), Food and Drug Administration (1906), Benadryl (1946), Chlorpromazine (1952), Dextromethorphan (1958).

An early member of the phenothiazine class of drugs, which includes chlorpromazine, Phenergan is used to prevent and control nausea and vomiting associated with motion sickness. Because it causes marked sedation, however, it is not recommended for use by drivers.

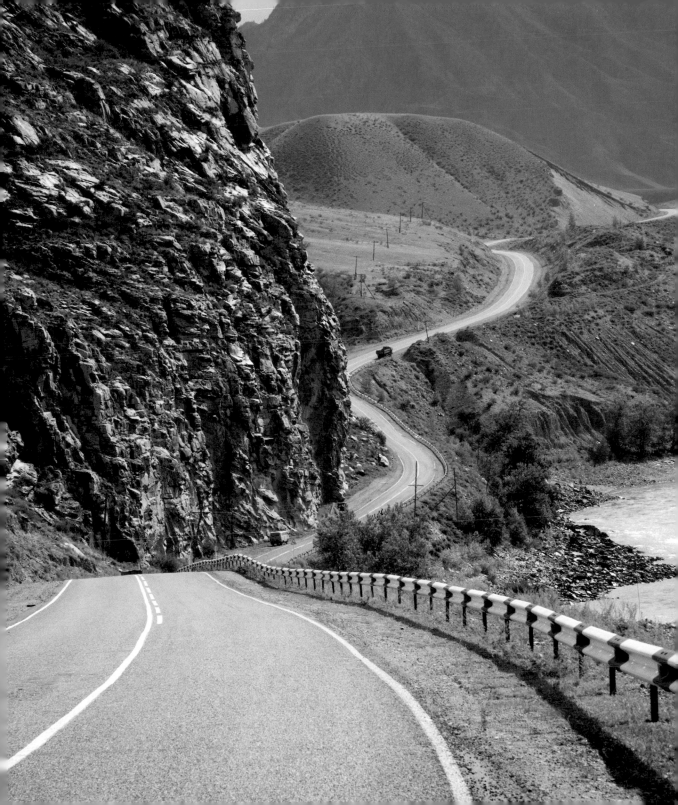

Benemid

Karl H. Beyer Jr. (1914–1996)

In 1941, soon after **penicillin** had been extracted from the *Penicillium* mold, its potentially lifesaving effects were first demonstrated in a human patient: a policeman dying of blood poisoning. At three-hour intervals, he was given intravenous injections of penicillin G. Because only meager amounts of penicillin were available then, each day penicillin was extracted from his urine and reinjected. It worked, and after five days, he appeared to be on his way to recovery . . . until the penicillin supply became depleted. His medical condition deteriorated, and he died one month later.

In 1951, Karl Beyer, a research pharmacologist at Merck, discovered that probenecid (Benemid) greatly slowed the loss of penicillin in urine. This enabled the antibiotic to attain much higher levels in the body for much longer periods, more effectively fighting severe bacterial infections. Although penicillin G is now plentiful, Benemid continues to be used for this purpose.

Beyer recognized that Benemid's effects on the kidney had another important medical application for the treatment of gout. Excessive levels of uric acid in the blood cause gout. Uric acid, a breakdown product of purines from meat, is normally eliminated in urine, but when urate levels build up in individuals predisposed to gout, hard crystals form and are deposited in the joints. Intermittent gouty attacks occur, in which the patient experiences sudden, intense burning pain, swelling, and redness, most commonly in the big toe.

While Benemid retards the elimination of penicillin, it promotes the loss of uric acid by the kidney (a uricosuric effect). As the blood levels of uric acid decrease, the crystals in the joints dissolve and the frequency of debilitating attacks decrease. While **colchicine** and anti-inflammatory drugs such as ibuprofen (Motrin) or **cortisone**-related steroids are used to treat an acute attack, Benemid was the first drug that could prevent acute gouty attacks from occurring in the first place.

SEE ALSO Colchicine (c. 70), Penicillin (1928), Cortisone (1949), Zyloprim (1966).

Hans Holbein the Younger painted this portrait of Henry VIII (1539–40). This English king (1491–1547) was a classic gout sufferer whose condition was brought on by gluttony and drink. As a young man, he had an athletic build, reaching 6'3" (190.5 cm), while in his last years he weighed 300–320 pounds (135–145 kg) and had a waist measuring 58–60 inches (147–152 cm).

ANNO·ETATIS· SVE·XLIX·

Chlorpromazine

Jean Delay (1907–1987), **Heinz Lehmann** (1911–1999), **Henri Laborit** (1914–1995), **Pierre Deniker** (1917–1998)

Chlorpromazine, the progenitor of several dozen phenothiazine derivatives, was originally intended for surgical use but has had the greatest impact as the most significant treatment for the mentally ill, replacing psychosurgery, **insulin shock therapy**, and electroconvulsive shock therapy. In 1964, one decade after its introduction, 50 million people around the world used chlorpromazine. It and related antipsychotic drugs were instrumental in progressively reducing the patient count in U.S. state psychiatric hospitals from 559,000 in 1955 to 110,000–120,000 in 1990.

In 1949, Henri Laborit, a French naval surgeon, was testing a series of antihistamines to prevent surgical shock. One of the compounds, developed in the Rhône-Poulenc Company laboratory located near Paris and tested by Laborit, was chlorpromazine. Patients receiving this drug were remarkably calm before surgery and did not experience surgical shock. Recognizing its psychiatric potential, in 1952 Pierre Deniker and Jean Delay at Sainte-Anne Hospital in Paris gave chlorpromazine to schizophrenic patients and found them less aggressive and less delusional. Deniker's findings excited Heinz Lehmann at the Verdun Protestant Hospital in Montreal, who replicated and extended Deniker's dramatic findings. Chlorpromazine was marketed in France as Lacgactil by Rhône-Poulenc in 1952, and in the United States as Thorazine by Smith Kline & French in 1954, for schizophrenia and nausea.

Chlorpromazine is far from perfect. While some 70 percent of schizophrenics show improvement and can return to more normal lives, the remainder fail to benefit. Nor are patients cured. Within one year after discontinuing medication, 75–95 percent experience a return of symptoms. While the majority of mentally ill patients can leave psychiatric hospitals and reside in a community, many individuals become homeless or go to prison.

Phenothiazines are "dirty" drugs because they lack specificity. Their antipsychotic effects have been attributed to the blocking of dopamine receptors in the brain, which also accounts for their Parkinson-like effects. Newer atypical antipsychotics, such as **clozapine** (1989), are not necessarily more effective but have fewer adverse effects.

SEE ALSO Insulin Shock Therapy (1927), Phenergan (1951), Reserpine (1952), Tofranil and Elavil (1958), Clozapine (1989), Zyprexa (1996).

Thanks to chlorpromazine and other related anti-schizophrenic drugs, inpatient psychiatric facilities no longer resemble Bedlam (Bethlem Royal Hospital), as depicted in A Rake's Progress (1763) by William Hogarth. This hospital, founded in 1247, is said to be the oldest institution specializing in mental illnesses.

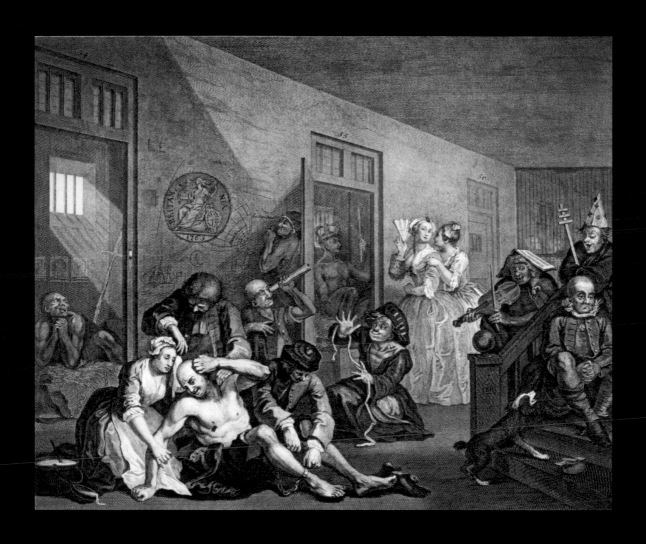

Reserpine

Ram Nath Chopra (1882–2002), **Robert Wallace Wilkins** (1906–2003), **Rustom Jal Vakil** (1911–1974), **Nathan S. Kline** (1916–1982)

The snakeroot plant, *Rauwolfia serpentina*, was long an integral component of Indian Ayurvedic medicine. During the 1930s and 1940s, scientific and clinical studies conducted in India by Ram Nath Chopra and Rustom Jal Vakil focused attention on the effects of the root on high blood pressure (hypertension) and mental disorders—in particular, schizophrenia. In addition to the clinical studies by these respected scholars, interest in **rauwolfia** was heightened by the paucity of safe and effective drugs for these conditions in 1950. That year, studies by Robert Wallace Wilkins at Massachusetts General Hospital first established in Western medicine rauwolfia's effectiveness for mild hypertension. However, early enthusiasm waned when far better antihypertensive drugs, with fewer side effects, appeared during the 1960s.

In 1952, the Basel-based pharmaceutical company Ciba announced the isolation of reserpine (Serpasil), the primary **alkaloid** responsible for rauwolfia's effects. Extensive clinical trials by Nathan S. Kline at Rockland State Hospital in New York established reserpine's ability to reduce symptoms in schizophrenic patients, and for several years during the mid-1950s, it enjoyed considerable popularity for this condition. However, the timing of its introduction was inopportune. **Chlorpromazine** (Thorazine), which had made its appearance for the treatment of schizophrenia in 1952, was a more effective and efficient drug. And unlike reserpine, it did not cause depression.

Reserpine-induced depression, which led to suicide in some patients, spelled the drug's demise as an anti-schizophrenic drug. Instead, reserpine embarked on a noncommercial career as a tool in the formulation of theories on the biochemical bases of depression and schizophrenia. Studies in animals showed that reserpine depleted serotonin, norepinephrine, and dopamine, **neurotransmitters** collectively called biogenic amines. Depression has been hypothesized to be associated with a deficiency of norepinephrine and serotonin, while schizophrenia may involve excessive dopamine. Thus, the research tool has superseded the medicine in importance.

SEE ALSO Rauwolfia (c. 500 BCE), Alkaloids (1806), Neurotransmitters (1920), Chlorpromazine (1952), Prozac (1987).

The goal of Ayurvedic medicine—of which rauwolfia and its primary alkaloid, reserpine, are an integral component—is to prevent disease by achieving balance of the three energy types (doshas). This pharmacy in Rishikesh, the gateway to the Himalayas, is located in northern India.

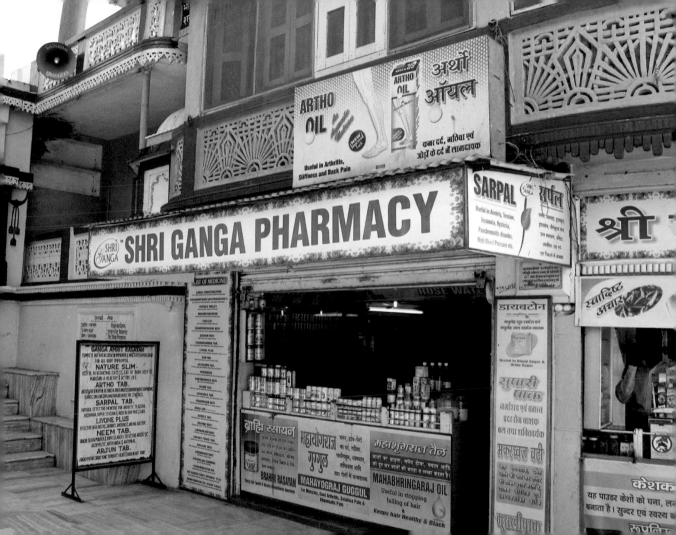

Iproniazid

Nathan S. Kline (1916–1982)

With the realization that **isoniazid** had revolutionized the treatment of tuberculosis (TB), scientists at Hoffman La Roche Laboratories altered its chemistry in efforts to find a comparable drug. The most promising of these new compounds was iproniazid. Early trials were conducted on patients at Sea View Tuberculosis Hospital in New York, which, when it opened in 1912, was considered the finest TB hospital in the country.

The results were dramatic. TB hospitals were not known for their joyful ambience in 1952, yet, after receiving iproniazid, the patients were clearly happy, with robust appetites leading to weight gain. They were even photographed dancing! Lung x-rays failed to show any improvement in their TB, however, and trials ended when the drug was found to cause disturbing side effects, including excessive stimulation.

In unrelated laboratory tests conducted in 1952 by E. Albert Zeller at Northwestern University Medical School, iproniazid was found to block monoamine oxidase (MAO), an enzyme normally responsible for inactivating norepinephrine and serotonin. When MAO is blocked, there is a resulting increase in the levels of these neurotransmitter compounds in the brain.

THE FIRST ANTIDEPRESSANT. In the mid-1950s, newly available drugs treated schizophrenia and anxiety but not depression. Nathan S. Kline, Director of Research at Rockland State Hospital, was aware of Zeller's findings and theorized that iproniazid, an MAO inhibitor, might have potential as an antidepressant. In 1957, Kline administered the drug to fourteen depressed patients and obtained favorable results in twelve. The psychiatric community enthusiastically embraced iproniazid (Marsilid) as a *psychic energizer* (Kline's term). The glow dimmed in 1961, when the drug was withdrawn from the market after its use was associated with fifty-four fatalities caused by liver toxicity. The search was on for a safe(r) MAO inhibitor.

SEE ALSO Neurotransmitters (1920), Streptomycin (1944), Isoniazid (1951), Monoamine Oxidase Inhibitors (1961), Prozac (1987).

Depression is the most common mental-health disorder affecting teens in the United States, and suicide is one of the leading causes of death among American high school students. Iproniazid, an MAO inhibitor, was among the first widely used antidepressants.

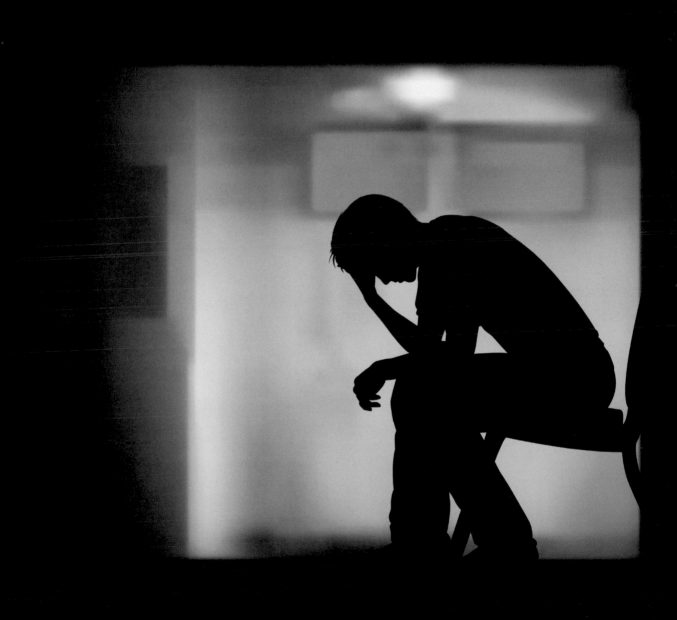

Erythromycin

Abelardo Aguilar (1917–1993)

In July 1976, some 4,000 World War II veterans who were members of the American Legion assembled in Philadelphia to participate in the bicentennial celebration of the signing of the Declaration of Independence. Some 600 of these veterans were staying at the landmark Bellevue-Stratford Hotel, the convention headquarters. Within days, 221 conventioneers experienced fever, cough, and breathing difficulties, with 34 subsequently dying. From an influenza epidemic seen six months earlier to conspiracy theories involving Communists trying to kill American veterans, there was no shortage of speculation regarding the cause of the mysterious disease.

In December 1976, Joseph McDade, a Centers for Disease Control scientist, determined the cause of Legionnaires' disease: *Legionella* bacteria, previously identified in 1947 but only associated with animal illnesses. The microbe resided in the water of cooling towers of the hotel's central air conditioning system and was spread as an aerosol on the unsuspecting conventioneers. Subsequent outbreaks of Legionnaires' disease have occurred in the United Kingdom (1985), the Netherlands (1999), Australia (2000), and most extensively in Spain (2001), affecting some 650 individuals. Legionnaires' disease is still with us: There are 10,000–50,000 cases each year in the United States, and the fatality rate ranges from 5 to 30 percent.

Among the earliest and still most effective treatments for Legionnaires' disease is erythromycin. In 1949, Abelardo Aguilar, a Filipino scientist, sent soil samples to his employer Eli Lilly for testing. From one sample, erythromycin was isolated from the *Streptomyces* mold by a research team lead by J.M. McGuire and marketed as Ilosone in 1952. Although erythromycin does not resemble **penicillin** in its chemistry or mechanism of action, it is useful in combating similar microbes. Erythromycin is considered one of the safest antibiotics and is a common alternative for individuals who are allergic to penicillin.

The first member of the *macrolide* class of antibiotics—so-called because of their large, bulky chemical structure—erythromycin is preferred for the treatment of such conditions as diphtheria, pneumonia, and whooping cough.

SEE ALSO Penicillin (1928), Tetracyclines (1948), Ampicillin (1961).

The cause of Legionnaires' disease was found to be Legionella *bacteria, spread as an aerosol via a hotel's air-conditioning system. Erythromycin is its most effective treatment.*

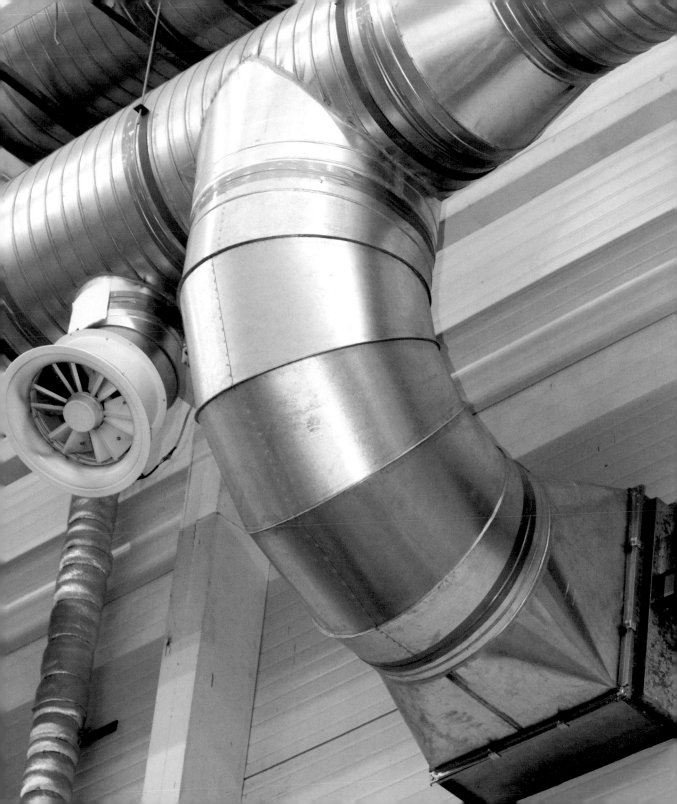

Diamox

Soon after the antibacterial drug **sulfanilamide** appeared in the late 1930s, it was noted that even normal doses modified the acid-base balance in the body, leading to the loss of large volumes of alkaline urine. The imbalance was caused by sulfanilamide blocking carbonic anhydrase, an enzyme required for transforming carbon dioxide and water to carbonic acid in the body.

Following this discovery, the search for chemical variations of sulfa drugs that were more potent carbonic anhydrase inhibitors and more effective diuretics (increasing the outflow of urine) began. The most promising of these was acetazolamide, marketed by Lederle Laboratories in 1952 as Diamox. Diamox was never a very impressive diuretic, particularly when used alone, but happily, it was not shelved. Its chemical cousin **Diuril** is the first of the thiazide diuretics.

Diamox's most important current use is for the treatment of glaucoma, one of the major causes of blindness. Glaucoma is associated with increased pressure within the eye that results from more fluids being formed inside the eye than leaving it. Diamox and related drugs, when taken by mouth or as eye drops, decrease the production of this fluid.

Diamox is the most widely used drug for the prevention and treatment of acute mountain (or altitude) sickness. Whereas there is considerable variation in our susceptibility to altitude sickness, early flu-like symptoms may occur at 8,000 feet (2,500 meters). Severe symptoms are not experienced until heights of over 12,000 feet (4,000 meters) are reached.

At 8,000 feet, the air contains 25 percent less oxygen than at sea level. This causes blood to leak from the smallest blood vessels (capillaries) into surrounding tissues. Even modest fluid buildup in the brain causes symptoms of acute mountain sickness. Diamox is thought to work by increasing the acidity of the blood, stimulating the breathing center in the medulla region of the brain, which increases ventilation, including during periods of sleep. The most effective method of preventing altitude sickness remains the gradual acclimatization to altitude when climbing.

SEE ALSO Sulfanilamide (1936), Diuril (1958).

With increasing altitude, there is a drop in atmospheric pressure and a corresponding drop in oxygen pressure. At the summit of Mount Everest (29,021 feet/ 8848 meters), the pressure of inspired oxygen is only 29 percent of that at sea level. This sign, warning of altitude sickness, is posted at Mount Evan (14,265 feet/4348 meters) in Colorado.

1952

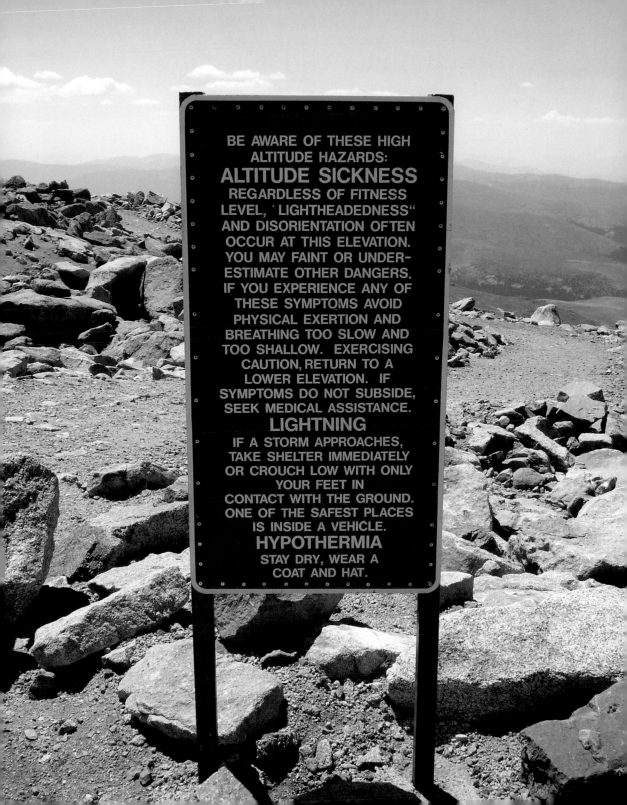

Acetaminophen/Paracetamol

Charles Frederic Gerhardt (1816–1856), Harmon Northrop Morse (1848–1920)

Called acetaminophen in the United States, Canada, and much of Latin America, and paracetamol almost everywhere else, acetaminophen/paracetamol is among the world's most widely used drugs, contained in more than one hundred products. The drug's unceremonious discovery in 1852 by the French chemist Charles Frederic Gerhardt, its fade into oblivion, its rediscovery by the American chemist Harmon Northrop Morse in 1873, and its eventual marketing and blockbuster success in the 1950s are worthy of note.

The story begins in 1886, when acetanilide was mistakenly given to a patient, whose fever unexpectedly dissipated. Physicians viewed an effective antipyretic (fever-reducing) drug such as acetanilide to be a significant medical advance. Its pain-relieving (analgesic) effects were an additional benefit. Acetanilide was used for decades despite causing methemoglobinemia, an impairment of the oxygen-carrying hemoglobin in the blood. Seeking an antipyretic that did not cause this problem, acetaminophen was tested in humans in 1893. It was effective but reported to have a modest tendency to cause methemoglobinemia, so it was shelved for six decades.

After its association with methemoglobinemia was disproved, acetaminophen was marketed by Sterling-Winthrop in 1953 as safer for children and adults with stomach ulcers than **aspirin**. In 1955, McNeil Laboratories sold acetaminophen as Tylenol; the following year, paracetamol was marketed by Frederick Stearns & Co. as Panadol. Apart from causing severe liver toxicity or failure when taken in overdose, it is a relatively safe aspirin substitute, especially for children.

To date, Tylenol contamination has resulted in two noteworthy drug recalls. In 1982, seven individuals in Greater Chicago died after ingesting Tylenol to which cyanide had been added intentionally. McNeil assumed responsibility and recalled 31 million bottles within a week. Fresh supplies were issued in tamper-proof containers. It was a public relations victory for McNeil, and virtually all lost sales were regained. By contrast, on multiple separate occasions in 2010, McNeil's parent company Johnson & Johnson was obliged to recall Tylenol and forty other nonprescription medicines because of chemical and bacterial contamination resulting from grossly substandard manufacturing procedures.

SEE ALSO Hydrogen Cyanide (1704), Aspirin (1899).

The Sick Girl is an 1882 oil painting by Danish painter Michael Ancher, a leading member of the Skagen artists. This nineteenth-century girl might have taken antipyrine (phenazone) to relieve pain and reduce fever, but this was a far more toxic drug than acetaminophen.

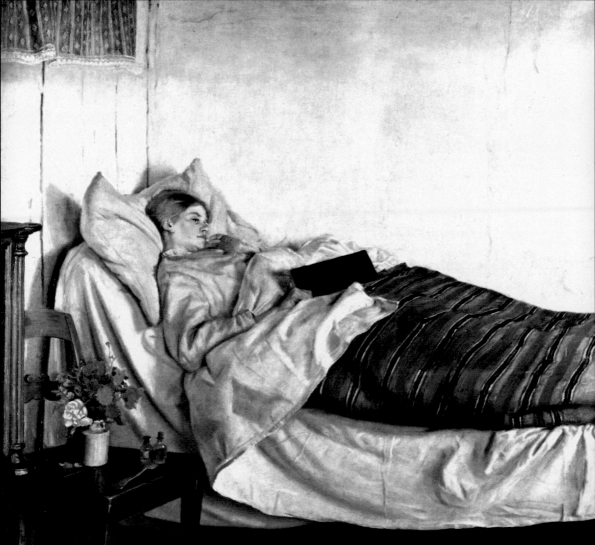

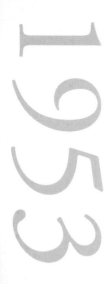

Mercaptopurine

George H. Hitchings (1905–1998), Gertrude B. Elion (1918–1999)

One of the great collaborations in science led to the development of highly significant and innovative drugs used for the treatment of cancer, bacterial and viral infections, malaria, and gout, as well as to prevent the rejection of transplanted organs. For these accomplishments, George Hitchings and Gertrude Elion were awarded the Nobel Prize in Physiology or Medicine in 1988.

In 1942, Elion joined Hitchings's laboratory at Burroughs Wellcome in Tuckahoe, New York (now GlaxoSmithKline in Research Triangle Park, North Carolina). Hitchings had earned a doctorate in chemistry at Harvard; Elion had a master's degree, but financial pressures prevented her from completing a PhD program. Over the years, Elion's career rapidly progressed from Hitchings's assistant to a fully equal collaborator.

TRICKING CANCER CELLS WITH COUNTERFEIT BUILDING BLOCKS. Studies by Hitchings and Elion focused on chemical modifications of natural purines and pyrimidines, building blocks in DNA synthesis. The development of their chemotherapeutic agents—medicines used to combat bacteria, viruses, and cancer—was based on the use of antimetabolite drugs. Antimetabolites are false building blocks that insert themselves into biochemical reactions. Once there, they substitute themselves for the normal purine or pyrimidine building block (the metabolite) used in the microbial or cancer cell; and because the cell cannot utilize them to synthesize DNA, the cell cannot divide and grow.

Hitchings and Elion's first significant drug was 6-mercaptopurine (Purinethol), a purine antimetabolite that Elion synthesized in 1950. It was further evaluated in New York City at the Sloan-Kettering Institute and then clinically tested at Memorial Hospital. Mercaptopurine produced complete remissions of leukemia in children, but these victories were temporary and followed by relapses within one year. Later, with a better understanding of the biology of the cell and cancer chemotherapy, other clinicians began to treat leukemias with mercaptopurine as a component of a combination of drugs. Leukemia cure rates now approach 80 percent.

SEE ALSO Sulfanilamide (1936), Amethopterin and Methotrexate (1947), Zyloprim (1966), Acyclovir (1982).

The cell-division cycle is a series of phases that occur in a cell and lead to its division and replication. In the illustration, the outer ring shows a long interphase (I), followed by cell division (M). Following the Gap 0 resting phase (G_0), the interphase consists of four phases, depicted in the inner ring: Gap 1 (G_1) prepares the cell for DNA synthesis (S), then Gap 2 (G_2) prepares the cell for mitosis (M). A major characteristic of cancer is the loss of normal control during cell proliferation, resulting in the growth of malignant tumors. Anticancer drugs such as mercaptopurine act at specific points in the tumor-cell cycle.

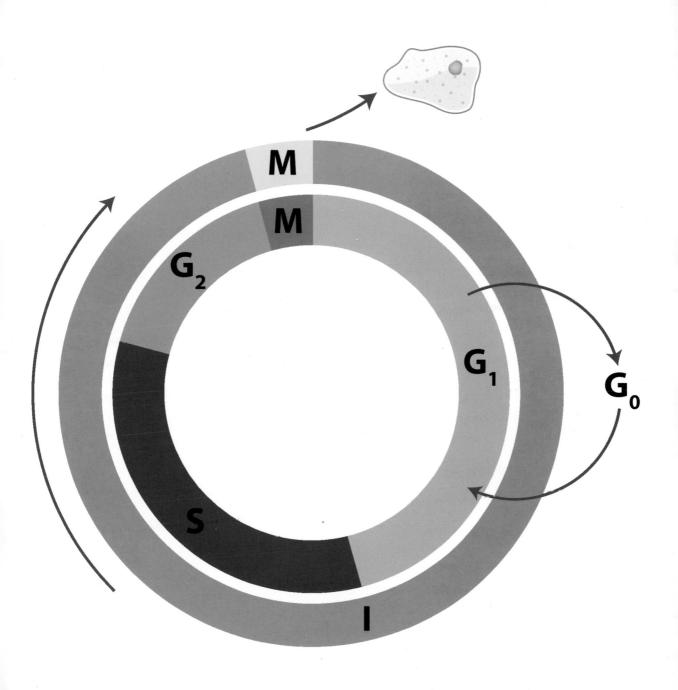

Nystatin

Elizabeth Lee Hazen (1885–1975), Rachel Fuller Brown (1898–1980)

Fungi such as *Candida* are normal inhabitants of the skin, intestines, and mucous membranes of the mouth and vagina. They rarely cause any health problems because their growth is limited by bacteria that share the same neighborhood. However, fungal infections can occur after certain antibiotics are taken, such as the broad-spectrum **tetracyclines** that affect a wide range of microbes. When the delicate balance between bacteria and fungi is disrupted, *Candida* grows unchecked, which can result in candidiasis (yeast infection) or thrush when the infection is in the mouth. Fungal overgrowth is also seen in individuals whose immune system is depressed, such as AIDS patients, cancer patients receiving chemotherapy, and organ transplant patients receiving immunosuppressive drugs.

Working for the New York State Department of Health, chemist Rachel Fuller Brown, in Albany, and microbiologist Elizabeth Lee Hazen, in New York City, shared samples of potential antifungal antibiotics found in the soil. This long-distance scientific collaboration was made possible through the U.S. mail. In 1949, nystatin was isolated from the soil bacterium *Streptomyces* and named after their employer.

In the Petri dish, nystatin (Mycostatin, Nilstat), the first antifungal antibiotic, was found to be active against a wide range of fungi. Clinically introduced in 1954, it is effectively and safely used to treat fungal infections of the skin, mouth, and vagina. However, its usefulness for the treatment of systemic infections is limited because nystatin is poorly absorbed and does not enter the blood after being taken orally. Brown and Hazen turned down the $13.4 million in royalties from the sales of Squibb's Mycostatin, assigning half this money to the Research Corporation of New York for grants to support scientific research. The other half was used to establish the Brown-Hazen Fund, which from 1957 until 1978 supported research programs, with emphasis on microbiology, and encouraged women to embark on careers in science.

SEE ALSO Streptomycin (1944), Tetracyclines (1948), Amphotericin B (1956), Griseofulvin (1958), Cyclosporine/Ciclosporin (1983).

This digital illustration shows Candida albicans, *a frequent cause of yeast infections and thrush. Fungi such as* Candida *are distinct from plants, animals, and bacteria, but they are more closely related to animals than plants.*

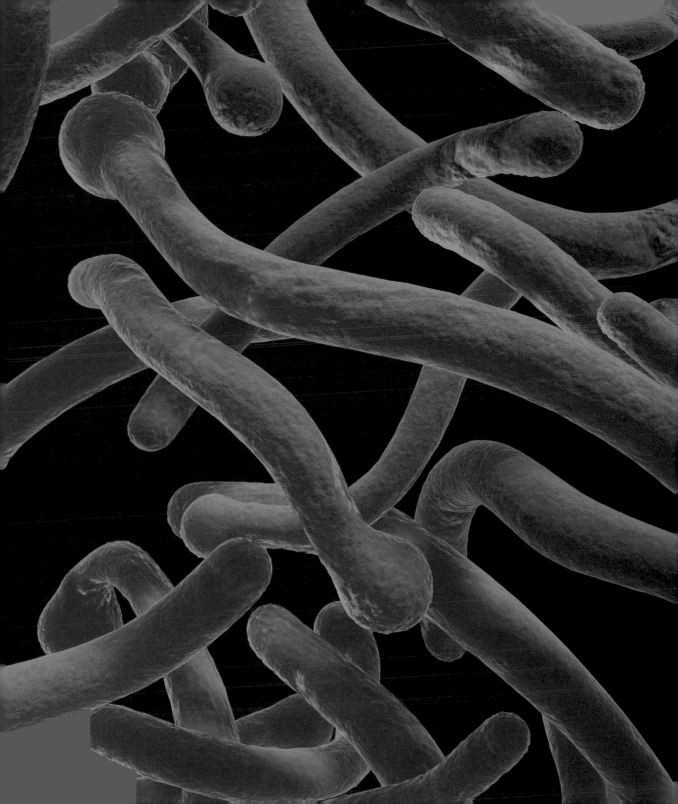

Polio Vaccine

John F. Enders (1897–1985), **Albert B. Sabin** (1906–1993), **Jonas E. Salk** (1914–1995), **Thomas H. Weller** (1915–2008), **Frederick C. Robbins** (1916–2003), **Hilary Koprowski** (b. 1916)

During the 1940s and 1950s, polio was the greatest public health threat. Movie theaters and public swimming pools emptied when periodic outbreaks of polio occurred, and the "iron lungs" lining hospital wards became its symbol. With the widespread adoption of polio vaccines, these are now historic memories. For the past decade, polio has been eradicated in all but four countries. Worldwide cases of polio precipitously fell from 350,000 in 1988 to 1,652 in 2007.

The pivotal breakthrough in the development of an effective vaccine to prevent poliomyelitis (polio) came in 1948, when American virologists John Enders, Thomas Weller, and Frederick Robbins at Children's Hospital, Boston, grew the poliovirus in tissue cultures outside the body; they were jointly awarded the Nobel Prize in Physiology or Medicine in 1954. Using funding support from the National Foundation for Infantile Paralysis (now the March of Dimes), founded by President Franklin D. Roosevelt, Jonas Salk at the University of Pittsburgh developed and, in 1954, successfully field-tested an injectable, killed-virus vaccine that was clinically introduced the following year.

In 1958, Albert Sabin at the University of Cincinnati developed another polio vaccine—this one using a live, attenuated (weakened) virus. Sabin's oral vaccine provided longer-lasting immunity against all strains of polio and required no booster shots, yet it had the potential to cause vaccine-associated paralytic polio.

"Victory has a thousand fathers," and this was the case for claimants of the polio vaccine. Salk was internationally acclaimed for his discovery, which he made no attempt to patent, but he failed to acknowledge the pioneering contribution of Enders, Weller, and Robbins. Sabin initially attacked the safety and effectiveness of the Salk vaccine, and for years his vaccine was preferentially used in the United States. Virtually forgotten is the Polish-born virologist Hilary Koprowski who, while working at Lederle Laboratories in 1950, developed the first orally effective, attenuated vaccine.

For the past decade, only Salk's vaccine has been used in the United States and United Kingdom, while Sabin's is preferred in developing countries.

SEE ALSO Smallpox Vaccine (1796), Gardasil (2006).

In 1921, Franklin Delano Roosevelt (1882–1945) contracted an illness that resulted in permanent paralysis below the waist. The condition was originally diagnosed as polio, but some believe that it was actually Guillain-Barré syndrome. Roosevelt founded the March of Dimes in 1938 to support polio research and education.

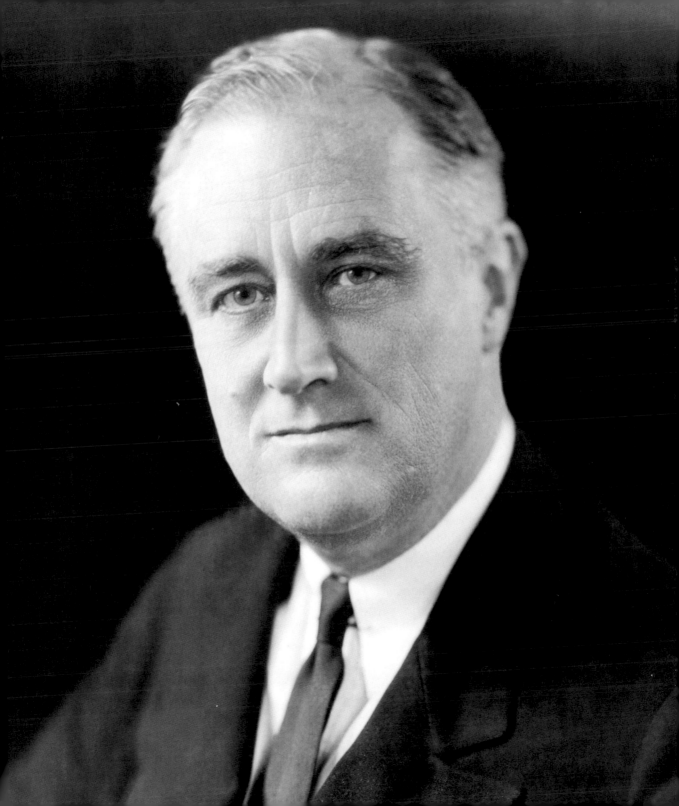

Meprobamate

Frank Milan Berger (1913–2008)

The phenomenal marketplace success of meprobamate, a rather ordinary drug, can be attributed to creative and aggressive publicity and its timely introduction. Its humble beginning can be traced to a British research laboratory in the mid-1940s, where Frank Berger, a medically trained scientist from what is now the Czech Republic, was investigating possible preservatives for **penicillin**. One of these compounds was mephenesin, which upon further testing showed muscle-relaxing effects and, as he termed it, a "tranquilizing" effect in rodents. It was, however, too weak and too short-acting.

FIRST BLOCKBUSTER "TRANQUILIZER." Berger was Director of Research at Wallace Laboratories when, in 1950, he and chemist Bernard Ludwig synthesized meprobamate, a compound that was more potent and longer-acting than mephenesin. Marketed as a "tranquilizer" for the relief of anxiety, tension, and muscle spasms under the trade name Miltown (a village in New Jersey), it was an immediate success. Within months of its introduction in 1955, it was the best-selling drug in the United States, and by 1957, one out of three prescriptions was written for Miltown or Equanil, the Wyeth Laboratories brand of meprobamate. Supplies in pharmacies could not keep up with demand. The first TV star in the United States, Milton Berle, called himself "Miltown Berle."

By 1960, the balloon burst! The drug was not as safe and abuse-free as it was purported to be. Doses not greatly in excess of those used for medical purposes were found to cause dependence, and the symptoms associated with meprobamate withdrawal were similar to withdrawal from barbiturates and **alcohol**. Sales declined precipitously. In 1965, meprobamate was removed from a list of "minor tranquilizers" and, more appropriately, reclassified as a sedative. Federal restrictions were imposed on its prescribing and refilling. That same year, Johnny Cash was arrested returning from Mexico with 655 **amphetamine** and 475 Equanil tablets in his guitar case. He was fined and given a 30-day suspended jail sentence.

Meprobamate's decline was also hastened by the arrival of the benzodiazepines **Librium** (1960) and **Valium** (1963). These drugs had tranquilizing effects that could relieve anxiety without the excessive sedation.

SEE ALSO Alcohol (c. 10,000 BCE), Nembutal and Seconal (1928), Penicillin (1928), Amphetamine (1932), Librium (1960), Valium (1963), BuSpar (1986).

Plate II from Charles Darwin's The Expression of the Emotions in Man and Animals *(1872), Chapter VII, "Low Spirits, Anxiety, Grief, Dejection, Despair." After their introduction, Miltown and Equanil (trade names for meprobamate) were the best-selling drugs in the anxiety-prone United States.*

PLATE II

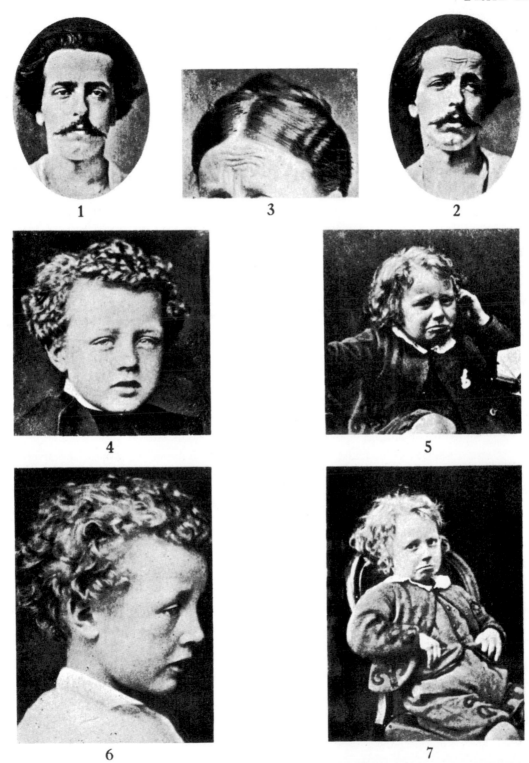

1   3   2

4   5

6   7

Placebos

Henry Beecher (1904–1976)

When physicians prescribe a medication, they are tacitly implying that the drug works, and the patient anticipates positive effects. There may be great truth to the French proverb, "The presence of the doctor is the beginning of the cure." However, must the prescribed medication be a "real" drug? A placebo (from the Latin "I will please") is any therapy, drug or nondrug, that objectively lacks activity for the condition being treated and whose effectiveness is predicated upon suggestions offered by the healthcare professional.

Are "sugar pills" or saline injections clinically effective? Henry Beecher, an American anesthesiologist and medical ethicist, served in North Africa and Italy during World War II and became interested in the subjective responses of patients and treatments. In his classic 1955 paper, "The Powerful Placebo," Beecher reported that placebos were effective in 35 percent of patients for the relief of such medical problems as severe postoperative wound pain, cough, depression, stomach ulcers, and anxiety and tension. Other investigators have seen favorable responses in conditions that include elevated blood pressure, insomnia, and schizophrenia. However, some scholars have challenged the magnitude and extent of these positive placebo effects. Beneficial effects are most likely to occur when measuring a change in behavior or a subjective sensation but are far less likely for such problems as widespread as cancers or joint changes in rheumatoid arthritis.

In view of the high proportion of patients who respond to placebos, particularly with antidepressants, drug trials most often compare a new or test medicine with a placebo for its relative effectiveness. To eliminate bias, double-blind studies are typically conducted in which neither the physician-investigator nor the patient is aware of whether an active drug or a placebo has been given.

RESEARCH TOOL OR PATIENT DECEPTION? Placebos are safe, effective (for many), and inexpensive, but a spirited debate exists as to whether the use of a placebo for the treatment of a medical condition is ethically justified or rather a deception that can undermine the physician-patient relationship.

SEE ALSO Clinical Testing of Drugs (1753), Kefauver-Harris Amendment (1962), Prozac (1987).

The infamous Tuskegee syphilis study conducted by the U.S. Public Health Service from 1932 to 1972 was intended to investigate the progression of untreated syphilis in black men. In the image, a doctor is injecting a placebo to a subject who believes that he is receiving active health care.

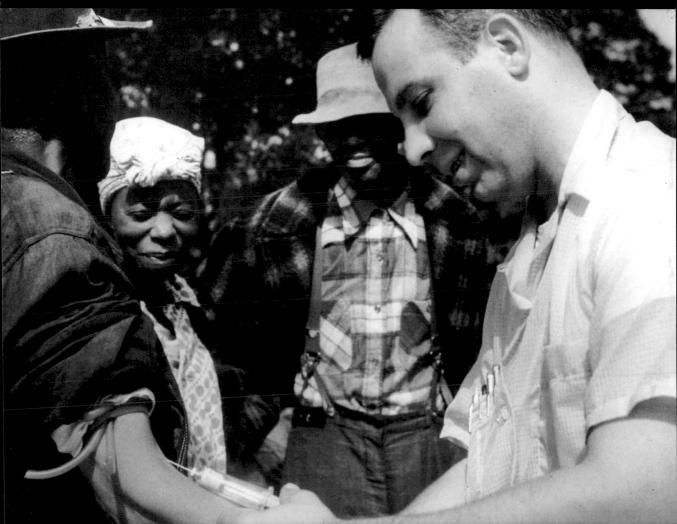

Ritalin

1955

Ritalin is a mild stimulant with **amphetamine**-like effects. With their seemingly energizing effects on the body, how can Ritalin and the amphetamines calm overactive children with attention deficit hyperactivity disorder (ADHD)? Before attempting to answer this question, let's briefly look at ADHD, for which the literature presents widely divergent perspectives.

ADHD, the most commonly diagnosed behavioral disorder in children, is a chronic disorder that may continue into adulthood. The hyperkinetic child is typically overactive, has a poor or short attention span, has problems completing tasks, and is impulsive. Roughly 5–10 percent of school-age children in the five- to eleven-year-old range are diagnosed with ADHD, and it is more than twice as common in boys as in girls. No single cause is responsible for ADHD, but genetic factors may play an important role. Other postulated causes include such environmental factors as exposure to lead, maternal smoking and alcohol use, brain damage by injury or infection, and food additives.

Methylphenidate (Ritalin, Concerta, Metadate), detroamphetamine (Dexedrine), and amphetamine salts (Adderall) are some of the drugs used to treat ADHD. Symptoms improve in 70–80 percent of children and in 70 percent of adults taking these drugs. Benefits derived from these drugs include a reduction in impulsive behavior and interrupting, greater goal-directed behavior, and improved attention.

How Ritalin and the amphetamines work in ADHD is not clear, although they are known to increase brain levels of dopamine, a **neurotransmitter** that is associated with attention. One of many complex (and confusing) explanations proposes that children with ADHD have a dopamine deficiency and that these drugs increase attention by increasing dopamine.

Although Ritalin and related amphetamines have abuse potential in adults, when used to treat ADHD in children, they are not thought to be habit-forming or to lead to drug abuse in adults. These drugs may suppress or delay the growth of some children, but studies suggest that the effect is only temporary.

ADHD is often observed in highly creative and talented individuals. A very partial and diverse list of people reported to have ADHD includes Ludwig van Beethoven, Tom Cruise, Albert Einstein, Benjamin Franklin, Bill Gates, Michael Jordan, Abraham Lincoln, John Lennon, Michael Phelps, and Steven Spielberg.

SEE ALSO Neurotransmitters (1920), Amphetamine (1932).

Children with ADHD exhibit one or more of the following symptoms: inattentiveness, hyperactivity, and impulsive behavior. While Ritalin and related drugs cannot cure ADHD, they can produce a significant calming effect on these children.

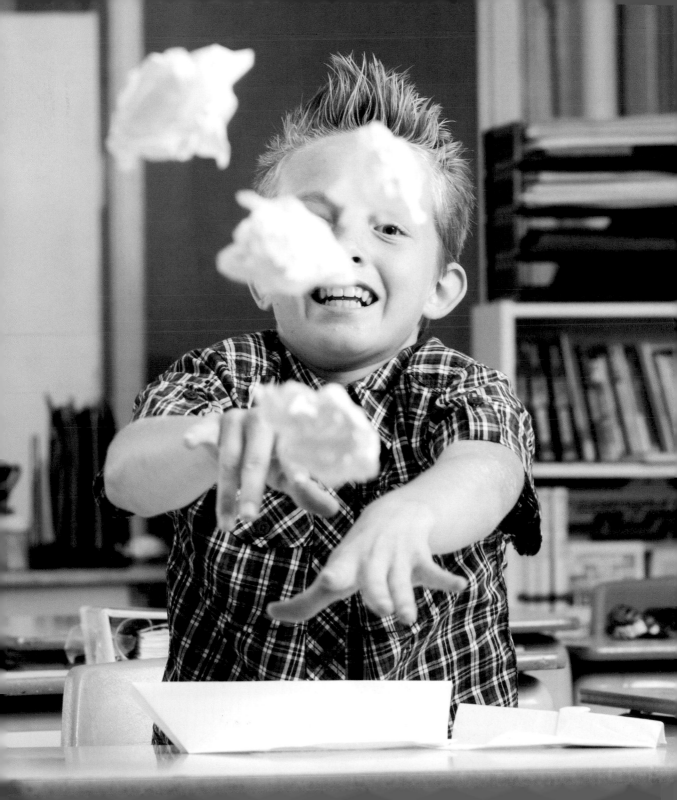

Dianabol

John Ziegler (1920–1983)

Within years after the isolation of **testosterone** and its synthesis in 1935, unconfirmed reports surfaced that German scientists were testing testosterone derivatives to improve the fighting capability of their soldiers. During and after World War II, these drugs were given by the Allies to promote weight gain in concentration camp survivors and malnourished soldiers. Testosterone was found to have two general effects: anabolic effects that increase muscle mass and decrease body fat and androgenic effects that promote sexual characteristics and function.

John Ziegler, a Ciba Pharmaceuticals physician, was instrumental in the development of Dianabol (methandrosterolone), a synthetic compound that had far greater relative anabolic effects than testosterone. The medals gained and records set by East German swimmers from the late 1960s to 1980s have been attributed to their use of Dianabol-like anabolic steroids (AS). In response to why many of their swimmers had deep voices, the East German coach replied, "We came here to swim, not sing." Although AS use has been banned in most sports, a number of outstanding athletes and body builders have been found using these drugs to enhance performance.

Illicit laboratories have attempted to design drugs, such as "The Clear" (tetrahydrogestrinone), that remain undetected in urine. There are six to eight AS on the legal market, including Anadrol, Durabolin, and Halotestin, but many more are manufactured in clandestine labs in the United States and abroad. Users obtain them from underground sources, websites, and health food stores.

Regular use of AS is not without hazard. They can elevate levels of LDL (bad) cholesterol, increasing the risk of cardiovascular problems, produce liver toxicity and masculinization of female users, and cause mood disorders and behavioral changes such as "roid rage" and depression.

AS are classified in Schedule II of the Controlled Substances Act, the most restrictive class for drugs with approved medical uses. Approved AS uses include increasing muscle mass in individuals with such wasting diseases as AIDS and cancer.

SEE ALSO Testosterone (1935), Off-Label Drug Use (1962).

Notwithstanding the potential danger they risk by using anabolic steroids, some body builders continue to supplement their weight training with Dianabol and related drugs.

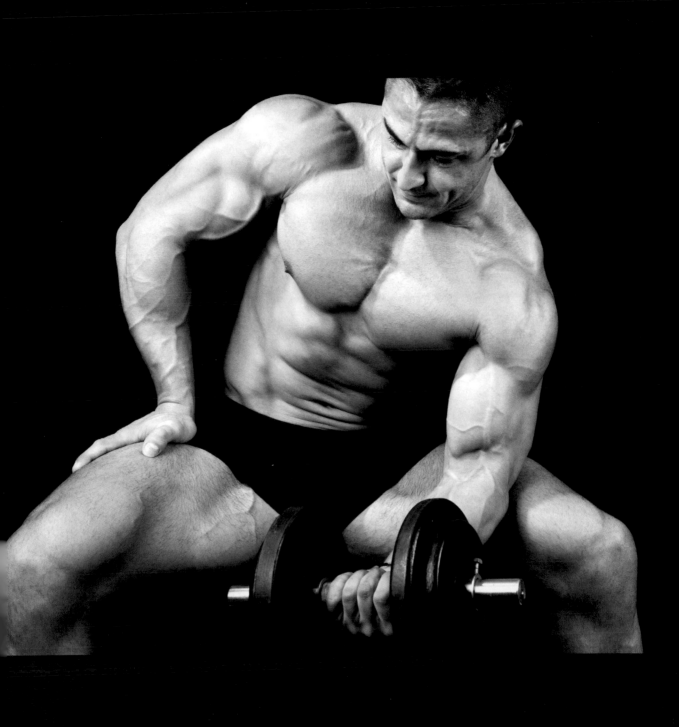

Amphotericin B

The use of any drug carries some level of risk. When evaluating a drug for market approval, the **Food and Drug Administration** (FDA) weighs its benefits and potential risks. Doctors must make similar evaluations when deciding to prescribe drugs for their patients. In both cases, the level of risk must be weighed against the severity of the condition being treated. For the treatment of minor disorders, we would expect the potential risks to be minimal. Not so for life-threatening conditions, such as certain systemic fungal infections, in which treatments such as amphotericin B carry a major risk of causing severe toxicity.

AMPHOTERRIBLE. Amphotericin B (Fungizone) is an exceedingly important drug, active against a very wide range of disease-causing fungi and the first pick in the treatment of most systemic fungal infections, which before its introduction in 1956 were invariably fatal. However, amphotericin B's downside is that it causes kidney toxicity and troubling adverse reactions associated with its intravenous infusion that may continue on a daily basis for two to four months. Referred to as *amphoterrible*, it may also cause liver, heart, and blood problems.

An obvious drug challenge is to maximize amphotericin B's antifungal effects while minimizing its damaging effects to the kidneys. A similar problem exists with certain anticancer drugs, which are also toxic to organs of the body. One of the newer approaches involves the use of liposomes—laboratory-prepared microscopic bubbles that are filled with drugs and that prevent the toxic drug from collecting in the kidneys. Liposomal amphotericin B (AmBisome) and similar products have been found to be as effective as the original drug while protecting the kidneys and other sites from its deleterious effects. However, these newer preparations are so expensive that their use is restricted to patients who cannot tolerate the conventional amphotericin product.

SEE ALSO Food and Drug Administration (1906), Nystatin (1954).

Physicians prescribing amphotericin B must weigh its potential success treating life-threatening systemic fungal infections, such as Cryptococcus neoformans *(pictured), against its potential for causing severe, multiple-organ toxicity, even at the recommended doses.*

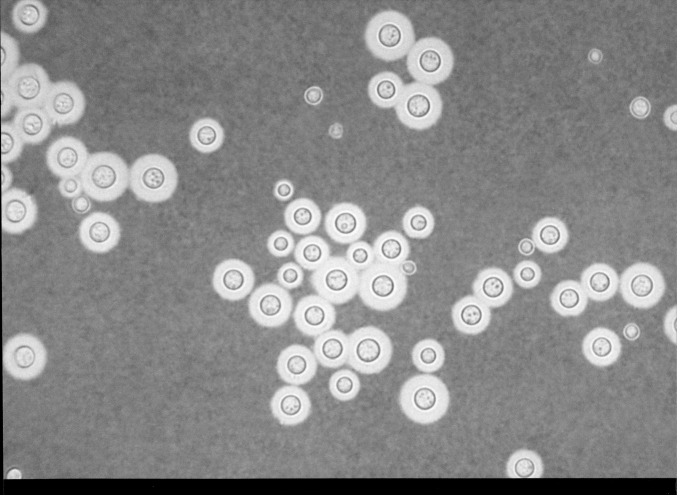

Orinase

Diabetics need insulin injections to live. But what about "prediabetics," typically older and heavier individuals, who have none of the symptoms and do not feel sick, but who, over the years, become diabetic? Today, we call them type 2 diabetics. To treat or not to treat was the challenge facing diabetes experts in the 1950s. For Upjohn, manufacturer of Orinase, the answer was obvious.

Insulin injections provide the insulin that cannot be manufactured by the diabetic's pancreas. Orinase, like insulin, lowers increased blood sugar levels, but it is not an oral insulin and does not help all diabetics. It works by stimulating the release of insulin, which the pancreas must first manufacture.

Orinase (tolbutamide), the first member of the sulfonylurea class of oral antidiabetic drugs and chemically related to **sulfanilamide**, was approved for marketing in the United States in 1957. Type 2 diabetics did not have to suffer the pain of injections, exercise, or strict diets; they only had to take a pill. Doctors were happy because the pills lowered their patients' blood sugar and supposedly reduced their long-term risks of diabetic complications, including heart disease, strokes, impaired vision, and kidney failure.

The story does not conclude on a happy note. In 1970, a ten-year study comparing the effectiveness of tolbutamide with a **placebo** unexpectedly found that tolbutamide-treated patients had a 2.5-fold greater risk of dying of heart disease. The results of this University Group Diabetes Program (UGDP) study was embraced by the **Food and Drug Administration** and the American Medical Association but savaged by the American Diabetes Association, many physicians using Orinase to treat their patients, and the pharmaceutical manufacturer, Upjohn.

Interpretation of the results of the UGDP study has been subject to criticism, and more than four decades later, a clear picture of Orinase's effect on the heart has yet to emerge. However, since 1984, all sufonylurea antidiabetic drugs must bear the warning of "increased risk of cardiovascular mortality." Although Orinase is no longer marketed, generic tolbutamide still is.

SEE ALSO Insulin (1921), Sulfanilamide (1936), Placebos (1955), Glucophage (1958), Human Insulin (1982), Avandia (2010).

Type 2 diabetes is becoming increasingly common in young people, probably due to lack of exercise and obesity, the latter resulting in part from excessive consumption of soft drinks. One twelve-ounce can of a popular cola beverage contains forty grams (about 9.4 teaspoons) of sugar!

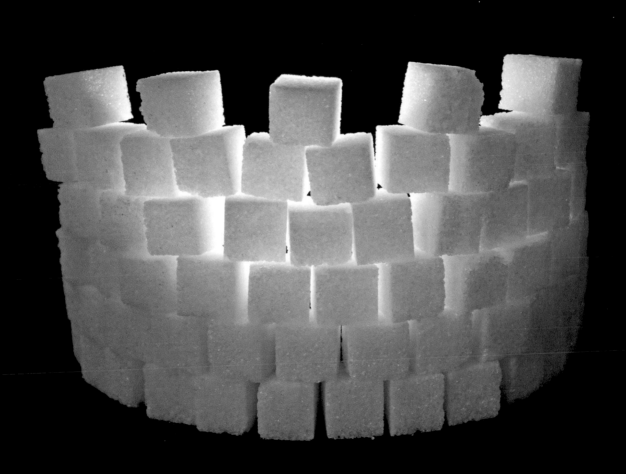

Thalidomide

Frances Oldham Kelsey (b. 1914), **Widukind Lenz** (1919–1995), **William McBride** (b. 1927)

A MONUMENTAL MEDICAL TRAGEDY. When thalidomide was introduced in 1957 to promote sleep and treat morning sickness, it seemed remarkably safe. The following year, it was approved in the United Kingdom and, by 1961, was marketed in Canada and more than twenty countries in Europe and Africa. In 1960, Richardson Merrell aggressively sought approval to market thalidomide (Kevadon) in the United States and distributed 2.5 million tablets, which were received by 20,000 patients; by 1961, seventeen cases of birth defects were reported. Frances Kelsey, an FDA pharmacologist, reviewed the application. Her concerns about the drug's safety led her to recommend its rejection, and in 1962, she received the President's Award for Distinguished Federal Civilian Service from John F. Kennedy for "sparing the nation a human tragedy."

Working independently in 1961, William McBride in Australia and Widukind Lenz in Germany established the linkage between thalidomide and the birth defects. By the time thalidomide was withdrawn that year, more than 10,000 babies worldwide were born with major birth defects. The most extreme were very rare malformations of the limbs—known as phocomelia—often characterized by flipper-like hands extending from the shoulder. These dramatic effects occurred after women took as little as one dose during the first three months of pregnancy.

The thalidomide tragedy focused attention on the effectiveness of the "placental barrier." The placenta serves as a respiratory, circulatory, and excretory organ for the fetus, and we now know that this barrier is ineffective in protecting the fetus against most drugs taken by the mother. As a result of this disaster, an essential component of testing now includes an evaluation of drug effects on the developing fetus during pregnancy. Among the drugs *known* to be teratogenic (from Greek *terat* or *monster*, in reference to birth defects) are remedies for acne (**Accutane**), seizures (**Dilantin** and **valproic acid**), and cancer (**methotrexate**), with many others suspected of causing defects.

Thalidomide (Thalomid) returned in the late 1990s for the treatment of multiple myeloma (a blood cell cancer) and complications of leprosy.

SEE ALSO Dilantin (1938), Amethopterin and Methotrexate (1947), Kefauver-Harris Amendment (1962), Valproic Acid (1967), Accutane (1982).

Frances Oldham Kelsey was singularly responsible for averting a thalidomide birth-defect disaster in the United States. In recognition, John F. Kennedy presented her with the President's Award for Distinguished Federal Civilian Service in 1962.

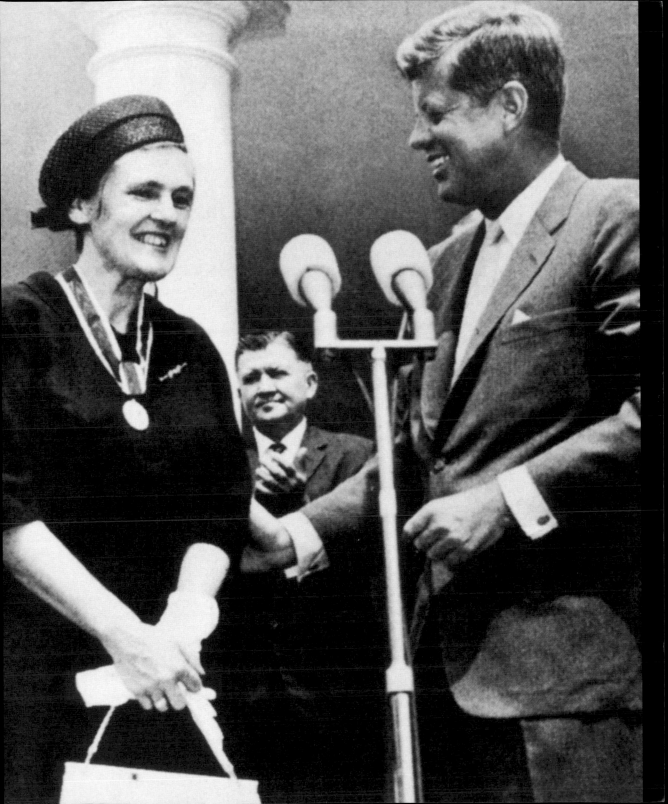

Tofranil and Elavil

Roland Kuhn (1912–2005)

The medical and financial success of the anti-schizophrenic drug **chlorpromazine** (Thorazine) was a compelling incentive for pharmaceutical companies to modify the drug's chemistry and develop similar drugs. One of the first "potential anti-schizophrenic" drugs developed by Geigy (now Novartis) was imipramine. Contrary to the expectations of Swiss psychiatrist Roland Kuhn, his psychotic patients failed to improve, and some even grew worse. However, his depressed patients benefited—in some cases, dramatically.

Imipramine was marketed as Tofranil in 1957, and in 1961, Merck's chemists subtly modified imipramine's chemistry to give us amitriptyline (Elavil). Tofranil and Elavil were the first members of the *tricyclic antidepressant class*—so-called because their chemical structures have three rings. In time, they were joined by some twenty other tricyclics and related drugs.

How do these drugs relieve depression? Many experts believe that depression results from a deficiency of either norepinephrine (noradrenaline), serotonin, or both in mood-influencing areas of the brain. Antidepressants reverse this deficit. Some tricyclics increase norepinephrine, while others increase serotonin; most affect both **neurotransmitters**. Which tricyclics are most effective? This cannot be predicted in advance and can only be determined by trial and error. The theory of how antidepressants work seems simple, but questions remain. Among the most puzzling is why several weeks pass after starting medication before positive changes in mood begin to occur and the dark clouds of depression begin to lift.

Not sensing quick, positive mood changes after taking their antidepressant, some patients lose hope of ever feeling "good" again and may attempt to end their misery with a drug overdose. Suicide attempts with tricyclics are sometimes successful, and when not successful, the symptoms of poisoning are always difficult to treat.

Prozac and related selective serotonin-reuptake inhibitors (SSRIs) have replaced tricyclics because they are safer when intentionally taken in overdose and have fewer side effects. However, SSRIs are not necessarily more effective than tricyclics, and some evidence suggests that neither class of antidepressants is much better than a **placebo** in reversing depression.

SEE ALSO Neurotransmitters (1920), Chlorpromazine (1952), Monoamine Oxidase Inhibitors (1961), Prozac (1987).

Sarah Bernhardt (1844–1923) is shown here in her role as Hamlet. Hamlet's depression has been attributed to his father's murder and his mother's hasty marriage to Claudius, his dead father's brother and murderer.

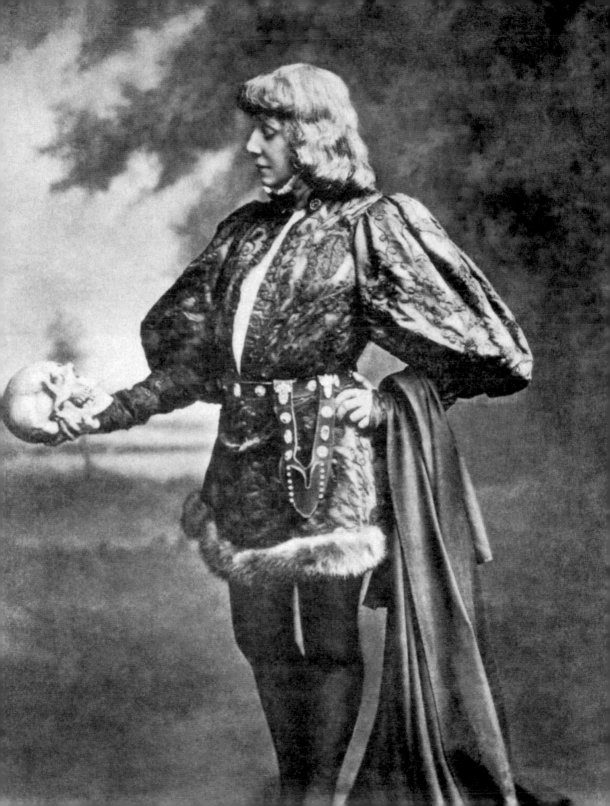

Griseofulvin

Infections caused by fungi are categorized as being systemic or superficial. Systemic infections are less common but far more serious, even life-threatening. Among the most common superficial infections are ringworm infections of the skin, hair, and nails. *Ringworm* refers to the circular shape of the infected area. Before the 1958 introduction of griseofulvin, the first orally administered antifungal drug, a variety of topically applied products were used, with questionable success. Alternative approaches to dealing with ringworm infections included removal of hair from the scalp with x-rays or surgical removal of infected nails.

Griseofulvin was first isolated from the mold *Penicillium griseofulvin* in 1939, but since it lacked activity against bacteria, the primary interest of scientists at the time, it was put aside. Several years later, when it was found to have a stunting and curling effect on certain fungi, it was first used for the treatment of fungal diseases in plants, but it was not until 1958 that griseofulvin was used to treat fungal infections in humans and animals. Trade names include Fulvicin P/G, Grisactin, and Gris-PEG.

Unlike antibiotics that aggressively and rapidly attack bacteria, griseofulvin is far more deliberate and slow moving against fungi. After the drug is absorbed, it is deposited in keratin, a protein that is an essential building block in the manufacture of the horny outer layers of skin, hair, and nails. Once present in the keratin, griseofulvin prevents new infections and actively growing fungi from reproducing. Thus, the first signs of improvement are seen in new growths of hair or nails. The speed with which griseofulvin clears up a fungal infection is determined by how quickly the cells grow in a given area. Ringworm of the skin and hair can be successfully treated in one to two months, while infections of the toenails require six to twelve months of drug treatment. Ringworm infections are highly contagious and may be spread from animals to humans.

SEE ALSO Nystatin (1954), Amphotericin B (1956).

This image is of a hair follicle from a patient with a ringworm infection, which can be effectively treated with griseofulvin. Ringworm infections are becoming increasingly common because of the rising population of immunocompromised patients with such conditions as AIDS, diabetes, and cancer.

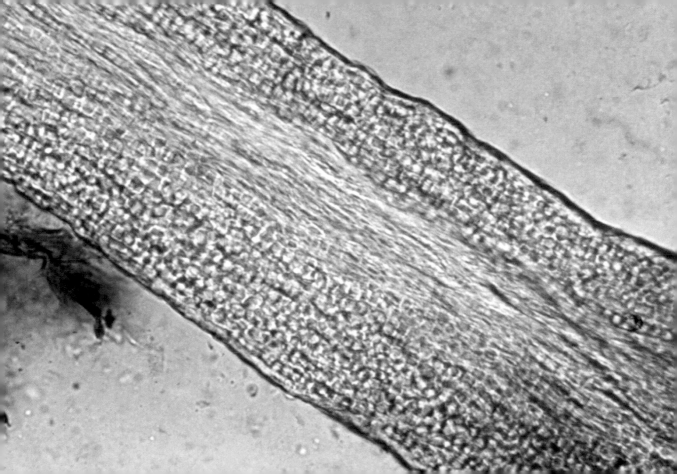

Glucophage

Jean Sterne (1919–1997)

One the world's most widely used antidiabetic drugs has its roots in the Middle Ages, when *Galega officinalis* (French lilac or goat's rue) was taken to treat this disease. The plant contains guanidine, found in 1918 to be responsible for the plant's blood-sugar–lowering (hypoglycemic) effects, but it and several chemical derivatives were too toxic for use as medicines. In the 1920s, the derivative metformin produced hypoglycemic effects in rabbits, but the diabetes treatment world was focused on a far more dramatic drug: **insulin**.

In the 1940s and 1950s, several factors led to renewed interest in metformin. **Orinase** (tolbutamide), among the first oral hypoglycemic drugs effective in humans, generated considerable enthusiasm in medical and financial circles, and when used for the treatment of influenza, metformin was found to lower blood sugar with few toxic effects. Follow-up studies on these chance observations by the French diabetologist Jean Sterne—who named it Glucophage, or glucose eater—validated its potential usefulness as an antidiabetic drug. Glucophage was approved for use in Great Britain in 1958 and in Canada in 1972. Finally in 1995, it became available in the United States.

Type 2 diabetes is the most common and fastest growing form of diabetes, occurring increasingly in children and adolescents, with obesity and lack of exercise as major contributory factors leading to its development. With proper management, the progression of type 2 to type 1 diabetes (which requires insulin injections) and long-term complications can be delayed or even prevented.

FIRST CHOICE FOR TYPE 2 DIABETES. In a highly authoritative ten-year study in the United Kingdom reported in 1998, metformin (Glucophage) was the only oral drug shown to decrease the risk of diabetic complications and the death rate resulting from heart attack and stroke in type 2 patients. Use of this drug may also decrease the likelihood of developing type 2 diabetes in patients at risk, although vigorous exercise and diet are even more effective. Experts recommend that metformin—said to be the world's most widely prescribed antidiabetic drug and one of only two oral antidiabetic drugs on the World Health Organization's Model List of Essential Medicines—be included in the treatment of all type 2 diabetic patients.

SEE ALSO Insulin (1921), Orinase (1957), Human Insulin (1982), Avandia (2010).

During the late 1800s, goat's rue (Galega officinalis, pictured) was thought to have potential as a fodder crop in Europe. It didn't taste good, as perceived by cattle and horses, and it is now listed as a Federal noxious weed, but Glucophage—the medicine derived from it—is widely used for the treatment of diabetes.

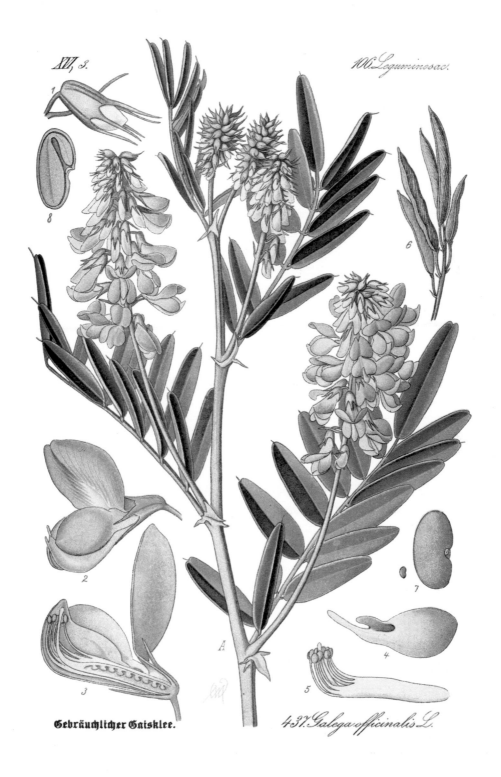

Gebräuchlicher Gaisklee.

437. Galega officinalis L.

Diuril

Karl H. Beyer Jr. (1914–1996), **Edward D. Freis** (1912–2005)

The introduction of Diuril in 1958 was not only a major advance in the evolution of diuretics (drugs that promote the flow of urine), but also, and far more significantly, it revolutionized the treatment of hypertension. Before Diuril, organic mercury-containing diuretics were the most effective drugs for the elimination of excessive body fluids, but their use required injections and was associated with severe toxicity. In addition, the treatment of hypertension was limited to severe cases, and all the available drugs produced a high incidence of undesirable side effects at their usual doses.

Karl Beyer at Merck, Sharp & Dohme (MSD), sought to develop a safe, orally effective diuretic that could reduce fluids in heart failure and edema, and he initially envisioned Diuril (chlorothiazide) to be that drug. Rather unexpectedly, clinical studies revealed that it not only reduced edema but also decreased blood pressure. Older drugs decreased blood pressure in all patients, but Diuril only did so in hypertensive patients. It was a specific antihypertensive drug.

Not surprisingly, the thrust of MSD's marketing campaign expanded beyond diuresis and focused on Diuril's antihypertensive effects, a far more lucrative market. Many articles proclaimed Diuril to be the biggest medical breakthrough in recent years.

QUIETING THE SILENT KILLER. Until the 1950s, only "severe" hypertension was treated, as medical experts were divided as to whether "mild" hypertension—present but without discernable symptoms—should be. Unlike older antihypertensives, Diuril could be used safely, with little risk to the patient, which shifted the tide toward routine drug treatment of mild hypertension. By 1970, hypertension researcher Edward Freis, conducting nationwide studies in Veterans Administration hospitals, demonstrated that treatment of even mild-to-moderate hypertension significantly reduced the risk of heart attack, heart failure, stroke, and other complications of hypertension.

Today, Diuril-like thiazides and related diuretics, used alone or in combination with other antihypertensives, are the most commonly used drugs for the treatment of elevated blood pressure.

SEE ALSO Merbaphen (1920), Sulfanilamide (1936), Diamox (1952), Propranolol (1964), Lasix (1966), Captopril (1981).

Diuril promotes the elimination of excessive water and salt. The first step in this process is the filtration of blood by the kidney, involving the passage of blood through the glomerulus. The human glomerulus, magnified here 100x, resembles tiny tubules.

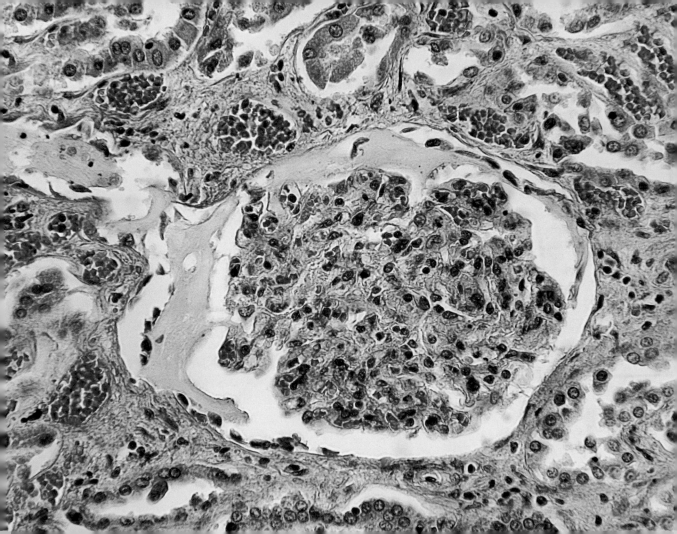

Haldol

Paul Janssen (1926–2003)

Several years after the 1954 introduction of **chlorpromazine** (Thorazine), a drug that revolutionized the treatment of schizophrenia, Paul Janssen synthesized haloperidol. This was among the most important drugs to be developed at Janssen Pharmaceutica, which he founded in 1953 in Beerse, Belgium, with the vision of a totally independent and self-supporting research laboratory. Discoverer of more than eighty medicines, four of which are on the World Health Organization Model List of Essential Medicines, Janssen was the runner up to "Apostle of the Lepers" Father Damien as The Greatest Belgian in a 2005 poll organized by Flemish media.

Haloperidol (Haldol) was originally intended to be a chemical modification of meperidine (pethidine, Demerol), a narcotic painkiller. Although devoid of analgesic effects, Haldol proved to be an extremely active anti-schizophrenic drug, with 1 mg of haloperidol equivalent to 50 mg of chlorpromazine. Haloperidol and chlorpromazine drugs are essentially equivalent in their clinical effectiveness but have different side effects. Haloperidol is primarily used for manic and highly agitated patients.

Haloperidol was approved for use in the United States in 1967, almost a decade after it was available in Europe. In addition to an oral dosage form, it is also available for long-acting use as an injection given every four weeks to patients who frequently relapse or who fail to take their medication.

CHEMICAL CONTROL OF DISSENT. Haloperidol was an ancillary tool of repression during the last decades of the former Soviet Union. In lieu of being deported to labor camps, mentally healthy political dissidents were interned in psychiatric hospitals, in isolation, for extended periods of detention. Many were said to have received high doses of haloperidol to treat their "sluggish schizophrenia," a classical symptom of which was the desire to reform the political system. Apparently selected because it was one of the few anti-schizophrenic drugs available in sufficient quantities in the Soviet Union at the time, haloperidol was used to crush dissidents' will to resist by converting them into zombies.

SEE ALSO Chlorpromazine (1952), Reserpine (1952), Clozapine (1989), Zyprexa (1996).

Schizophrenia ranks among the top ten causes of disability in developed countries worldwide, with rates ranging from 0.5 to 1 percent of the population. At least 200,000 of the 600,000 homeless people in the United States suffer from either schizophrenia or bipolar (manic-depressive) illness.

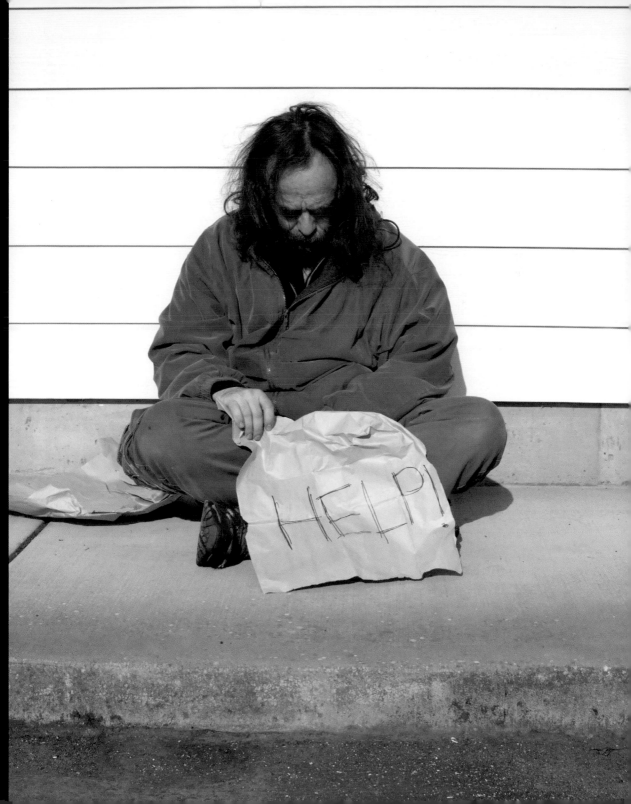

Vinca Alkaloids

Robert L. Noble (1910–1990), **Charles T. Beer** (1915–2010), **Gordon H. Svoboda** (1922–1994)

The discovery of the vinca **alkaloids** is rife with controversy, including a Canadian-American rivalry. It is clear, however, that the alkaloids vinblastine and vincristine, discovered some six decades ago, continue to remain important drugs in the treatment of cancer—vinblastine (Velban) for testicular cancer and Hodgkin's disease, and vincristine (Oncovin) for non-Hodgkin's lymphoma and leukemia.

Scientific studies on vinca began in the early 1950s. At the University of Western Ontario, Robert Noble investigated claims that a Jamaican tea brewed from the leaves of the ornamental Madagascar periwinkle (formerly known as *Vinca rosea*) was effective in treating diabetes. In Noble's laboratory studies, periwinkle extracts had no effect on blood sugar in rats and, thus, were not the sought-after oral insulin. Rather unexpectedly, the extract dramatically altered the blood, depressing white blood cells and bone marrow, the site of blood-cell production. In 1958, Charles Beer, a British-born chemist working with Noble, isolated vinblastine, the active alkaloid responsible for the fall in white blood cells, from periwinkle.

Contemporaneously, Gordon Svoboda at Eli Lilly in Indianapolis, Indiana, was testing some 5,000 plant materials a year in search of antitumor drugs and issued a rival claim for the first discovery of vinblastine's antitumor effects. The drug worked in animals, but what about in humans? Eli Lilly was able to produce large quantities of the antitumor compound, and a race ensued as to whether the earliest human trials would be undertaken in Canada or the United States. In 1961, vincristine was isolated from periwinkle and marketed by Eli Lilly two years later.

The debate continues as to which side of the border can claim the bragging rights for the discovery and clinical testing of vinblastine. In Canada, the issue has been settled. In 1997, Noble and Beer were inducted into the Canadian Medical Hall of Fame for their "discovery of vinblastine, the first major advance in chemotherapy originating in Canada."

SEE ALSO Alkaloids (1806).

In addition to its wide assortment of medical uses over the centuries, the Madagascar periwinkle (pictured) was used in medieval Europe in love potions, to exorcise evil spirits, to protect the bearer from sudden harm, and for wreaths placed on the gravestones of infants.

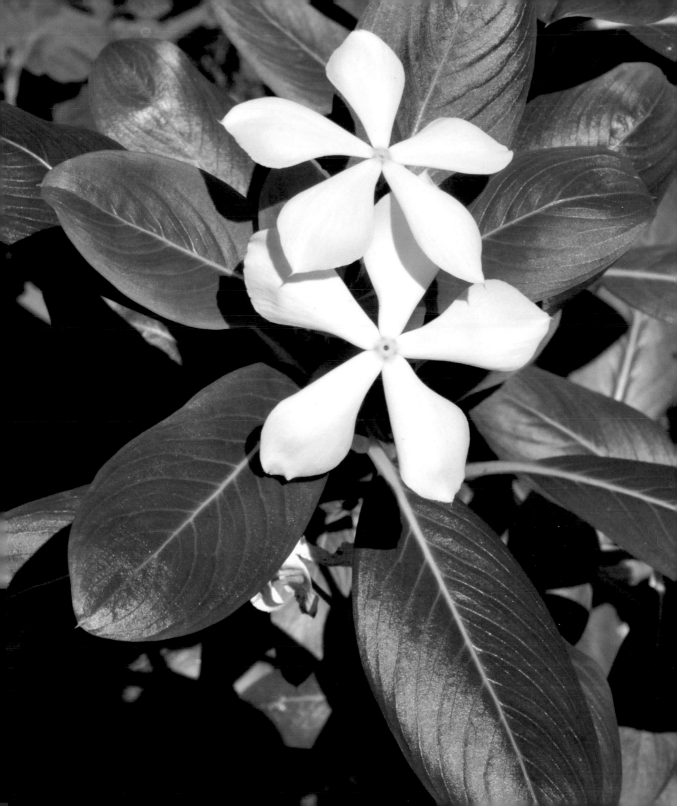

Dextromethorphan

Most readers will be familiar with DM. Even if they do not know DM's full name, they have undoubtedly seen these initials appended to the trade names of the numerous cough and cold products lining their pharmacy's shelves. Dextromethorphan or DM is an antitussive that reduces cough by blocking the cough center in the brain.

Scores of DM-containing products are available, alone or in combination with such ingredients as an expectorant that promotes the removal of mucus from the respiratory tract, a decongestant that relieves nasal congestion, a pain reliever and fever reducer, and even an antihistamine. Although widely used for decades to suppress coughs in adults and children, more recent studies have shown that DM is not only ineffective in children but also may be harmful.

DM emerged from a 1954 U.S. Navy– and Central Intelligence Agency–funded project that was intended to develop a "nonaddictive substitute for **codeine**." For well over a century, codeine had been widely used to reduce cough. While it was a highly effective antitussive, it suffered from a number of significant problems of particular military significance: it produced sedation and was subject to both misuse and abuse. In 1958, DM (Romilar) was introduced as a nonprescription, chemical second-cousin of codeine. Although it lacked pain-relieving properties, it causes less constipation and no physical dependence.

In an all-too-familiar story, much higher than recommended doses of DM produce mind-altering effects, described as occurring in dose-related "plateaus." These include an intense euphoria, an excessively vivid imagination, and hallucinations. At still higher doses, users encounter very unpleasant alterations in consciousness and out-of-body experiences. These effects—referred to as dissociative general anesthesia—have been likened to those produced by ketamine and **phencyclidine** (PCP). Notwithstanding the problems associated with its recreational use, few restrictions have been placed on the sale of DM-containing nonprescription products.

SEE ALSO Codeine (1832), Phencyclidine (1967).

Dextromethorphan (DM) is a common ingredient in cough and cold products. This photograph, taken in 1894, is an Edison kinetoscopic record of Fred Ott's sneeze in progress.

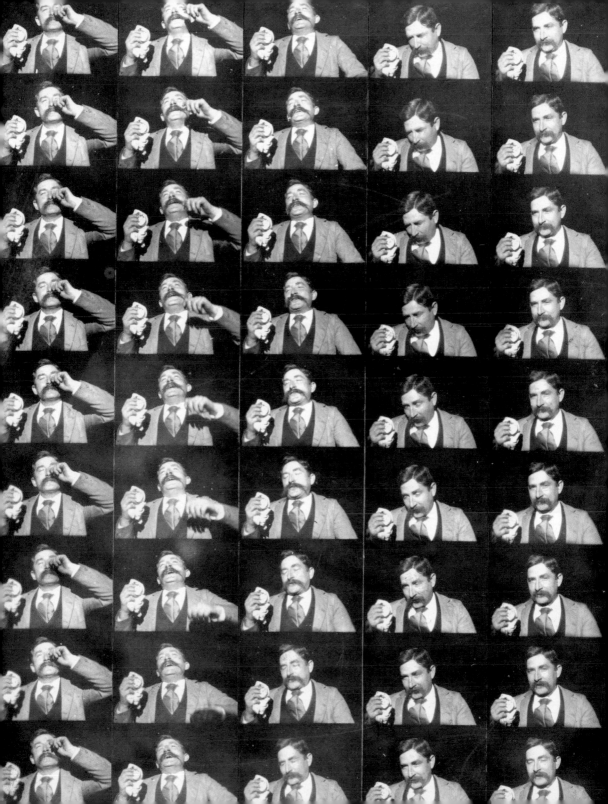

Flagyl

Flagyl was initially developed to treat parasitic infections but was later found to be effective in combating bacteria. It is one of those rare drugs that is a very affordable, available worldwide, and capable of curing a very common sexually transmitted infection (STI) and a diarrheal disease that afflict many in the developing world.

Trichomoniasis (trich) is among the most widespread STIs, with some 170–180 million new cases annually worldwide. Caused by the single-celled protozoan *Trichomonas vaginalis*, trich is associated with problems in pregnancy and infertility and may increase the risk of spreading HIV. While women often have uncomfortable symptoms affecting the vagina and urethra, men often don't show symptoms, so the condition frequently goes undetected and untreated. Flagyl (metronidazole) produces cure rates of approximately 95 percent in men and women often after a single dose.

Giardiasis is the most common intestinal disease caused by a parasite, and some 20 percent of the world's population may be chronically infected. One of the causes of "traveler's diarrhea" that develops where there is inadequate sanitation or safe drinking water, it is also acquired from food that has been contaminated by feces harboring the parasite and in day-care centers. Flagyl eradicates giardiasis in more than 85 percent of cases after five to ten days of treatment. It is also the most effective drug for treating amebic infections of the intestinal tract (amebic dysentery) and liver.

Half the world is infected with *Helicobacter pylori*, most commonly in regions where crowded, unsanitary conditions exist. Flagyl is an inexpensive component of a combination therapy used to cure most cases of peptic ulcers and chronic inflammation of the stomach (gastritis) caused by the bacterium.

Previously, medical authorities warned that alcoholic beverages should not be imbibed until three days after Flagyl is stopped in order to avoid the nausea, vomiting, headache, flushing, and galloping heartbeat thought to result from the interaction. While the combination is not advised, recent evidence has disproved this long-held belief.

SEE ALSO Prilosec (1989).

Giardia, a genus of flagellated protozoan parasites that causes giardiasis, is protected by an outer shell that permits its survival outside the body for long periods, even in the presence of chlorine disinfectant in water.

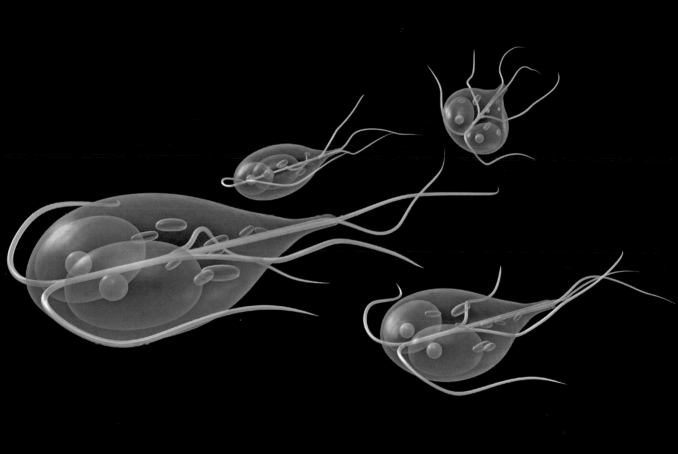

Librium

Leo Sternbach (1908–2005), Lowell Randall (b. 1910)

The discovery of Librium, the first benzodiazepine, is among the most fortuitous and profitable findings in the history of drug development, although it involves as many mistaken identities as a comic opera. In 1954, the Polish chemist Leo Sternbach, working at Hoffmann-La Roche in Nutley, New Jersey, was examining compounds he had prepared twenty years earlier while a PhD student at the University of Krakow. From them, he synthesized forty new compounds that were found to be biologically inactive. The fortieth compound, however, was chemically altered and put aside. Before pitching it in 1957 during a lab cleanup, by chance Sternbach decided to send it to Lowell Randall, Roche's Director of Pharmacology, for a battery of biological screening tests in mice and cats.

The results were startling. Like **phenobarbital** and **meprobamate**, the test compound had sedative, antiseizure, and better muscle-relaxing activity, but unlike these older drugs, the animals that received the injection remained calm and alert. With its specific "tranquilizing" effects that could not be attributed to mere sedation, relatively low toxicity, and few side effects, the newly discovered chlordiazepoxide was marketed for the treatment of anxiety in 1960 as Librium.

Librium's financial potential was obvious, and hundreds of benzodiazepines were synthesized. Several marketed derivatives include **Valium** (diazepam, the most successful), Ativan (lorazepam), Dalmane (flurazepam), Halcion (triazolam), Klonopin (clonazepam), Restoril (temazepam), **Rohypnol** (flunitrazepam), Serax (oxazepam), and **Xanax** (alprazolam). Benzodiazepines relieve anxiety, cause sedation to treat insomnia, attenuate muscle spasms, suppress seizures, and possibly interfere with the formation of new memories (anterograde amnesia). Small differences exist among the drugs in their effects, with the most variation in how long they continue to work.

The great acceptance of and reliance on the benzodiazepines by physicians and patients alike led to their use over extended periods for even trivial disorders. In such cases, dependence develops and discontinuation becomes difficult, as withdrawal effects can be very severe and include convulsions.

SEE ALSO Phenobarbital (1912), Meprobamate (1955), Valium (1963), Rohypnol (1975), Xanax (1981), BuSpar (1986).

Librium was the first drug to effectively relieve stress, anxiety, and tension with minimal sedation and very low mental and physical impairments. It also became the progenitor of dozens of benzodiazepine derivatives.

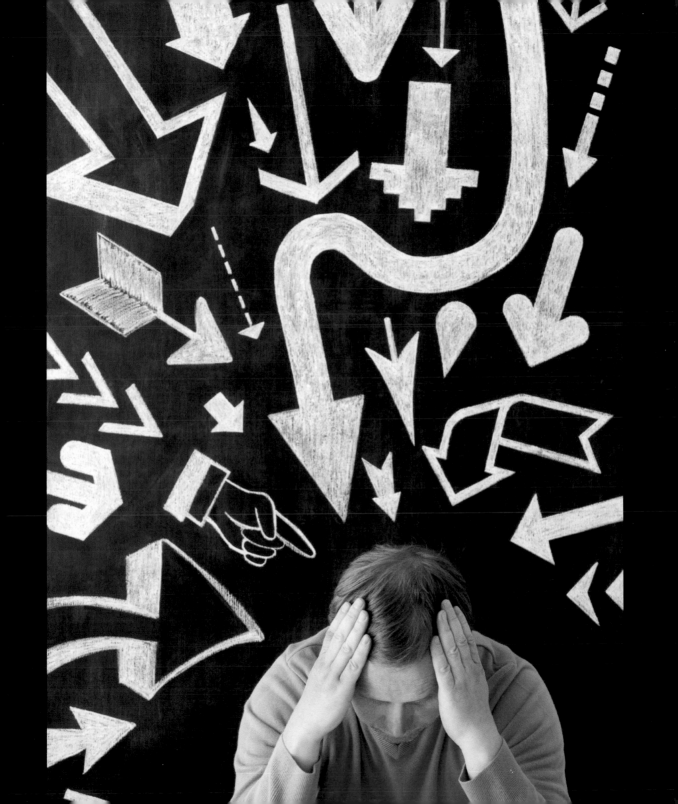

Enovid

Margaret Sanger (1879–1966), **John Rock** (1890–1984), **Gregory Pincus** (1903–1967)

MOTHER OF THE SEXUAL REVOLUTION. Although *The Drug Book* is replete with examples of drugs that have saved countless individuals, reduced pain and suffering, and improved the quality of our lives, Enovid arguably had the greatest impact on society. For the first time, in 1960, women had a safe, highly effective, reversible birth-control drug that could be used privately and independent of intercourse. As *Sex and the City* reveals, the Pill has enabled women to advance their educational, career, and financial objectives by determining if and when they become pregnant. Not surprisingly, the development and approval of Enovid, the first clinically available oral contraceptive, was confronted with legal and religious challenges.

The passage of the Comstock Laws in 1873 made the sale and use of any method of birth control illegal in many states for almost a century. Under the leadership of Margaret Sanger, a New York nurse and founder of the Planned Parenthood Federation of America, these laws were overturned in many states. She was also instrumental in securing private funding for the American biologist Gregory Pincus to pursue research on developing the Pill.

In 1951, Pincus showed that **progesterone** injections inhibited ovulation and, thus, prevented pregnancy in animals. Three years later, working with Harvard obstetrician and gynecologist John Rock, Pincus ran the first human clinical trial using an oral synthetic progesterone. None of the fifty women became pregnant, and the trials were expanded using Searle's Enovid. Because of anti-birth–control laws in Massachusetts and other states, the trials were conducted in Puerto Rico where, once again, the results were conclusively positive.

Enovid was approved in 1957 to treat menstrual disorders and in 1960 for contraceptive purposes. It left the market in 1988, with the vacuum amply filled by several dozen other oral contraceptive products, as well as hormonal contraceptive injections, implantable pellets, patches, and rings. Worldwide, some 100 million women use oral hormonal contraceptives, (of whom more than 10 million are in the United States). A 2012 study estimated that meeting contraceptive demands by women in developing counties could reduce maternal mortality worldwide by one-third.

SEE ALSO Estrone and Estrogen (1929), Progesterone and Progestin (1933), Mifepristone (1988), Plan B (1999).

Margaret Sanger, nurse and founder of the modern birth-control movement, opened the first birth-control clinic in the United States and in 1921 established what is now called Planned Parenthood Federation of America.

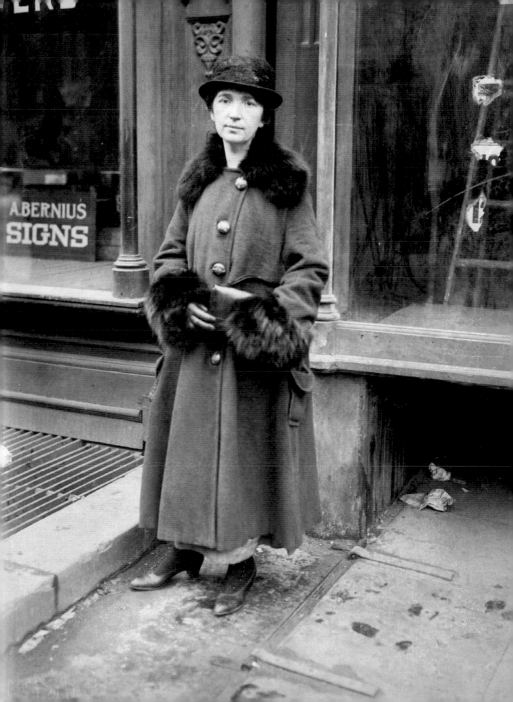

Ampicillin

Hans Christian Gram (1853–1938)

Bacteria are single-celled organisms surrounded by a protective cell wall. Faced with the challenge of visualizing bacteria under a microscope, in 1884 (one year after his graduation from medical school), Danish bacteriologist Hans Christian Gram devised a stain that has since been used to differentiate the two primary groups of bacteria. One group stains purple (Gram-positive), the other pink (Gram-negative). This difference is based on the chemical and physical properties of their cell walls, which in turn determines their sensitivity to different antibiotics.

The first **penicillin**, penicillin G, is active against most Gram-positive and many Gram-negative bacteria. This natural product, isolated from the *Penicillium* mold, kills bacteria by interfering with their ability to manufacture cell walls, which are essential for their survival. Penicillin is an unusual drug because, apart from allergic reactions (which affect one in ten of us), it produces very few toxic effects.

PENICILLIN BY MOUTH. Penicillin G is by no means perfect, however. When taken orally, it is inactivated by acids in the stomach and, therefore, can only be given by injection. By modifying its chemistry, in 1961 scientists at Beecham Laboratories in England produced ampicillin, one of the first penicillin derivatives able to withstand attack by these acids. In addition, ampicillin proved effective treating infections caused by a wider range of Gram-negative microbes than penicillin G, including many very common urinary-tract infections.

Notwithstanding ampicillin's amazing success in the marketplace—where it has been sold as Penbritin, Omnipen, Polycillin, and Principen—it has one major shortcoming that it shared with many other penicillins. Ampicillin is susceptible to breakdown by penicillinase, an enzyme produced by some bacteria. Penicillinase is responsible for the resistance of these bacteria to many penicillins. To overcome this problem, ampicillin and its first cousin amoxicillin (Amoxil) have been packaged in combination with drugs (e.g., Augmentin) that can inactivate penicillinase.

The penicillins are the oldest group of antibiotics, but, with continual facelifts, they are looking as young as ever.

SEE ALSO Penicillin (1928), Tetracyclines (1948).

The Gram stain is used to stain and differentiate bacteria. The Gram-positive Bacillus cereus *appears violet, while the Gram-negative* Escherichia coli *appear in small pink clusters in the background.*

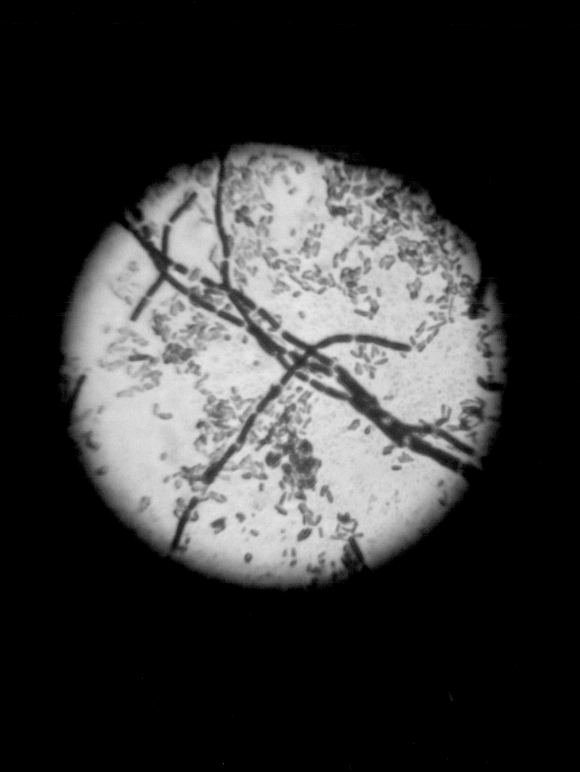

Hexachlorophene

During the 1960s, hexachlorophene was among the most widely used antibacterial antiseptics available to the consumer without a prescription. The ubiquitous use of this wildly successful drug abruptly ended in 1972, when a manufacturing error led to the death of several dozen infants.

Hexachlorophene first appeared in the early 1940s, used as a preservative in cosmetics at low concentrations (0.1 percent). In 1961, it reappeared in much higher concentrations (1–3 percent) in cleansing products (pHisoHex) used for babies and in hospitals and operating rooms to protect patients and healthcare workers against staphylococcus infections. Soon after, it was included in literally hundreds of nonprescription cosmetic and medicinal products, including antibacterial soaps (most notably, Dial deodorant soap) and gels, baby powders and lotions, shampoos, toothpastes, shaving creams, anti-acne products, and even vaginal and underarm deodorants.

Although hexachlorophene was clearly effective in reducing the population of disease-causing Gram-positive bacteria, many extravagant claims, unsubstantiated by fact, were made about its benefits. The high degree of effectiveness of hexachlorophene against Gram-positive microbes after repeated applications, and its ineffectiveness against their Gram-negative competitors, led to a disruption in the normal bacterial balance on the skin. Overgrowth of Gram-negative bacteria and difficult-to-treat infections resulted.

Late in the 1960s, hexachlorophene was found to be absorbed across injured skin—a finding later extended to the skin of premature infants—causing nervous system toxicity. In 1972, several dozen infants in France between one and fifteen months of age showed signs of twitching and seizures and died after being treated with talcum powder containing hexachlorophene. The powder was supposed to contain 3 percent of the drug, but because of an innocent manufacturing error, it contained twice this concentration. Abnormalities in the brains of these children were seen on autopsy.

Hexachlorophene was withdrawn from use in maternity wards, and outbreaks of staph infections rapidly ensued. Nevertheless, regulatory officials in many countries have imposed restrictions on its use, including requiring a prescription for purchase.

SEE ALSO Phenol (1867), Ampicillin (1961).

For decades, hexachlorophene was used in nurseries and homes to clean and powder newborns. After it was removed from the market because of nervous system toxicity, outbreaks of staph infections have ensued.

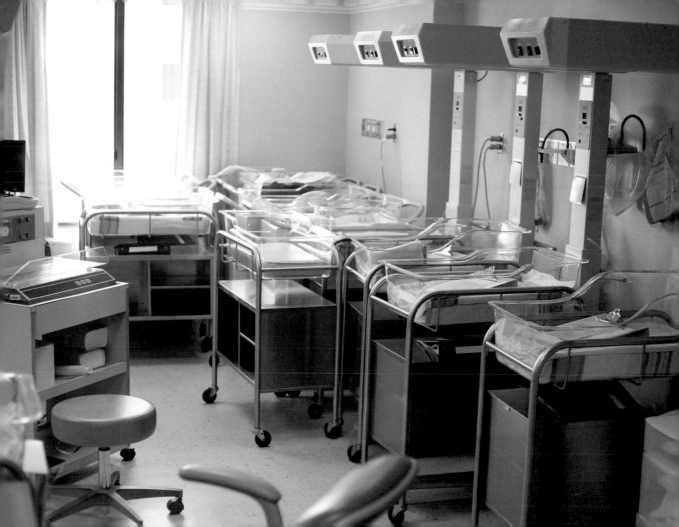

Monoamine Oxidase Inhibitors

During the 1950s, two chemicals that attracted keen interest in understanding normal and abnormal behavior were serotonin and norepinephrine. These neurotransmitters permit nerves to communicate with one another and play a role in regulating our mood. Monoamine oxidase inhibitors (MAOIs) inhibit the action of monoamine oxidase (MAO), an enzyme that breaks down these monoamine neurotransmitters, thereby increasing the brain levels of these neurotransmitters—a process thought to be responsible for their ability to relieve depression.

Iproniazid, the first marketed antidepressant, was toxic to the liver and withdrawn from the market. Appearing several years later, in 1961, the safer MAOIs phenelzine (Nardil) and tranylcypromine (Parnate) are not liver toxic and are still used today. While effective for severe depression, these drugs may cause a sharp drop in blood pressure when the patient suddenly stands (orthostatic hypotension), leading to light-headedness or fainting. More interesting and troubling problems arise when they are taken with other drugs or foods—problems that led to the temporary recall of Parnate in 1964.

Since many of us take more than one drug, awareness of interactions between different drugs is essential. Sometimes one drug increases the effects of another, potentially causing toxicity, while other drugs may reduce or cancel out a second drug's effects. MAOIs inhibit not only MAO, but also other drugs that are broken down by MAO. The consequences can be fatal.

Far more unusual are drug-food interactions, and here MAOIs are the poster child. Tyramine is a naturally occurring chemical found in generous concentrations in beers and wines (particularly Chianti), fava beans, aged cheeses, beef and chicken liver, pickled and smoked fish and meats, and other delicacies. Normally, these foods present no problems because MAO keeps tyramine levels in check by rapidly breaking it down. When taking an MAOI, however, tyramine levels increase, which can cause blood pressure to rise high enough to cause a stroke! Moreover, the risk of drug and food interactions can persist for up to two weeks after the last MAOI dose is taken.

The MAOIs are now used as backup drugs when patients with severe depression fail to respond to simpler and safer **Tofranil**-like and **Prozac**-like drugs.

SEE ALSO Neurotransmitters (1920), Iproniazid (1952), Tofranil and Elavil (1957), Prozac (1987).

Although rarely used today, the MAOIs are about as effective as newer drugs in alleviating depression, but their clinical usefulness as medicines is limited by a wide array of problematic drug-drug and drug-food interactions. Their use is especially troublesome in conjunction with red wines or aged cheeses, both of which contain high concentrations of tyramine.

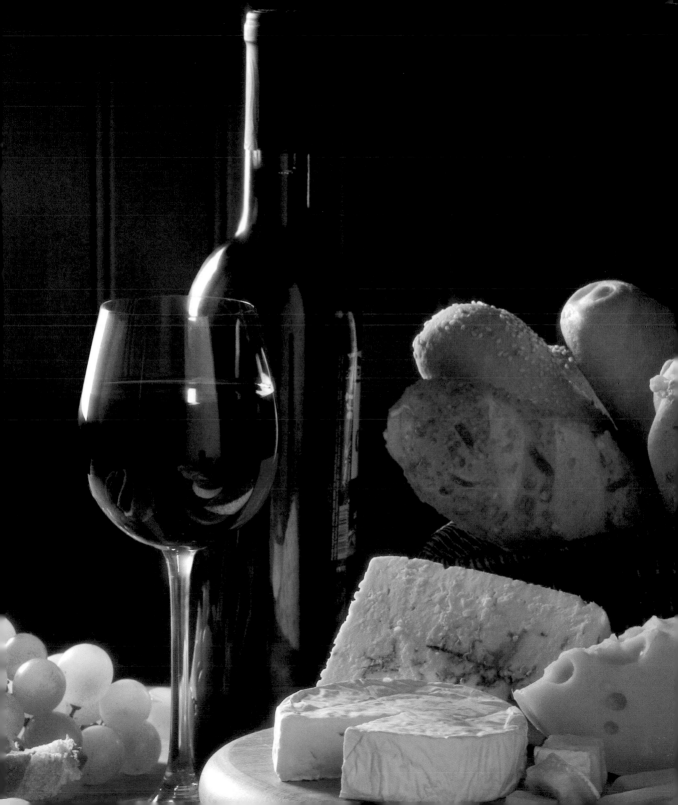

Kefauver-Harris Amendment

Estes Kefauver (1903–1963), **Oren Harris** (1903–1997)

As the dust began to settle on the **thalidomide** tragedy, in which more than 10,000 children were born with major birth defects, national attention was focused on drugs. Although far from perfect, legislation in 1906 established that drugs be free from misbranding and alteration and, in 1938, mandated that drugs be proven to be safe before being marketed. Safe, maybe . . . but there was no requirement that they be effective.

In 1962, hearings in the U.S. Senate chaired by two-time presidential contender Estes Kefauver (D-TN) and in the House of Representatives by Oren Harris (D-AK) led to an amendment to the **Federal Food, Drug, and Cosmetic Act** of 1938. Kefauver-Harris required that every drug be demonstrated safe *and* effective for all claims made, with effectiveness demonstrated in carefully controlled studies. (The FDA has no authority to require evidence of safety or effectiveness of **dietary supplements** before their marketing.)

Beginning in 1966, the **Food and Drug Administration** (FDA) reviewed the 4,500 prescription and 512 nonprescription drugs marketed between 1938 and 1962. By 1984, of 3,443 drug products evaluated, 1,051 (30.5 percent) were found to be ineffective and removed from the market. Since the passage of the amendment, the FDA has been engaged in a delicate balancing act of ensuring that approved drugs are safe and effective without unduly delaying the marketing of important drugs. While new drugs were being approved in Europe, a "drug lag" was said to exist in the United States, allegedly resulting from the FDA imposing unreasonable roadblocks before approval. This issue intensified in the late 1980s, when AIDS activists demonstrated at the FDA headquarters, seeking approval of **AZT**. This drug received "fast track" approval, within twenty-four months of its discovery.

Although the FDA's approval process has been markedly expedited, tension continues between the FDA's conservative approach and the push for rapid approval by the pharmaceutical industry and its allied disease activists.

SEE ALSO Clinical Testing of Drugs (1753), Pure Food and Drug Act (1906), Food and Drug Administration (1906), Federal Food, Drug, and Cosmetic Act (1938), Placebos (1955), Thalidomide (1957), AZT/Retrovir (1987), Dietary Supplements (1994).

AIDS activists pressured the FDA to grant accelerated approval for anti-AIDS drugs and protested congressional budget cuts in HIV/AIDS prevention-and-care programs. Using a collage with horror-inspiring images, this poster seeks to promote AIDS awareness and prevent AIDS transmission.

AIDS EDUCATION CAN

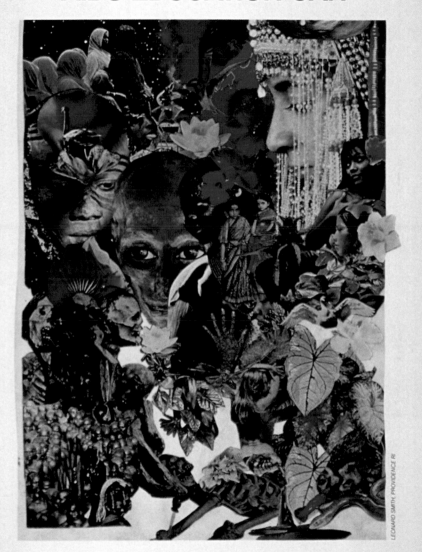

LEONARD SMITH, PROVIDENCE RI

PREVENT THE HORROR

Minority AIDS Prevention Program

John Hope Settlement House
7 Burgess Street, Providence, RI 02903
For further information call: 421-6993

"The Pulse of the Neighborhood"

Funded by RI Department of Health

Off-Label Drug Use

When receiving a doctor's prescription, you can assume that the drug has been approved for use by a federal regulatory agency (e.g., **Food and Drug Administration**). This approval process includes providing evidence that the drug is safe and effective for specified medical uses. But can you assume that your doctor is using this medicine for one of the approved uses?

OLD DRUGS, NEW USES. Once approved for *any* medical indication, a drug can be prescribed by licensed doctors in the United States and the United Kingdom for *any* purpose they professionally believe to be safe and effective. Off-label prescribing is the use of a drug for a non-approved use, and one in five of all prescribed drugs is off-label. This figure is far higher in pediatrics and for psychiatric, antiseizure, and cancer medications.

Advocates for off-label drug use argue that the approval process can take a decade, during which time patients do not benefit from a drug that has the potential for saving lives. The cost of bringing a new drug to market is said to approach $1 billion, and approval of a new use for an already approved drug can cost hundreds of millions of dollars. Why would a drug sponsor (pharmaceutical manufacturer) expend such funds to convince the FDA that an older generic drug is effective for a new condition when it's being already prescribed? Why invest in orphan drugs that are intended for conditions in a very small fraction of the population, when the costs of testing might never be recouped by sales?

Although off-label prescribing is legal and recognized by the FDA, it is illegal for a pharmaceutical manufacturer to actively promote a drug for an off-label use. Companies found to have done so have been fined many hundreds of millions of dollars—usually far less than the profits made from such sales.

Off-label prescribing raises a number of ethical questions: Should doctors inform patients that their prescribed drug is not FDA-approved for that use? In the absence of evidence that the drug is safe and effective for a condition, is the prescriber experimenting on patients? Should patients be offered the opportunity to consent to an off-label use?

SEE ALSO Clinical Testing of Drugs (1753), Food and Drug Administration (1906), Federal Food, Drug, and Cosmetic Act (1938), Kefauver-Harris Amendment (1962).

This doctor may be prescribing an FDA-approved medicine for an off-label use—that is, for a medical condition for which the drug has not been evaluated to be safe or effective by the FDA.

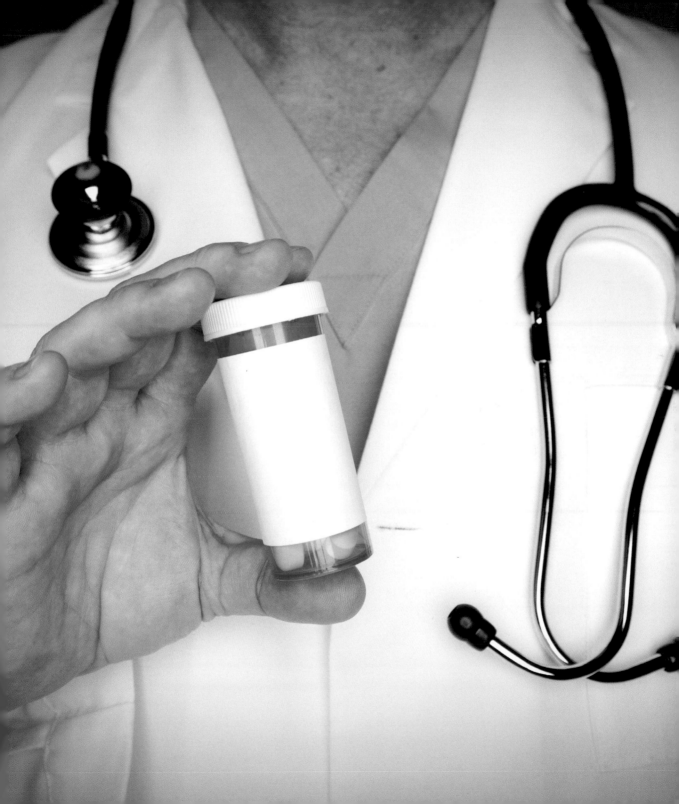

Valium

As an antianxiety drug, **Librium** was a great success. Three year later, in 1963, Valium appeared on the market. Not only the leading hitter in the benzodiazepine lineup, this drug also became one of the best selling of all pharmaceuticals ever! Valium (diazepam) extended its therapeutic uses beyond anxiety to insomnia, muscle spasms, acute alcohol withdrawal, and preoperative sedation, and, via injection, to control status epilepticus, a life-threatening condition in which seizures persist without letup for more than thirty minutes. For many of these conditions, it represented the first or second drug of choice.

The appearance of Valium and related benzodiazepines spelled the end of the decades-long reign of **phenobarbital** and its barbiturate cousins. In contrast to the barbiturates, Valium caused less drowsiness at normal therapeutic doses, thereby not impairing mental or physical function. More significantly, Valium has a wide interval between a safe therapeutic dose and the toxic consequences resulting from overdose.

However, even safe drugs have limits. When taken in overdose—in sharp contrast to the barbiturates—the benzodiazepines very rarely cause death, *except* when taken in combination with large amounts of alcohol or other depressants. This was sadly the case for Heath Ledger (1979–2008), who played leading roles in the films *Brokeback Mountain* (2005) and *The Dark Knight* (2008). His death, just months before the release of the latter film, was ruled an accidental overdose caused by a lethal combination of several narcotics and benzodiazepines, including Valium and an antihistamine.

The relative safety of Valium led to a false sense of security that it could be used without risk. Not surprisingly, when doses escalated over extended periods, dependence developed. However, we now know that when Valium and related drugs are used at the *normal* doses for a period of more than six weeks, dependence still develops. If the drug is abruptly withdrawn or the dosage precipitously reduced, such withdrawal symptoms as extreme anxiety and panic attacks may occur. These generally appear within 24–48 hours of the last dose and may persist, with reduced intensity, for up to a year. So-called benzodiazepine withdrawal syndrome is particularly intense for users quitting **Xanax**.

SEE ALSO Phenobarbital (1912), Nembutal and Seconal (1928), Librium (1960), Xanax (1981), BuSpar (1986).

This sign in a Mandeville, Louisiana, restaurant summarizes the way many individuals cope with demands for both energy and calm in their personal and professional lives.

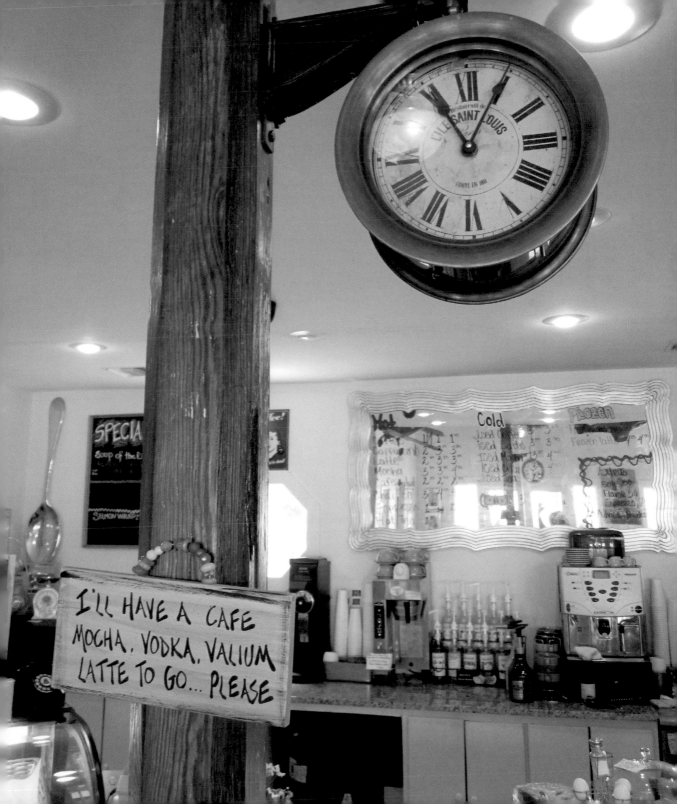

Gentamicin

Streptomycin was the forebear of the aminoglycoside family of antibiotics, and gentamicin (Garamycin) is one of its illustrious descendents, preferred because of its effectiveness and low cost. Injected for the treatment of very serious infections—most commonly caused by Gram-negative bacteria—the medical uses and unusual adverse effects of aminoglycosides are similar. There is a relatively thin margin between doses that effectively kill bacteria and those that cause major toxicity, so the dose must be carefully calibrated.

In addition to causing kidney toxicity, aminoglycosides can cause inner ear damage. The inner ear plays a critical role in hearing and in maintaining balance. The aminoglycosides cause ototoxicity by killing inner ear hair cells that play a critical role in these sensory functions. Of the six aminoglycosides, some preferentially affect hearing, while others disrupt balance.

Hearing involves the transduction or conversion of sound waves into electrical signals that travel to the brain. This auditory conversion takes place at sensory hair cells. Dead hair cells are incapable of regenerating, and hearing loss caused by aminoglycosides is permanent. The extent of this loss depends upon the number of hair cells killed and may affect up to 25 percent of patients taking these drugs. Aminoglycosides initially impair high-frequency sounds, progressing to the lower frequencies, but profound deafness can occur after a single injected dose.

Aspirin and cisplatin also commonly cause hearing deficits. High doses of aspirin can cause temporary hearing impairment and tinnitus, a ringing in the ears, but problems disappear when the dose is reduced. By contrast, the anticancer drug cisplatin can cause permanent hearing loss in between 30 and 100 percent of patients receiving high doses.

The vestibular organ hair cells of the inner ear maintain balance by detecting the rotations and movements of the head. Unlike auditory hair cells, the vestibular variety can partially recover after aminoglycoside damage.

SEE ALSO Aspirin (1899), Streptomycin (1944), Ampicillin (1961).

This anatomical drawing of the inner ear is from Bourgery & Jacob's Traité de l'Anatomie Humaine (1862). Gentamicin's effects on the inner ear can cause problems in hearing and balance.

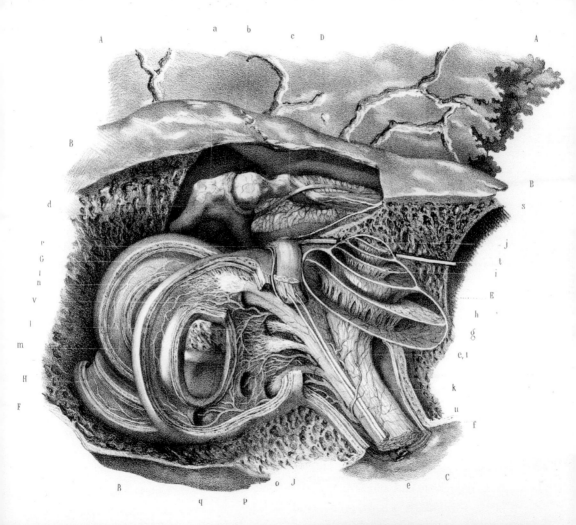

Propranolol

Raymond P. Ahlquist (1914–1983), James W. Black (1924–2010)

Propranolol ranks with the greatest discoveries in twentieth-century medicine and is the most important heart drug developed since the discovery of **digitalis** almost 200 years earlier. It was originally developed to relieve the chest pain of angina pectoris but was soon being used for the treatment of heart-rhythm abnormalities, heart attacks, and high blood pressure, in addition to migraine headaches and anxiety.

Raymond Ahlquist, professor of pharmacology at the Medical College of Georgia, planted the seeds of propranol's discovery in a 1948 publication. Armed with experimental evidence, he postulated that drugs such as **epinephrine/adrenaline** acted on two related receptor types, which he designated alpha- and beta-adrenergic receptors. The impact of this concept on the biomedical world was a resounding thud until Ahlquist was given the opportunity to write a chapter in a 1954 textbook of pharmacology.

In 1958, Scottish physician-pharmacologist James Black, working at ICI Pharmaceuticals (now AstraZeneca), read Ahlquist's chapter with keen interest. Black theorized that adrenaline stimulated the beta-adrenergic receptor, leading to an increase in heart rate, which in turn boosted the heart's requirements for oxygen in excess of the available supply and provoked an anginal attack. If this were the case, slowing the heart rate by blocking the beta-adrenergic receptor could treat angina.

Black's propranolol (Inderal) rapidly became the world's best-selling drug, until it was replaced by cimetedine (**Tagamet**), another Black-developed pharmaceutical. Both discoveries contributed to his 1988 Nobel Prize in Physiology or Medicine. Black (a laboratory physician) is said to have relieved more human suffering than thousands of practicing physicians could have while attending their patients for a lifetime.

Propranolol was the first beta-blocker, a class of drugs that now numbers around twenty. Many of these are preferred to propranolol because of their more specific effects on the heart. Because they reduce heart rate and tremors and relieve anxiety, beta-blockers are sometimes used by entertainers and musicians before performances and auditions to curb stage fright.

SEE ALSO Digitalis (1775), Digitoxin (1875), Nitroglycerin (1879), Epinephrine/Adrenaline (1901), Drug Receptors (1905), Quinidine (1912), Neurotransmitters (1920), Tagamet (1976).

For the past half-century, propranolol and its beta-blocker progeny have been associated with the heart and its disorders.

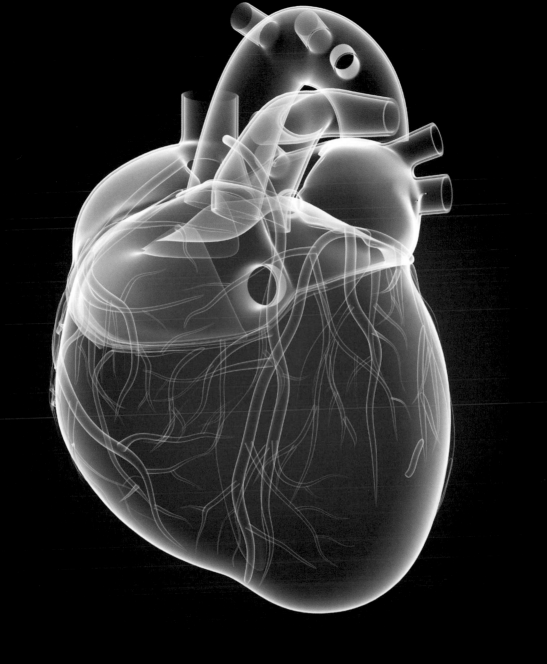

Cephalothin

Giuseppe Brotzu (1895–1976), **Howard Florey** (1898–1968), **Edward Abraham** (1913–1999), **Guy Newton** (1919–1969)

Giuseppe Brotzu, professor of hygiene at the University of Cagliari in Italy, had many accomplishments. The most noteworthy of these were his work with the Rockefeller Foundation and his use of **DDT** to eliminate malaria from the island of Sardinia. But it is his discovery of the cephalosporins, among the most widely used antibiotics, that interests us here.

Typhoid fever is a disease spread by bacterial contamination of water supplies and inadequate treatment of sewage. Contaminated water was an endemic problem in Sardinia, and yet individuals bathing in it or eating shellfish from the sea in the vicinity of a sewage outlet seemed unaffected. This observation led Brotzu to speculate that a mold in the sewage might be producing a substance that killed the typhoid-causing bacteria. He sampled the water, isolated a mold, and found that it prevented the growth of many bacteria in both petri dishes and patients—findings he published in 1948.

FROM SEWERS TO THE CLINIC. Samples of the mold were sent to Howard Florey, professor of pathology at Oxford, who in 1945 shared the Nobel Prize in Physiology or Medicine with Alexander Fleming for his work leading to the introduction of **penicillin** into medical practice. Over the next dozen years, Florey's colleagues Edward Abraham and Guy Newton worked to isolate and identify the chemistry of the active antibiotic, cephalosporin C.

In 1964, Eli Lilly marketed cephalothin (Keflin), the first of some twenty cephalosporins that bear the revealing prefix cef-. To differentiate them, they are commonly grouped into four "generations." The classification, while not perfect, is based on their relative activity against Gram-positive and Gram-negative bacteria. The cephalosporins act in a manner similar to penicillin and are often used to combat the same types of microbes, but they can be used in many patients who are allergic to penicillin.

Cephalosporins—often used in agriculture to treat infections in cattle and other animals—are injected into the eggs of broiler chickens. The **Food and Drug Administration** has expressed concern that such uses pose a threat to humans by contributing to the development of bacterial infections that are resistant to antibiotic treatment.

SEE ALSO Food and Drug Administration (1906), Penicillin (1928), DDT (1939), Ampicillin (1961).

Mold found in a sewage system like this one was the source of cephalosporins, one of the world's most widely used classes of antibiotics.

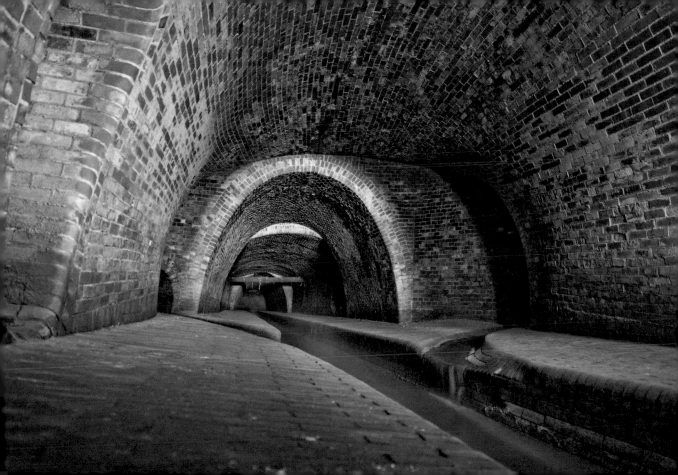

Lasix

Lasix and related "loop diuretics," are the most powerful and effective diuretics (water pills) available, and can be lifesaving drugs in the treatment of heart failure. There is a direct connection between heart function and fluids in the body. When the heart fails, it cannot adequately pump blood throughout the body. Two critical organs affected by this paucity of blood flow are the kidneys and the lungs.

Among the kidneys' main functions are filtering the blood of waste materials and maintaining its volume and contents. When the heart begins to fail, less blood is filtered, and the output of urine decreases. Fluid builds up in the body, causing swelling (edema) in the lower limbs and abdomen, and fluid collects in the lungs. Fluid in the lungs interferes with the oxygen supply to the tissues, leading to shortness of breath — first during periods of exercise and later at rest. This life-threatening emergency is called pulmonary edema.

Lasix (furosemide or frusemide) can produce rapid and massive fluid and salt loss from the body in the form of urine, thereby greatly decreasing the load imposed on the heart by reducing the amount of fluid it must pump. Lasix is also used in other conditions involving edema, including disorders of the liver and kidneys and in the treatment of high blood pressure (hypertension) that does not benefit from milder diuretics, such as **Diuril** and other thiazides.

Lasix is referred to as a *loop diuretic* because it acts at a segment of the kidney called the loop of Henle. Here, a substantial amount of salt is normally returned to the blood. By blocking this reabsorption, Lasix allows salt and water to remain in the kidney tubules and be excreted as urine. However, if too much salt is lost from the body, dehydration and serious electrolyte imbalances can result.

SEE ALSO Merbaphen (1920), Diuril (1958).

Urine formation and the conservation of water and salt are two of the most important kidney functions. As urine flows through the loop of Henle (depicted here), water, sodium, and chloride ions are reabsorbed into the blood and retained in the body. The remaining urine becomes increasingly concentrated (hypertonic) with waste materials, such as urea, which are eliminated from the body.

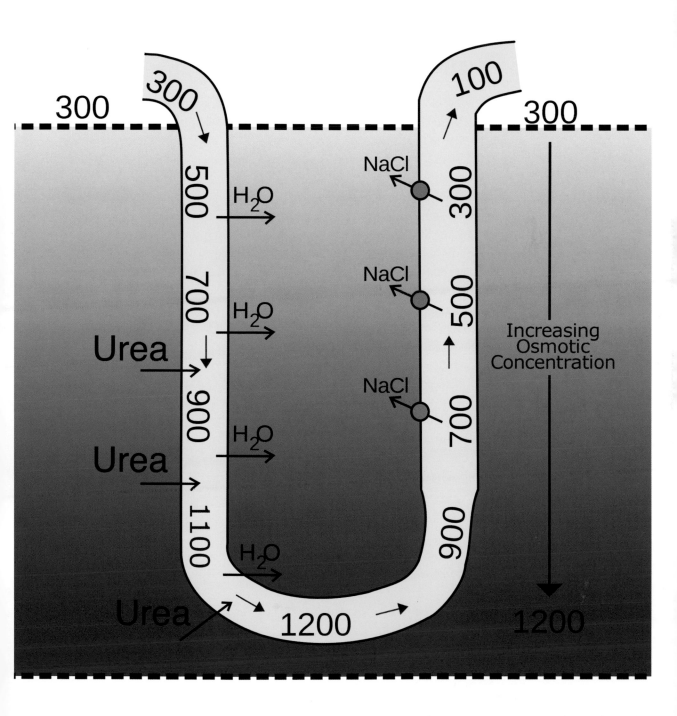

Zyloprim

George H. Hitchings (1905–1998), Gertrude B. Elion (1918–1999)

During the 1950s and 1960s, future Nobel laureates George Hitchings and Gertrude Elion were testing hundreds of chemicals at Burroughs Wellcome Laboratory, looking for a better way to treat chronic leukemia in children. In 1953, their **mercaptopurine** (Purinethol) was among the first drugs found to be clinically useful for the treatment of this cancer.

Mercaptopurine is broken down and inactivated by the enzyme xanthine oxidase, and Hitchings and Elion sought to improve the effectiveness of their anticancer drug by blocking this enzyme. Allopurinol (Zyloprim) did just that. In spite of this, mercaptopurine's antileukemic effects were not enhanced.

Hitchings and Elion did note, however, that allopurinol's ability to block xanthine oxidase reduced uric acid levels, which are normally elevated in the blood of patients treated with mercaptopurine. When excessive levels of uric acid deposit into the joints of predisposed individuals, gouty attacks occur. Hitchings and Elion's research direction took a sharp detour, and they began investigating allopurinol for its uric-acid–lowering effects. In 1966, it was marketed as Zyloprim, the most effective drug for the treatment of gout. Almost one-half century later, it remains the drug of choice for the long-term management of this metabolic disorder and is taken on an ongoing basis by predisposed patients.

Although it helps prevent gouty attacks, Zyloprim does not provide relief in the event of an acute attack. However, it can also prevent the formation of urate kidney stones in patients with leukemias and other cancers, particularly when they are being treated with anticancer drugs or radiation therapy.

SEE ALSO Colchicine (c. 70), Benemid (1951), Mercaptopurine (1953).

The U.S. Mint issued Benjamin Franklin $100 bills beginning in 1928 to celebrate one of America's greatest statesmen. Zyloprim treats gout — a condition Franklin suffered — by reducing urate levels in the body.

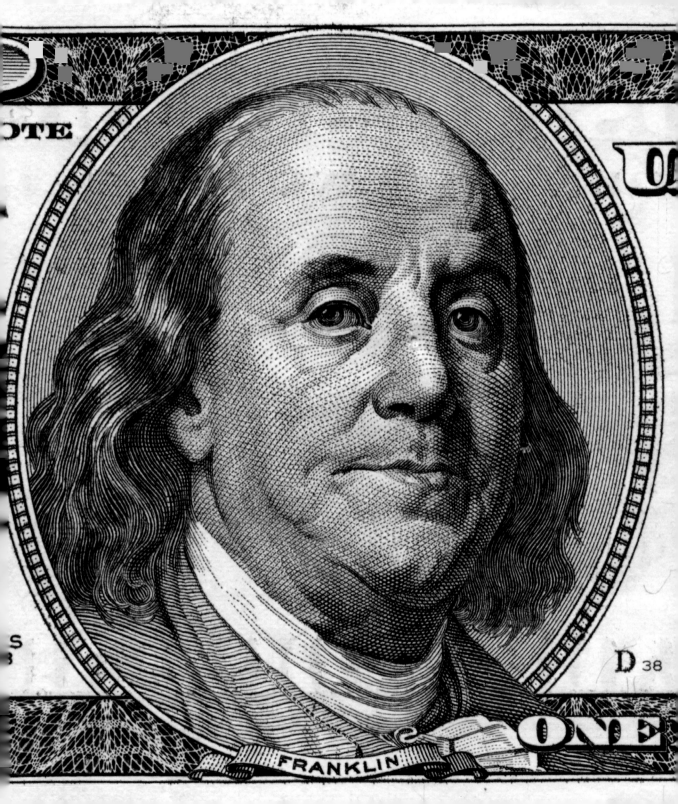

Rifampin

Piero Sensi (b. 1920)

During a 1957 screening program for Dow-Lepetit Research Laboratories of Milan, Piero Sensi isolated a series of chemicals with antibacterial activity from a pine forest near Nice, France. He designated these compounds rifamycins, based on the English title of the highly acclaimed 1955 French jewelry-shop-heist film noir *Rififi* (originally titled *Du rififi chez les hommes*), which he loved.

The most promising of the rifamycins was designated rifampin in the United States and rifampicin internationally. A structurally complex semisynthetic derivative of naturally occurring rifamycin, it is classified as a broad-spectrum antibiotic. Among the wide range of bacteria against which rifampin is active are the slow-growing mycobacteria that cause tuberculosis (TB) and leprosy.

Tuberculosis has been in and out of the public health spotlight. For many centuries, particularly during the nineteenth, it was a major killer. With the introduction of new anti-TB drugs, including **streptomycin**, **isoniazid**, and rifampin, it appeared as though this old killer was vanquished, but resistant and more aggressive bacterial strains have emerged in recent decades. Once again, TB is considered a "global emergency."

Rifampin's primary therapeutic use is for the treatment of TB, for which it is one of the most effective drugs available. To slow the development of bacterial resistance, it is always used in combination with isoniazid. These drugs are given for six months for sensitive bacterial strains and for twelve to twenty-four months for resistant bacteria.

Rifampin is also the most effective drug available for the treatment of leprosy (Hansen's disease). In combination with other anti-leprosy drugs, such as **dapsone**, it is administered once monthly for three months. Use of rifampin frequently causes the urine, sweat, saliva, and tears to assume a harmless red-orange discoloration. Liver toxicity is the most serious adverse effect associated with its use.

SEE ALSO Dapsone (1937), Streptomycin (1944), Isoniazid (1951), Ampicillin (1961).

This ribbon representation is of pyrazinamidase, an enzyme present in the tuberculosis bacterium. Pyrazinamide and rifampin are used in combination to treat dormant TB. To work, pyrazinamide must be activated by pyrazinamidase.

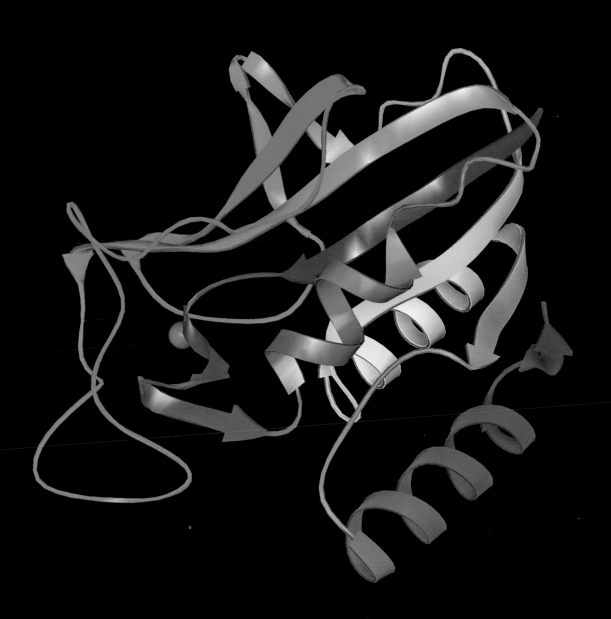

Clomid

Infertility is the inability to become pregnant after one year of unprotected sex. It is estimated to affect 8–10 percent of couples worldwide and approximately 15–20 percent in the United States, the United Kingdom, and France. The causes of infertility are many and may be caused by problems in either partner. Sperm defects in a man or fallopian tube defects in a woman are causative factors, but increasingly, advanced age is playing a role.

For a variety of reasons, including economic and career-related considerations, couples are waiting longer to have a child. A woman's chances of becoming pregnant decline significantly after age 35, as she is born with a finite number of eggs; the number decreases with age, along with the "quality" of the eggs (i.e., their ability to become fertilized). Ovulation, the release of the egg from the ovary, slows down and occurs less frequently with advancing age.

TURNING BACK THE BIOLOGICAL CLOCK. Clomid (serophene, clomiphene, or clomifene) is used for the treatment of infertility resulting from a failure of ovulation. It acts by increasing the release of gonadotropins from the pituitary gland, which leads to ovulation. At times, women treated with Clomid have multiple births—usually twins. The normal instance of multiple births is about 1 percent, but with Clomid, it ranges from 5–12 percent. Clomid is inexpensive, easy to take and to monitor, and most important, highly effective. After six to nine monthly cycles of taking Clomid, 80 percent of women ovulate and 70–75 percent become pregnant.

Far more controversial and problematic is the widespread and off-label use of Clomid to treat male infertility when the man is producing an inadequate number of sperm. While this drug increases testosterone levels and sperm counts, it has not been shown to increase the pregnancy rate. Because of its ability to increase testosterone levels, it has been banned as a performance-enhancing drug.

SEE ALSO Estrone and Estrogen (1929), Testosterone (1935).

From ancient times, societies across the globe offered sacrifices and supplicated to mythological fertility deities. This statue depicts a mother who has had a multiple-birth delivery, which is frequent among 5–12 percent of Clomid-treated women who become pregnant.

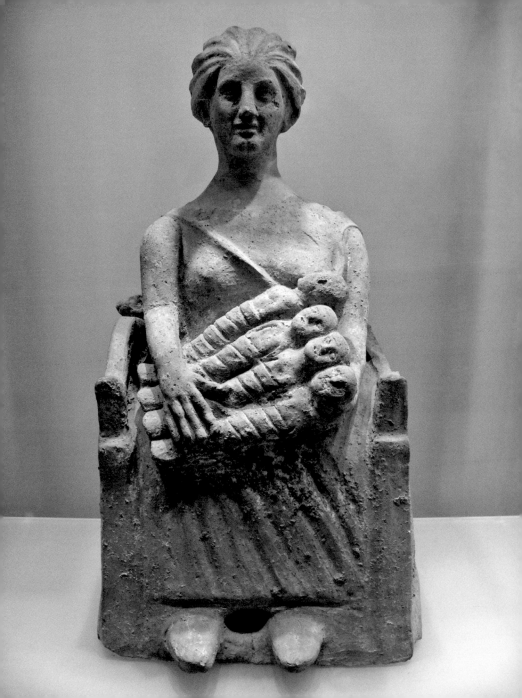

Valproic Acid

Not all significant drug discoveries arise from the application of theoretical principles, complex experimental designs and analyses, or years of animal and human testing. Valproic acid, a highly significant drug for the management of seizures and mood disorders, was discovered quite by chance.

During the course of doctoral research at the University of Lyon in France, graduate student Pierre Eymard needed a solvent for his newly synthesized chemicals in order to evaluate their potential antiepileptic effects. He selected valproic acid, which was synthesized in 1881. Rather unexpectedly, the compounds tested all had similar antiseizure effects in animals, thanks to the seemingly inactive solvent. Clinical trials were initiated in 1964, and the drug was approved for marketing as an antiepileptic drug in France in 1967, in the United Kingdom and other European countries in 1974, and in the United States in 1978.

Unlike other antiseizure drugs, valproic acid is effective against a wide range of seizure types in both children and adults. Although it works in ways that are not yet determined, because it causes minimal sedation and few serious side effects, it is often the first drug selected for these conditions. But its choice as a "go-to" drug does not suggest that the administration of valproic acid (Depakene, among other trade names) is without danger. In rare instances, its use has been associated with fatal liver toxicity—a risk that is greatly magnified in children under the age of two.

Valproic acid also effectively controls manic excitement in bipolar disorders and is used as a mood stabilizer to prevent recurring episodes of mania and depression. Additionally, it has been approved for the prevention of migraine headaches. Early studies published in 2010 suggest that valproic acid may be effective for the treatment of retinitis pigmentosa, a severe neurodegenerative disease of the retina that ultimately results in blindness.

SEE ALSO Phenobarbital (1912), Dilantin (1938), Lithium (1949).

Jacques-Louis David created this oil painting, Napoleon Crossing the Alps *(1800). Many medical experts believe Napoleon had psychogenic attacks brought on by stress and epileptic seizures due to chronic uremia associated with gonorrhea.*

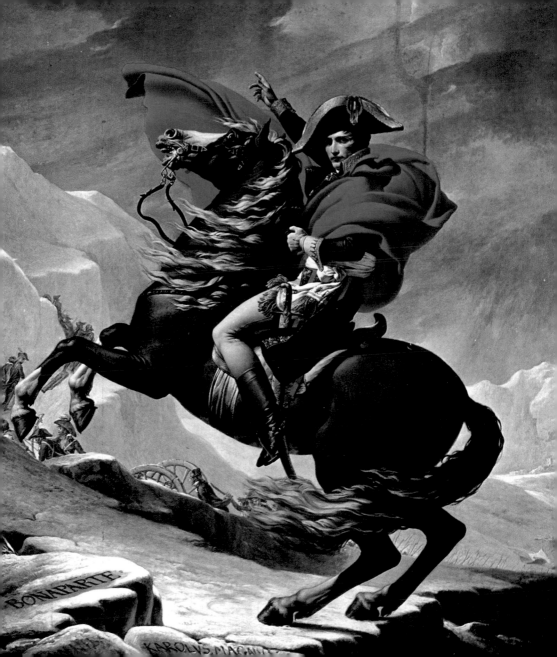

Phencyclidine

During the 1950s, Parke, Davis & Company was looking for an intravenously administered, short-acting anesthetic that would enable a patient to remain conscious yet pain free throughout an operative procedure. Phencyclidine (PCP), with the trade name Sernyl, initially looked promising for use in brief procedures: It appeared to be safe, and patients reported that they had no memory of what had transpired.

Some patients, however, upon recovering from anesthesia, became highly agitated, were severely confused, had hallucinations, and reported experiencing changes in the size of their body or body parts. Sernyl had little future as an anesthetic for human use, but in 1967 it was re-branded as Sernylan for veterinary use in monkeys and other primates, as well as to immobilize zoo animals; hence, its street name, "animal tranquilizer."

Starting in 1967 and throughout the 1970s, PCP used alone or in combination with marijuana (**cannabis**), made its appearance as "hog," "peace pill," and "angel dust" throughout the United States. It was inexpensive, readily available, and popular. PCP has been most commonly smoked, but can also be taken orally, snorted, or injected.

Low doses of PCP produce alcohol-like effects, and interest in its recreational use has reemerged in recent years. As the dose increases, changes in body image, hallucinations, extreme aggressiveness, and psychotic behavior resembling schizophrenia—effects that can persist for weeks—occur. Some users have attempted suicide. However, street reports that users have committed extreme acts of violence to themselves or others or that they have been endowed with PCP-induced superhuman strength have rarely been substantiated.

Very high doses of PCP can cause a coma that persists for seven to ten days, seizures, depressed breathing, marked elevations in body temperature, and a breakdown of muscle tissues. No specific antidotes exist to counteract PCP toxicity. Treatment involves supporting the patient, controlling the symptoms, and attempting to hasten the drug's removal from the body via the urine.

SEE ALSO Alcohol (c. 10,000 BCE), Cannabis (c. 3000 BCE), Mescaline (1897), LSD (1943).

When phencyclidine was being tested as a potential anesthetic, it produced very frightening nightmares, hallucinations, delusions, and delirium.

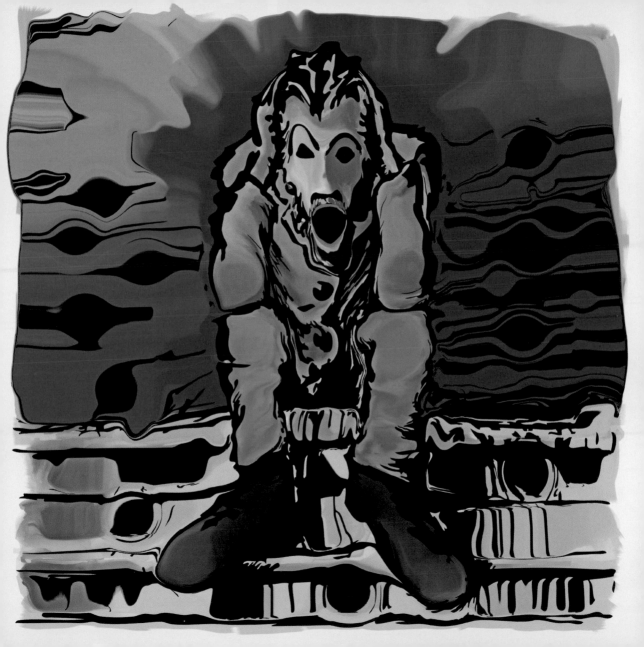

Levodopa

James Parkinson (1755–1813), **George Cotzias** (1918–1977), **Arvid Carlsson** (b. 1923), **Oleh Hornykiewicz** (b. 1926)

Parkinson's disease (PD) has been brought to the public's attention thanks largely to the efforts of actor Michael J. Fox, who has spearheaded major fundraising activities seeking a cure. Heavyweight champion Muhammad Ali, the "world's most famous Parkinson's patient" is the visible face of this neurological disorder. First described by British physician James Parkinson in 1817, its multiple symptoms include tremors when muscles are at rest, slowness of movements, and muscle rigidity. No drug can cure PD or slow its progression, but many drugs, most notably levodopa (L-DOPA), can produce dramatic improvements.

Levodopa is inextricably linked to dopamine, a natural biochemical first synthesized in 1910 and then put aside for more than four decades. In the 1950s, Arvid Carlsson at Lund University in Sweden found dopamine in the brain—in particular, in the basal ganglia, a region responsible for smoothing out muscle movements. In 1957 he proposed that dopamine was a neurotransmitter, and in 1959 speculated that it was associated with PD. The following year, Polish-born biochemist Oleh Hornykiewicz, at the University of Vienna, provided evidence that in patients with PD, muscle-controlling brain areas were markedly deficient in dopamine. Intuitively, the treatment of PD was simple: Why not simply administer dopamine to PD patients? Unfortunately, Hornykiewicz found that dopamine failed to enter the brain from the blood.

When dopamine is synthesized in the brain, its immediate precursor is levodopa, which enters the brain after being taken by mouth. This simple explanation belies the years of effort George Cotzias devoted to perfecting a suitable levodopa schedule of doses for PD at the Brookhaven National Laboratory, leading to the first successful trials of L-DOPA, published in 1968.

Levodopa is not the final answer to PD treatment. It initially benefits 80 percent of patients, but after five years its effectiveness becomes progressively diminished, with good responses rapidly alternating with no response (on-off phenomenon). Involuntary writhing movements and body spasms (dyskinesias) are common levodopa side effects, and these were memorably depicted in *Awakenings*, a 1990 film based on a 1973 memoir by the British neurologist Oliver Sacks.

SEE ALSO Scopolamine (1881), Neurotransmitters (1920).

A 1965 photograph of Spanish artist Salvador Dalí, with ocelot and cane, by Roger Higgins. In the early 1980s, Dalí (1904–1989) developed Parkinson's disease. Its debilitating effects caused him to abandon painting and contributed to his loss of joie de vivre.

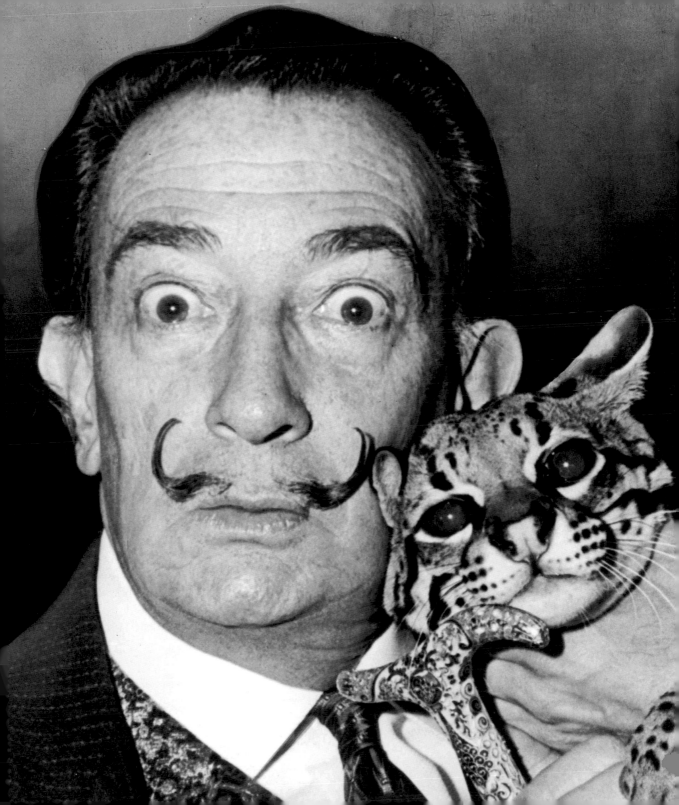

Albuterol/Salbutamol

Imagine that your breathing tubes, called bronchi, temporarily narrow or collapse, reducing the flow of air into your lungs. As a result, you experience wheezing, coughing, shortness of breath, and chest tightness. These are the symptoms of an asthmatic attack. Not only is such an attack frightening, it can also prove fatal—each year, globally, some 250,000 deaths result. Rates of asthma have been increasing since the 1960s to its current incidence of 300 million worldwide, with its highest prevalence seen in developed countries.

Experts have established guidelines for the treatment of asthma based on the frequency of such attacks and their severity. Bronchodilators are drugs that open the airways. Quick-relief or rescue medications, such as albuterol (United States)/ salbutamol (international), marketed as Ventolin, begin acting within minutes after inhalation and can be lifesaving by stopping an attack in progress, although effects wear off within three to six hours. Such drugs are also used to protect against shortness of breath and other symptoms brought on by exercise.

By contrast, drugs such as salmeterol (Serevent), which appeared in 1988, are intended to control asthma over the long term, preventing and reducing the frequency of symptoms. After being inhaled on a daily basis, these drugs open airways for up to twelve hours, working through the night and thus permitting undisturbed sleep. However, the considerable delay before these long-acting drugs begin to work—about twenty minutes—make them of little value when frantically gasping for air. Inhaled steroids, such as **Beclovent** (beclomethasone), also prevent symptoms but, because they cannot open airways, are not helpful in acute attacks.

Thanks to drugs such as albuterol, asthmatics can participate at the highest levels of athletic competition. Jackie Joyner-Kersee, who was first diagnosed with asthma at age eighteen, survived a near-fatal attack. Taking both long-acting and rapid-acting drugs, she was the winner of six gold medals in four consecutive Olympic games during the 1980s and 1990s, a world record holder in the woman's heptathlon, and *Sports Illustrated's* Female Athlete of the 20th Century.

SEE ALSO Theophylline (1888), Cortisone (1949), Beclovent (1976), Ephedra/Ephedrine (1994).

This illustration shows bronchial anatomy in detail. The bronchi lead to small sacs called alveoli. Within the alveoli, oxygen is obtained from inhaled air, and carbon dioxide is eliminated via exhaled air.

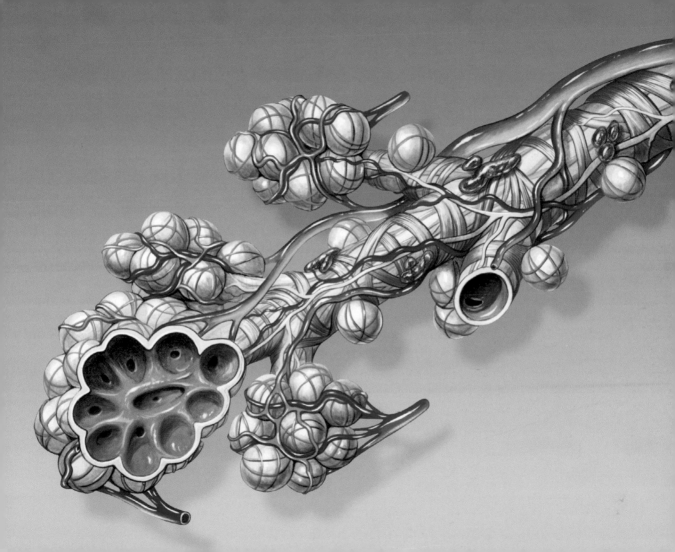

RhoGAM

Hemolytic disease of the newborn (HDN)—also called erythroblastosis fetalis—is a serious and potentially fatal blood disease that arises when there is an incompatibility between the blood types of the mother and baby. However, it can be completely prevented with two simple drug injections.

One in ten Caucasian pregnancies involves an Rh-negative (Rh–) mother and an Rh-positive (Rh+) father. If the baby's blood type is Rh+ and its red blood cells enter the mother's circulation, the mother's immune system views these cells as foreign, and she becomes "sensitized"—that is, she produces antibodies that seek to destroy the baby's red blood cells. A previous miscarriage, abortion, or amniocentesis can also sensitize the mother. In Caucasian populations, for example, 13 percent of Rh– mothers are sensitized during their first pregnancy with an Rh+ baby. These antibodies are kept in reserve for future use, putting Rh+ babies in subsequent pregnancies at risk for developing the disease.

When the mother's antibodies attack the newborn's red blood cells (hemolysis), the baby's blood cannot carry sufficient oxygen to its tissues and organs, leading to potentially fatal complications during pregnancy and after birth, including anemia and permanent brain damage. Severe, untreated HDN has a 70 percent mortality rate within the first week of neonatal life.

Since 1968, doctors have been able to prevent HDN by administering Rho(D) Immune Globulin (RhoGAM) to the mother during the twenty-eighth week of pregnancy and within seventy-two hours of the birth of a Rh+ baby. This product, introduced by Ortho-Clinical Diagnostics, a Johnson and Johnson subsidiary, contains anti-Rh(D) antibodies and suppresses the mother's normal production of antibodies upon exposure to Rh+ red blood cells. After treatment with RhoGAM, HDN has not been observed to occur in subsequent pregnancies.

SEE ALSO Ferrous Sulfate (1681), Epoetin (1989), 17P/Progesterone Injections and Gel (2003).

Karl Landsteiner (1868–1943) observed that blood transfused from one person to another could lead to red blood cell destruction in the recipient, leading to his classification of blood into groups A, B, AB, and O, for which he won the 1930 Nobel Prize in Physiology or Medicine. In 1940, he co-discovered the Rh blood factor, later shown to be responsible for hemolytic disease of newborns.

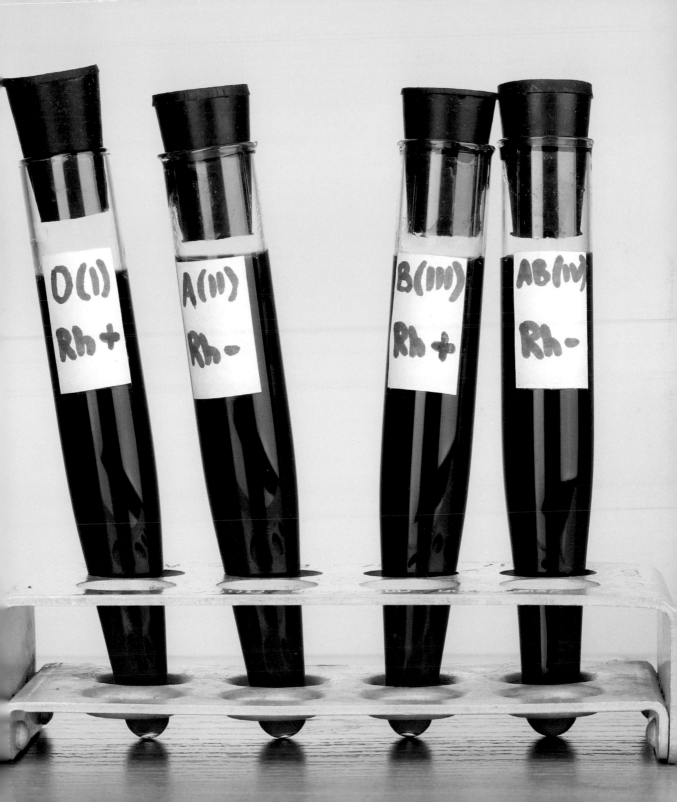

Fentanyl

A Drug for All Pains. Pain is a valuable protective mechanism, but some forms of pain can be physically and psychologically intolerable. No drug is more effective relieving pain than **morphine**, but there are occasions when similar drugs might be preferable because they can be administered in different ways. Fentanyl is a synthetic painkilling drug that has morphine-like (**opioid**) effects, but it works at a mere one-hundredth of the dose. While most opioid drugs can only be given by mouth or injection, fentanyl has been formulated into multiple dosage forms to deal with various types of pain.

Since fentanyl prevents pain within minutes after being injected, it is commonly used with other drugs prior to surgery to produce a state in which patients are pain free, partially conscious, and indifferent to their stressful surroundings. The effects wear off quickly after drug administration stops, and other less powerful drugs can be used to relieve postoperative pain.

In instances in which patients are likely to experience chronic, severe pain, as with cancer, it is desirable to relieve pain around-the-clock. Fentanyl can be administered as a transdermal product (Duragesic), in which a patch is applied to the skin, and the drug is slowly released and absorbed through the skin into the bloodstream. The patch produces sustained pain relief for up to forty-eight hours.

A high-dose fentanyl-containing "lollipop" (Actiq) is available for patients already using other opioids for severe pain but who still experience sudden pain for short periods. The lollipop allows fentanyl to be slowly absorbed across the membranes of the inner cheeks, tongue, and gums.

Fentanyl use is not without danger. Inadvertent exposure to high doses, such as those from defective patches, can result in overdose, respiratory failure, and death.

SEE ALSO Morphine (1806), Opioids (1973), OxyContin (1996).

Back pain is the most frequent cause of job-related disability and is second only to headaches as the most common symptom of a neurological ailment in the United States. A fentanyl patch may be prescribed to relieve acute and chronic pain.

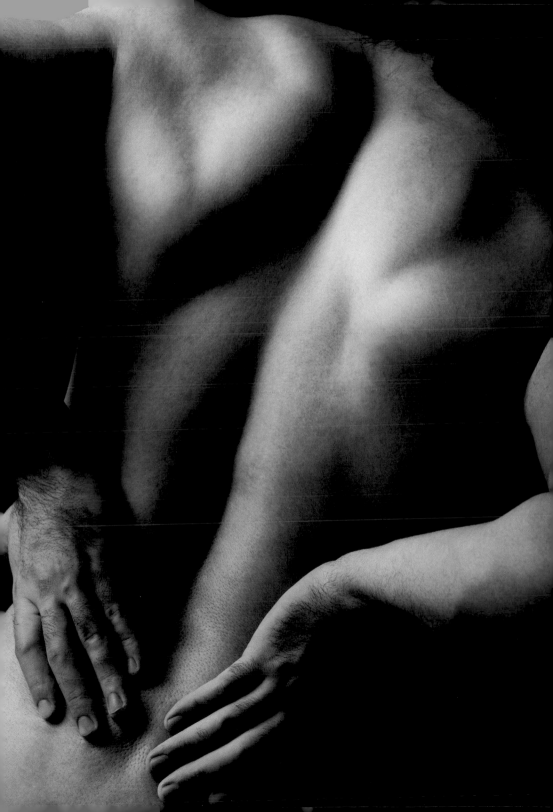

Butazolidin

Dancer's Image finished first in the 1968 running of the Kentucky Derby. Then, he had the dubious distinction of being the only winner in America's most famous horse race to be disqualified. Traces of Butazolidin (phenylbutazone), better known in racing circles as Bute, were found in the mandatory post-race urine test.

Six days before the race, the three-year-old stallion had, in fact, been given a Bute tablet to relieve the pain and inflammation in Dancer's sore ankles. The Kentucky Racing Commission ruled that the favored second-place horse, Forward Pass, be officially declared the winner of the 1968 Derby. While controversial to all racing devotees, to some the decision was viewed a travesty, and *Sports Illustrated* named it the sports story of the year.

Had the race been run at many other tracks throughout the United States, this drug's use would have been legal, but at Churchill Downs, it had not yet been sanctioned. The rules were to change, and in 1986, thirteen of the sixteen horses running were taking Bute. The doping of racehorses is not limited to those with swollen ankles; horses are commonly given painkillers to mask pre-race injuries. Many such horses have stumbled during the race, throwing their jockeys to the ground, with severe injury to both as an occasional consequence.

The first recipients of Butazolidin were not horses, but rather humans. In 1949, the Swiss pharmaceutical company Geigy (now Novartis) introduced this **aspirin**-like, nonsteroidal anti-inflammatory drug (NSAID). In addition to its anti-inflammatory and pain-relieving effects, it also promotes the excretion of uric acid and has been used for the treatment of gout. However, its many adverse effects have more than undermined these desirable properties, including bleeding peptic ulcers and life-threatening blood disorders. More than one-half century and thousands of drug-associated deaths later, and notwithstanding the availability of dozens of safer drugs, generic phenylbutazone is still on the market, bearing the warning that it should be used for the "shortest time possible."

SEE ALSO Colchicine (c. 70), Aspirin (1899), Benemid (1951), Celebrex and Vioxx (1998).

Horses are not raised as food animals in the United States, but horsemeat derived from American horses — including thoroughbred horses — is exported to various countries for human consumption. Some of these thoroughbreds have likely received phenylbutazone to relieve inflammation, and ingestion of their meat exposes humans to the drug's potentially dangerous adverse effects.

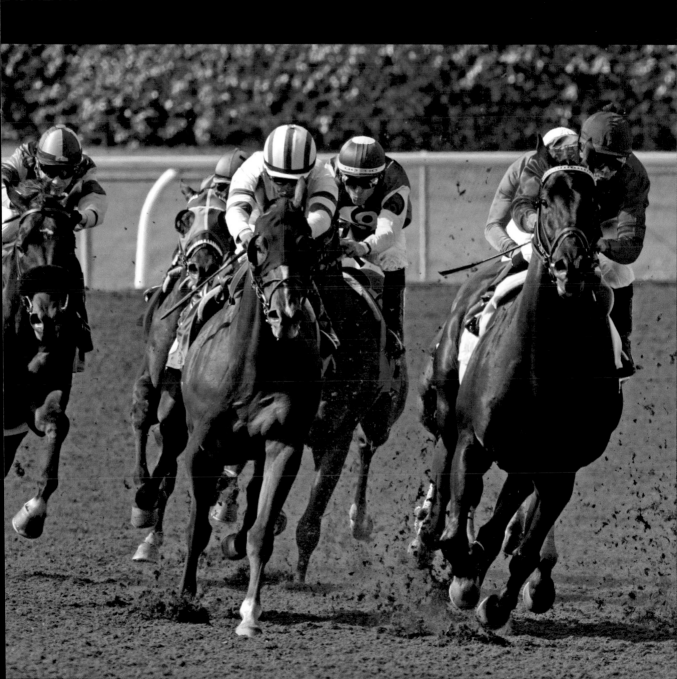

Praziquantel

Said to be second only to malaria as the most devastating tropical disease, schistosomiasis (snail fever) affects some 200 million people in seventy-four countries, with half the total cases in Africa and the rest in Asia and South America. The victims of this parasitic worm infection, caused by several species of schistosomes (blood flukes), are often children.

Schistosomiasis is acquired by bathing or swimming in fresh water containing snails that harbor these parasitic flatworms. The flukes multiply within the snails and are released into the water, where they remain until finding a human host's skin to penetrate. They then travel in the bloodstream and lodge in the bladder or intestines, potentially residing there for many years. Adult flukes lay eggs that can cause inflammation of these organs, blood loss, and bladder cancer.

The most effective approach to dealing with schistosomiasis is avoiding waters containing schistosomes. Once the disease is present in a human, it is most commonly treated throughout the world with praziquantel. This remarkable anthelmintic (parasitic worm–killing drug), effective against all species of schistosomes, was the product of a joint research effort between the Bayer Institute for Chemotherapy and E. Merck, both based in Germany.

Praziquantel (Biltricide, Droncit) is safe, inexpensive (18 cents/dose), and very highly effective when given as a single dose, once a year. It reverses 90 percent of the damage to internal organs caused by the schistosomiasis infection and is also used to treat tapeworm infections, including those caused by ingestion of beef, pork, and fish that are contaminated with tapeworm eggs.

Praziquantel's uses also extend to animals; it is given in tablet form to treat tapeworm infections in dogs and cats. Used as a topical solution (Profender) in combination with the antiparasitic drug emodepside, it is applied to a cat's shoulder to treat tapeworm, hookworm, and roundworm infections.

SEE ALSO Carbon Tetrachloride (1921), Hexylresorcinol (1924).

This frontal view of a male schistosoma showing both suckers has been magnified 100x. This parasitic worm is responsible for snail fever, which affects two hundred million people, half of whom reside in Africa.

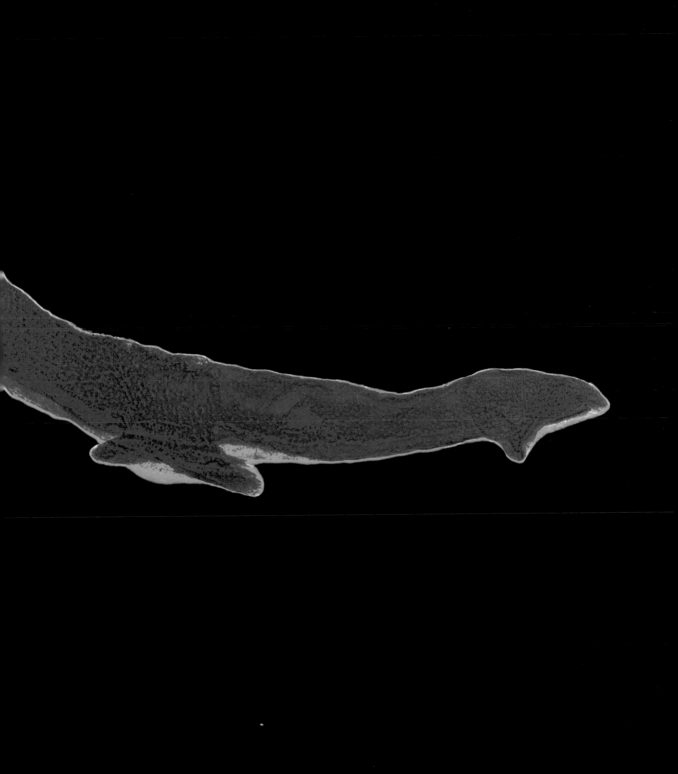

Artemisinin

Li Shizhen (1518–1593)

The most promising drug now used for the treatment of malaria dates back to 168 BCE in ancient China, when the weed *qing hao* (sweet wormwood, annual wormwood) was recommended for the treatment of hemorrhoids. Some five centuries later, in 340, the herb was an ingredient in a tea intended to reduce fevers. In 1596, the Chinese herbalist Li Shizhen recommended this tea for the relief of the chills and fever of malaria in his *Compendium of Materia Medica*.

In the late 1960s, Chinese scientists began a search for active drugs found in plants that had long been used in their traditional remedies. In 1972, they isolated *qinghaosu*—better known by its international name, artemisinin—from the leaves of *Artemesia*. Tests showed that the artemisinins, a collective term that includes derivatives of the natural chemical, very effectively clear the body of the malaria-causing *Plasmodium* parasites—in particular, *Plasmodium faciparum*, the most common and deadly strain.

The history of most antimalarial drugs teaches us that, as their use increases, so do drug-resistant strains of parasites. One of the greatest fears among the experts who treat malaria is the development of artemisinin resistance by currently susceptible plasmodia—fears confirmed in 2009 with reports of early signs of resistance. To forestall this possibility, the World Health Organization has urged that this drug only be used in combination with other antimalarial drugs.

In 2009, the United States joined more than eighty other countries worldwide and approved the use of Coartem, the first approved fixed-dose artemisinin combination therapy (ACT) for the treatment of malaria. A three-day treatment yields cure rates of more than 95 percent, even in areas where the parasite is resistant to multiple drugs.

Malaria, the most common parasitic infectious disease affecting humankind, kills more than 1 million people each year. Although malaria is not a problem in North America and western Europe, there are an increasing number of cases contracted by tourists and businesspersons when they visit the roughly ninety malaria-endemic countries.

SEE ALSO Quinine (1820), Chloroquine (1947).

This malaria-causing protozoan parasite is transmitted by a bite of the female Anopheles *mosquito. The head of a mosquito is shown here magnified 100x.*

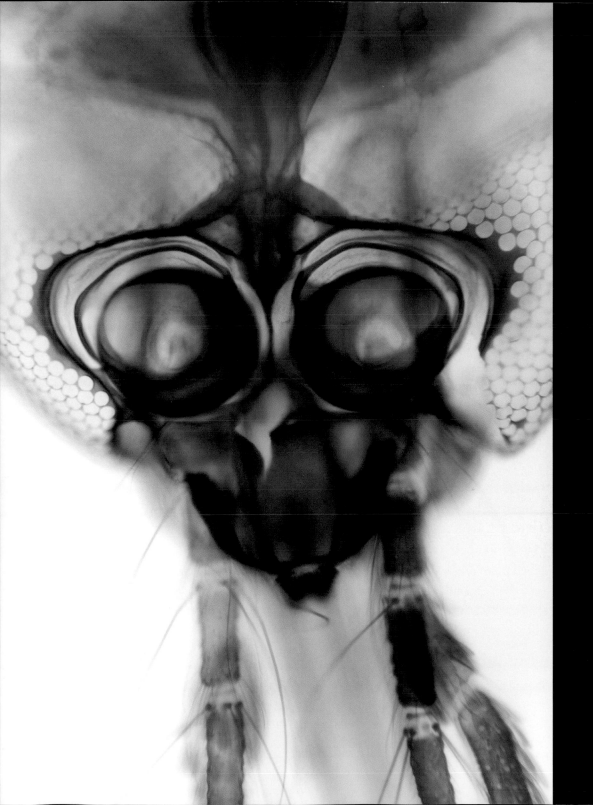

Opioids

Hans W. Kosterlitz (1903–1998), Solomon H. Snyder (b. 1938)

APPLYING RECEPTOR THEORY TO DRUG DEVELOPMENT. No drug is a more effective pain reliever than **morphine**, but scientists have long sought drugs that relieve pain as effectively without the potential for abuse. In 1973, results from Solomon Snyder's laboratory at Johns Hopkins University confirmed the suspicion that morphine and other morphine-related drugs relieved pain, diarrhea, and other common ailments by interacting with specialized receptors in the brain and elsewhere. Observations of the antagonistic effects of naloxone (Narcan), a highly specific and selective morphine blocker, strengthened the argument. The all-inclusive term *opioid* was used to classify both drugs that have effects like morphine and their antagonists and that act at this receptor.

Why should the body expend valuable resources producing these complex protein receptors unless they were present to interact with endogenous compounds (compounds produced within the body)? In 1975, Hans Kosterlitz and John Hughes, at the University of Aberdeen, isolated small peptides (proteins) from human and other mammalian brains that interact with opioid receptors and are blocked by naloxone. These enkephalins and related endorphins—collectively, endogenous opioid peptides—are thought to play a role in pain and mood. Moreover, multiple types of opioid receptors (mu, delta, kappa) are found in the brain, spinal cord, and gastrointestinal tract and are responsible for the multiple opioid actions, including their addiction potential.

Now knowing that morphine's pain-relieving effects and abuse potential result from its action at the mu receptor, scientists have developed drugs with complex actions at both mu and kappa receptors that are less likely to be abused. These include Buprenex, Stadol, and Talwin. The search for a totally abuse-free morphine continues.

Morphine and related natural drugs were not always classified as opioids. Since their effects were accompanied by sleepiness and stupor, they were called *narcotics*. With many newer semisynthetic derivatives, including **heroin**, Dilaudid, and **OxyContin**, scientists now use the all-inclusive term *opioid* to classify all drugs that act at the opioid receptors.

SEE ALSO Opium (c. 2500 BCE), Alkaloids (1806), Morphine (1806), Codeine (1832), Heroin (1898), Drug Receptors (1905), Methadone (1947), Fentanyl (1968), OxyContin (1996).

Originating in China more than 2,500 years ago, acupuncture is among the oldest and most commonly used medical practices in the world. It is thought to stimulate the central nervous system, releasing endogenous opioids that reduce pain.

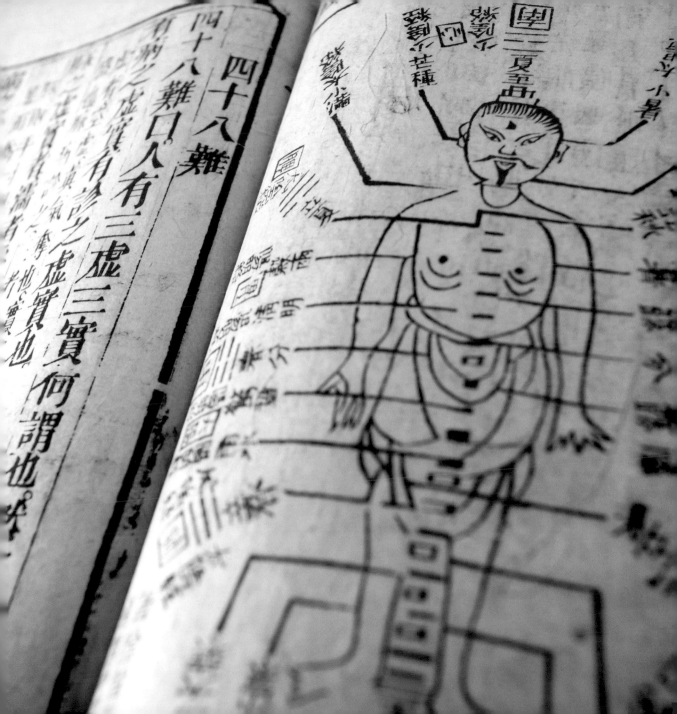

四十八難

四十八難曰人有三虛三實何謂也

然有脈之虛實有病之虛實有診之虛實也

Tamoxifen

Elwood Jensen (1920–2012)

Breast cancer is the most common cause of cancer deaths in women worldwide and the second-leading cause in the Western world. Today, tamoxifen (Nolvadex) is the most widely used drug for the treatment of early and advanced breast cancer in selected women of all ages, decreasing cancer recurrence by one-half and risk of death by 25 percent. Tamoxifen can also prevent the development of breast cancer in women at high risk.

Tamoxifen was originally synthesized in 1962 at ICI Pharmaceuticals (now Astra-Zeneca) in Cheshire, England. The compound, a nonsteroidal antiestrogen, was intended as a potential anti-fertility drug, although it stimulated ovulation instead of suppressing it in humans. A failed contraceptive didn't have much market potential, but after laboratory and human studies pointed to the compound's promise in preventing the development of breast cancer in high-risk women, it was approved for use in the United Kingdom in 1973 and in the United States in 1977.

Tamoxifen is not effective in all cases of breast cancer. Around the turn of the twentieth century, removal of the ovaries was shown to halt the growth of advanced breast cancer. In the 1960s, Elwood Jensen at the University of Chicago found that estrogen receptors (ER) were present in some breast cancer tumors, while not in others. If an ER receptor is present (ER+)—as it is in 50–70 percent of patients—these tumors require estrogen for their growth. Tamoxifen works by blocking the ER on the tumors, thus preventing their growth.

In addition to its anticancer actions, tamoxifen produces a complex array of effects—some bad, some good. It is generally accepted that tamoxifen therapy is most effective for a maximum of five years, but one of the potential problems associated with its long-term use is an increased risk of endometrial (uterine) cancer. On the flip side, tamoxifen reduces the loss of bone, and a pharmacologically related drug, **Evista**, is used to treat and prevent osteoporosis.

SEE ALSO Drug Receptors (1905), Estrone and Estrogen (1929), Clomid (1967), Evista (1997), Herceptin (1998).

The Chain Bridge across the Danube River in Budapest, Hungary, is lit pink in support of breast cancer awareness.

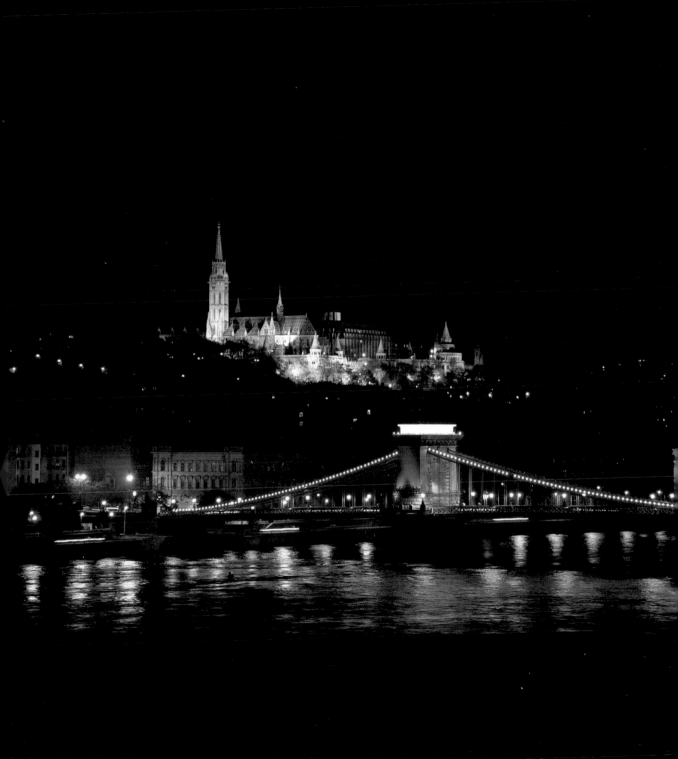

Rohypnol

Rohypnol is a highly effective sleep-producing drug. Some might suggest that it is *too* effective. Nevertheless, it is included among these entries because of its notorious reputation as a date-rape drug.

Flunitrazepine, a benzodiazepine related to **Valium**, was synthesized in the Roche Laboratories in Switzerland in 1972. It was marketed in Europe three years later and throughout many other countries in Asia and South America during the 1980s, most often bearing the trade name Rohypnol. It continues to be prescribed worldwide for the treatment of insomnia, but commonly with restrictions. Although Rohypnol was never approved for use in the United States, it has entered the country through illicit distribution channels with the common street name, "roofie."

During the mid-1990s, its use as a date rape drug became widespread. When added to an alcoholic beverage, it produces deep sedation and anterograde amnesia, so the victim has no memory of the events that transpired, including the assailant's identity, when under the drug's influence. Moreover, Rohypnol tablets are normally white, odorless, and tasteless, and readily dissolvable in liquids. To make their presence more visible to potential victims, reformulated tablets contain an inert dye that turns blue in liquids. The Drug Induced Rape Prevention Act of 1996 in the United States established harsh penalties for the distribution of such drugs associated with violent crimes, including sexual assault.

Rohypnol has been used as a recreational drug by itself and with other drugs, such as marijuana (**cannabis**), **MDMA/Ecstasy**, and **LSD**. More ominously, it has been a tool for intentional overdose suicides, especially when taken with alcohol. Nirvana lead singer and guitarist Kurt Cobain (1967–1994) used Rohypnol and champagne in his first suicide attempt. Weeks later, his self-inflicted shotgun wound proved successful.

SEE ALSO Cannabis (c. 3000 BCE), LSD (1943), Valium (1963), MDMA/Ecstasy (1976).

This image shows a man drugging a woman's drink in a bar—a possible prelude to date rape.

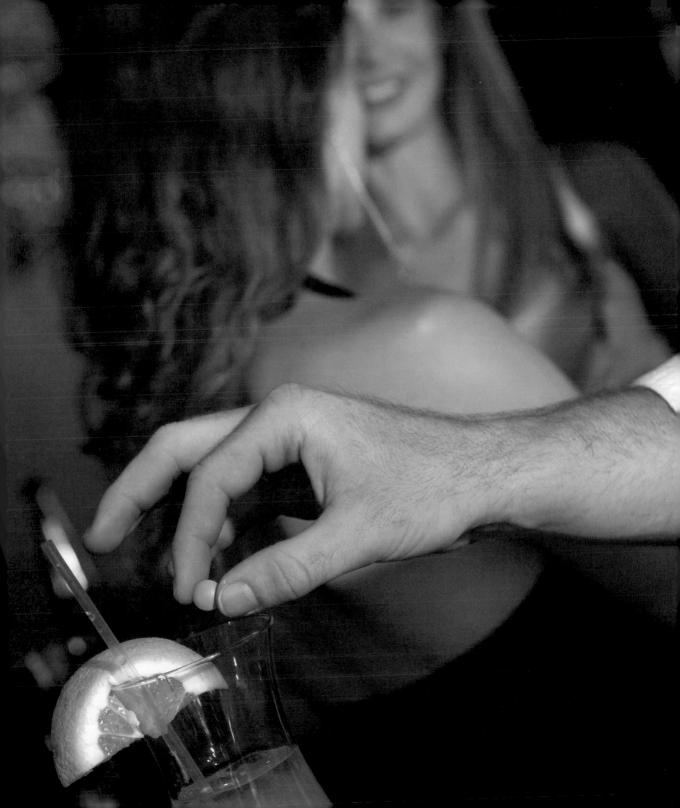

Beclovent

Since the 1950s, **cortisone** and related steroids, when taken by mouth, have been used to reduce inflammation in the airways. Drugs such as dexamethasone (Decadron) or methylprednisolone (Medrol) produce dramatic relief of symptoms in severe cases of chronic asthma, reducing the number of attacks and their severity. When used during the early stages of asthma, they can prevent the worsening of this respiratory disorder.

Because symptoms recur when these steroids are discontinued, they are commonly taken orally over extended periods, but such drugs can cause a very wide range of adverse systemic effects, some of which are quite dangerous. These include interference with the body's capacity to respond to infections or injury, alterations in the body's salt and water balance, abnormalities in metabolism that can lead to diabetes, and slowed growth in children. Sudden drug discontinuation after taking oral steroids for several weeks shuts down the body's normal production of hydrocortisone (cortisol), which impairs the immune response to stress and infections.

During the 1970s, beclomethasone (Beclovent) and similar steroids became available that could be effectively inhaled and delivered directly to the sites in the airways that were inflamed. The beneficial effects, fully comparable to those obtained when the drugs are taken orally, occur at a fraction of the oral dose. As a consequence, the frequency, extent, and severity of the systemic side effects are markedly reduced.

Since the 1950s, metered-dose inhalers (MDIs) have replaced squeeze-bulb nebulizers that were previously used to deliver inhaled drugs. MDIs are devices that use a propellant to deliver fixed and accurate doses of medication as a mist that is inhaled.

MDIs are now commonly used for the treatment of asthma and other respiratory conditions, and inhaled steroids are the first drugs doctors prescribe for the prevention of asthmatic attacks. However, these steroids should never be used as emergency antiasthmatics (as **albuterol/salbutamol** is) to arrest an imminent or ongoing attack, because they can irritate the airways and temporarily worsen the symptoms.

SEE ALSO Cortisone (1949), Albuterol/Salbutamol (1968), Ephedra/Ephedrine (1994).

Metered-dose inhalers (MDIs) are used to deliver fixed and accurate doses of many asthma medications. The patient obtains rapid relief from asthma symptoms when the drug is inhaled as a mist.

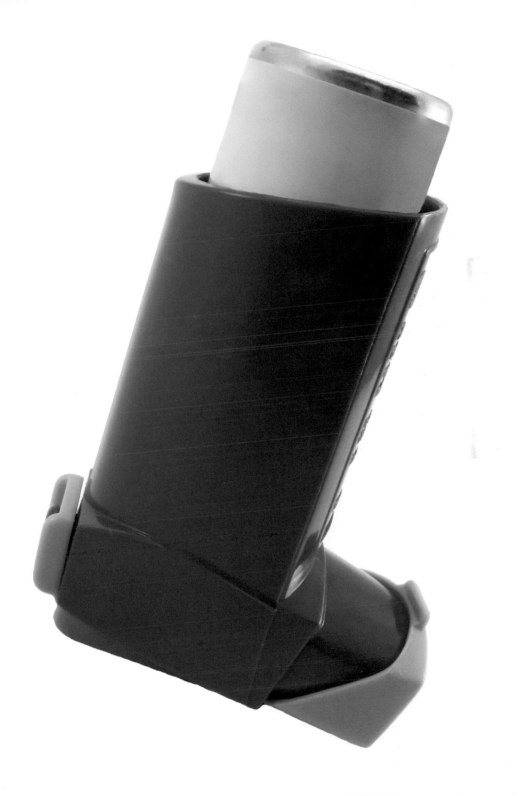

Tagamet

James W. Black (1924–2010)

Histamine attracted considerable scientific attention during the early decades of the twentieth century as a naturally occurring, highly active chemical. As the years progressed, a link was found between the release of histamine and allergic reactions; and in 1944, **Neo-Antergan**—the first antihistamine—appeared, followed by dozens of similar drugs.

To a greater or lesser extent, all these successors were comparable in treating allergic disorders, but none of them could block histamine's ability to stimulate gastric-acid release in the stomach—a cause of peptic ulcers. Scottish physician-pharmacologist James Black speculated that multiple histamine receptor types—one involved with the allergic response, another with acid secretion, for example—might underlie this anomaly. Thus, Black, then working at the Smith, Kline and French Research Institute in Hertfordshire, England, set out to develop a drug that could antagonize histamine's second receptor type.

In 1976, after twelve years of effort, Tagamet (cimetidine) was brought to market. The first member of a new class of drugs that rendered all previous ulcer and gastroesophageal reflux disease (GERD or heartburn) drugs obsolete, Tagamet not only reduced acid release but also promoted healing of gastric ulcers. With Tagamet's discovery, the designation *antihistamine* was now ambiguous and required additional specification. The classical antihistamines used to treat allergies were redesignated histamine H_1 receptor antagonists, while Tagamet-like drugs were classified as H_2 antagonists.

ONE SCIENTIST, TWO REVOLUTIONARY DRUGS. Tagamet became the world's best-selling drug in 1981, with annual sales exceeding $1 billion and displacing the heart drug Inderal (**propranolol**), another Black-developed medicine in the top spot. Tagamet, in turn, was displaced and relegated to the second slot in 1988 by Zantac (ranitidine), another H2 antagonist with fewer side effects. In recognition for his discoveries of Inderal and Tagamet, two revolutionary drugs, Black was named a co-recipient of the 1988 Nobel Prize in Physiology or Medicine.

SEE ALSO Drug Receptors (1905), Neo-Antergan (1944), Benadryl (1946), Propranolol (1964), Prilosec (1989).

Antihistamines are of two distinct types: those that treat allergic disorders (Neo-Antergan, Benadryl) and those that prevent the secretion of acid in the stomach. Tagamet was the first of the acid-inhibiting drugs, effectively combating heartburn (commonly caused by the consumption or overconsumption of spicy chilies, carbonated drinks, and various acid reflux–promoting food and beverages) as well as ulcers.

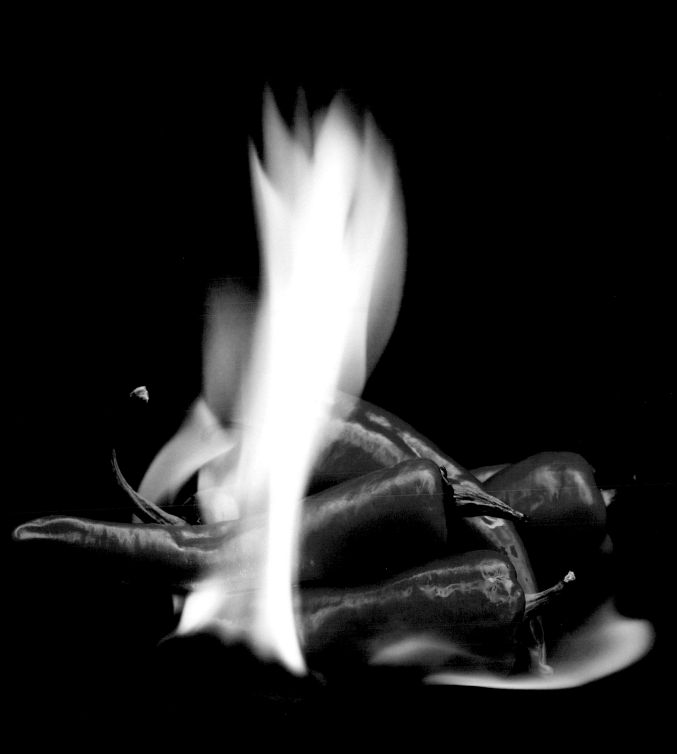

MDMA/Ecstasy

Anton Köllisch (1888–1916), Alexander Shulgin (b. 1925), Leo Zeff (1912–1988)

In the mid-twentieth century, **m**ethylene**d**ioxy-**m**eth**a**mphtamine was an obscure chemical synthesized in 1912 by Anton Köllisch, a Merck chemist. By the 1980s, MDMA was among the most widely used illicit drugs in the United States and Europe.

Active interest in MDMA dramatically increased in 1976, after the California pharmacologist-chemist Alexander Shulgin resynthesized MDMA, sampled it himself (as was his custom), and shared his enthusiasm for it with friends—one of whom was psychotherapist Leo Zeff. This amphetamine-like stimulant—now better known as "ecstasy"—produces euphoria and physical energy, increasing feelings of empathy and intimacy with partners and the perception that "all is right with the world." Zeff was so impressed with MDMA's ability to enhance patient-therapist communications and to relieve anxiety disorders that he was said to have trained some 4,000 therapists in its clinical virtues and use.

Enthusiasm for MDMA transcended psychotherapy circles. Devotees of clubs and raves (dance parties) embraced it. After nonstop frenetic dancing for hours in hot, crowded surroundings, some participants experience hyperthermia, a dangerous rise in body temperature that can cause kidney and liver failure. Drinking excessive volumes of water, coupled with dehydration due to sweating, can cause a steep drop in blood sodium levels, potentially resulting in confusion, delirium, and convulsions.

Objective assessment of MDMA's reported effects is complicated by the purity of street ecstasy, which commonly contains other psychoactive drugs responsible for adverse side effects, some quite dangerous. After MDMA use, some individuals report depression, anxiety, and fatigue. Conflicting reports have appeared as to whether it causes cognitive impairment.

MDMA is legally controlled in most countries and has been illegal in the United Kingdom since 1977 and the United States since 1985. Nevertheless, it remains among the most commonly used recreational drugs, taken by millions of people each year. Interest also continues among psychotherapists about its potential use in treating relationship disorders and to augment therapy for post-traumatic stress disorder.

SEE ALSO Amphetamine (1932), Methamphetamine (1944).

Ecstasy is the preferred drug at all-night dance parties (raves) that are commonly frequented by teenagers and young adults. "X" enables individuals to dance actively for long periods and it enhances emotional intimacy; hence, its nickname, "the love drug."

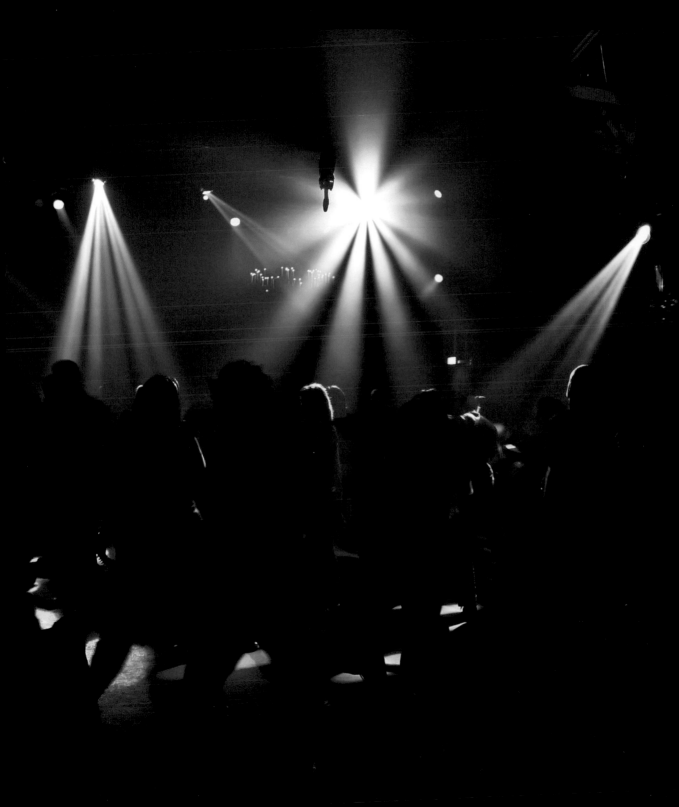

Lethal Injection

Capital punishment has been formally abolished in most countries and not imposed for many years in others. By contrast, it continues to be practiced in China, India, Indonesia, and the United States, where some two-thirds of the states and the federal government have death-penalty statutes. Lethal injection is the primary or an alternate method of execution in all but one state.

Lethal injection was introduced in the 1970s as a more humane and less expensive alternative to electrocutions or **cyanide** gas. In 1977, Oklahoma led the revolution, adopting a three-drug cocktail—sodium **thiopental**, pancuronium bromide, and potassium chloride—injected intravenously, in sequence. Originators envisioned that each drug would be lethal and that the combination would provide redundancy.

Sodium thiopental (Pentothal), an ultra-short-acting barbiturate used medically to induce anesthesia, causes loss of consciousness within thirty to forty-five seconds after a dose of 200–350 mg. By contrast, doses of 2 to 5 grams used in executions typically cause unconsciousness in ten seconds. The lethal dose of thiopental has not been determined and is variable. Next, pancuronium bromide (Pavulon) is injected. This **curare**-like muscle relaxant is used in conjunction with anesthetics during surgical operations. The high doses (100 mg) used in a lethal injection mixture paralyze the breathing muscles and cause respiratory failure within minutes. Finally, potassium chloride, when given intravenously at a dose of 100 milliequivalents, causes fatal paralysis of the heart.

HUMANE PRACTICE OR CHEMICAL ASPHYXIATION? Lethal injections have faced and withstood a number of challenges over the years. Difficulties have been encountered inserting needles into veins, and prisoners may die of suffocation while still conscious and in pain. In 2008, the U.S. Supreme Court ruled that the practice does not violate the Constitution prohibition against imposing "cruel and unusual punishment." In 2011, after a two-year delay in executions precipitated by the unavailability of Pentothal, some states have substituted pentobarbital (**Nembutal**) in the cocktail or have used this drug alone in high doses.

Capital punishment has long been practiced across the globe, and yet, it continues to remain an active subject of controversy between and within countries.

SEE ALSO Hydrogen Cyanide (1704), Curare (1850), Nembutal and Seconal (1928), Thiopental (1934), Tubocurarine (1935).

The lethal injection room at San Quentin State Prison in San Francisco Bay, California, is shown here. The condemned person is strapped to a gurney, and an intravenous line is inserted. While the drugs are administered, the person's heart rhythm is monitored. Death is generally deemed to have occurred within seven minutes, when heart activity stops.

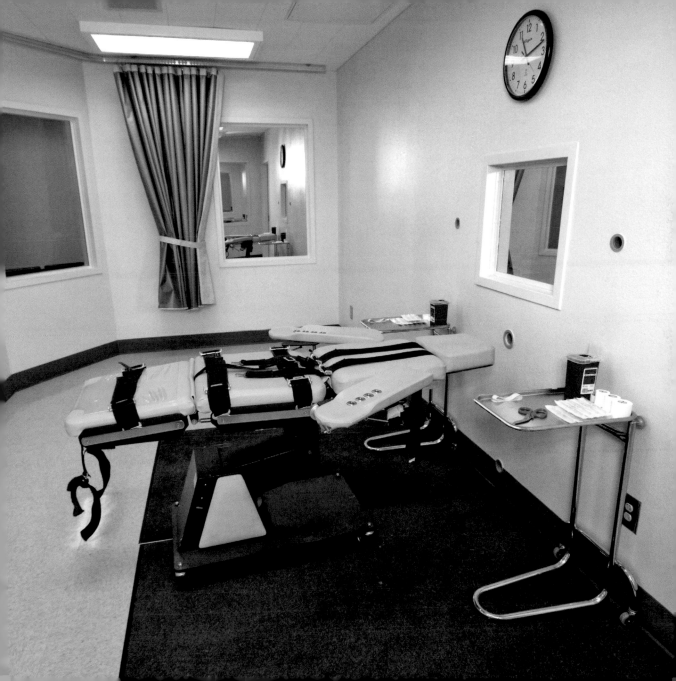

Timoptic

Glaucoma, the second leading cause of vision loss, affects 60 million people worldwide, causing blindness in more than 8 million. These numbers are expected to increase in the future, in part because of the rapidly aging population.

The eyeball is filled with the aqueous humor, which enables the eyeball to maintain its shape. This fluid is produced in the rear chamber of the eye, passing through it and entering the front or anterior chamber, where it normally drains from the eye at the same rate that it is being produced. When fluid drainage fails to keep pace with its buildup, intraocular pressure (IOP) builds up, compressing the optic nerve, which results in glaucoma.

There are several types of glaucoma. Open-angle glaucoma is the most common type and the leading cause of blindness among individuals of African origin. It develops slowly and without symptoms until vision becomes impaired. By contrast, angle-closure glaucoma is a painful condition that carries the risk of vision loss within days if not treated immediately. In this case, drainage from the eye is suddenly blocked, and the IOP abruptly rises.

Drugs can effectively control glaucoma, but they cannot cure it. Five classes of drugs are used to treat open-angle glaucoma by lowering the IOP. They act by reducing the production of fluid, by increasing its outflow from the eye, or by both mechanisms. Multiple drugs are often used in combination.

THWARTING THE SILENT THIEF OF SIGHT. Beta-adrenergic blocking agents, such as timolol (Timoptic), are usually the first class of drugs used to treat open-angle glaucoma by decreasing fluid production. Like **propranolol**, the classic beta-blocker, Timoptic is relatively nonselective in its beta-blocking effects. Hence, although Timoptic drops or gel are applied to the eye, the drug can enter circulation and exert effects on distant parts of the body. In susceptible individuals with a history of asthma or chronic obstructive pulmonary disease (COPD), Timoptic can cause constriction of the bronchi, resulting in severe shortness of breath. It can also interfere with heart function in patients with heart disease.

SEE ALSO Physostigmine (1875), Diamox (1952), Propranolol (1964).

This illustration depicts an approximation of what an individual with glaucoma might see when looking at a kitchen table. Glaucoma is a condition in which a person suffers irreversible loss of peripheral vision. In the absence of treatment, total blindness will occur.

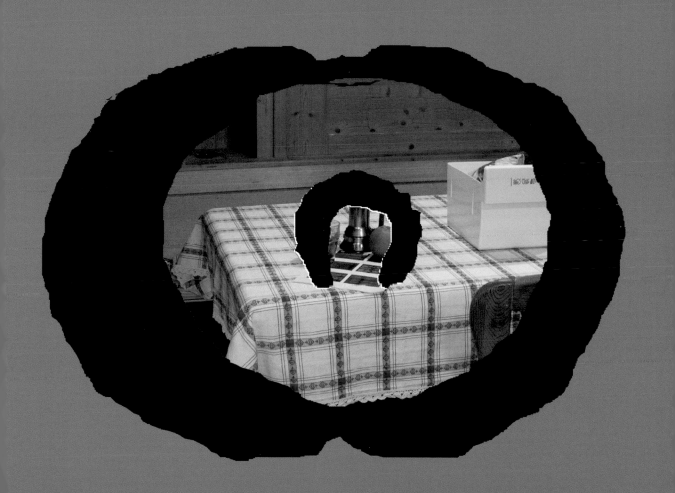

Captopril

Sergio Henrique Ferreiri (b. 1934), John Vane (1927–2004)

Should one experience a sudden drop in blood pressure or a reduction in blood volume, such as might occur after dehydration or bleeding, a sequence of compensatory events seeks to restore homeostasis, the normal state of balance in the body. Angiotensin II (Ang II), a highly active peptide formed in the liver, counters such drops in blood pressure by altering the activity of blood vessels to increase blood pressure and by prompting the kidney to retain body salt and water. The enzyme responsible for the formation of Ang II from the inactive Ang I is angiotensin-converting enzyme (ACE), first identified in the 1950s.

FROM PIT VIPER VENOM TO ACE INHIBITOR. A decade later, the Brazilian pharmacologist Sergio Ferreiri extracted a component from the venom of *Bothrops jararaca*, a South American pit viper, and brought it to the London laboratory of John Vane. The extract and its active chemical teprotide inhibited ACE and provided a novel approach for the treatment of hypertension (high blood pressure). Scientists at the Squibb Institute for Medical Research in New Jersey further evaluated teprotide and found it inactive by mouth. However, the discovery led Squibb scientists to synthesize captopril (Capoten), the first orally active ACE inhibitor, which they marketed in 1981. Approximately ten similar drugs are now available.

The ACE inhibitors have proved very important, not only for the treatment of mild-to-severe hypertension in patients experiencing other problems, but also for managing a range of cardiovascular conditions. When used for heart failure, in which they are considered integral to treatment, ACE inhibitors increase the ability of patients to function and reduce mortality rates.

Multiple clinical studies have shown that ACE inhibitors reduce the death rate when administered at the time of a heart attack. In addition, diabetes is the leading cause of end-stage kidney disease. ACE inhibitors help to prevent or delay the progression in such patients.

SEE ALSO Digitalis (1775), Diuril (1958), Propranolol (1964), Lasix (1966).

This poster provides valuable advice for people with hypertension: Maintain a healthy body weight, eliminate salt from the diet, kick the cigarette habit, take blood-pressure medication regularly, and monitor blood pressure.

IF YOU HAVE HIGH BLOOD PRESSURE...

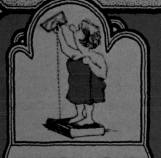

WATCH YOUR WEIGHT

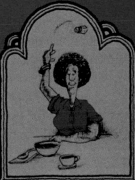

AVOID SALT

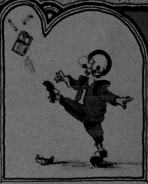

DON'T SMOKE

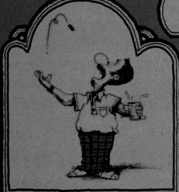

TAKE YOUR PILLS

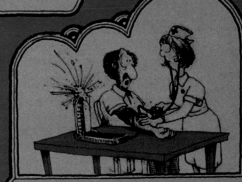

GET REGULAR CHECKS

N.Y.S. Health Department

1861

Xanax

Panic attacks come suddenly and without warning, at any time, and in the absence of any precipitating cause. The symptoms vary but are always frightening, including fear of dying, pounding heart, heartbeat racing out of control, chest pains perceived to be a heart attack, shortness of breath or the feeling of being smothered, and fear of losing control or going crazy. The intensity of these symptoms generally peak in about ten minutes and pass within about thirty minutes. Some individuals have only one or two attacks in a lifetime, while others have daily or weekly attacks—a condition termed *panic disorder*. Sufferers often have extreme anxiety about when the next attack will strike. Panic disorders are by no means rare, affecting 1.5–2 percent of the population in the United States every year.

Two groups of drugs are highly effective in reducing the frequency and intensity of attacks: different classes of antidepressants and several short-acting benzodiazepines, including Xanax (alprazolam). Both classes have shortcomings: They must be taken for extended periods (six to nine months) because quitting too soon often leads to a recurrence of attacks, and the preferred drug group, antidepressants, may have to be taken for six to twelve weeks before their full benefits kick in.

Xanax, which has both antianxiety and antidepressant effects, works after the first dose and causes few major side effects, but normal doses taken over only several months may lead to tolerance and physical dependence. These problems occur with other benzodiazepines but are much more pronounced with Xanax. When Xanax is abruptly discontinued or the dose is sharply reduced, hallucinations, delirium, and seizures may result.

More common during withdrawal is extreme anxiety and the return of symptoms reminiscent of the original panic disorder—symptoms that can continue for six months to several years. To prevent these problems, the dosage of Xanax must be gradually reduced over a period of many months, which often proves to be extremely difficult. All benzodiazepines are subject to recreational use, but Xanax leads the list for emergency-department visits.

SEE ALSO Tofranil and Elavil (1957), Librium (1960), Monoamine Oxidase Inhibitors (1961), Valium (1963), Prozac (1987).

Sufferers of panic attacks commonly say that Xanax has saved their life by rapidly alleviating their extreme anxiety with few noteworthy side effects. To retain its beneficial effects, Xanax must be taken continuously. If abruptly stopped, withdrawal effects occur, inducing a recurrence of extreme anxiety in addition to possible seizures.

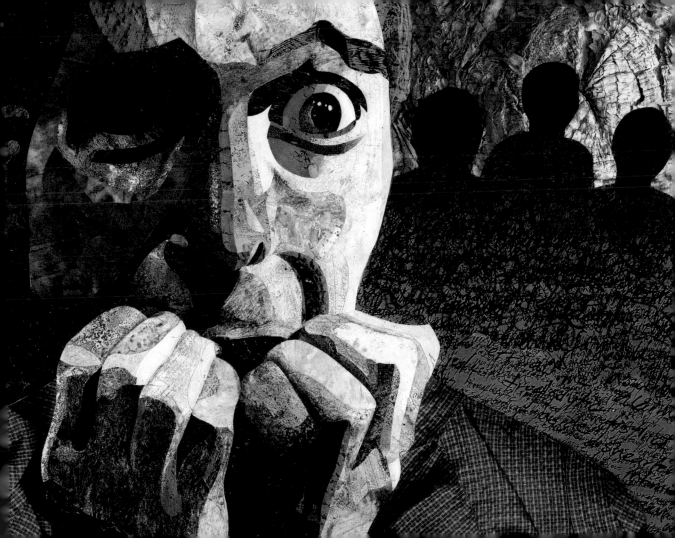

Acyclovir

Since the 1940s, tremendous advances have occurred in the treatment of bacterial infections—but advances in the fight against virus-causing diseases only began to occur four decades later. What took so long? Bacteria and viruses are fundamentally different. Bacteria are self-sustaining in their ability to reproduce. Antibacterial drugs attack a process or element in the microbe that is either absent or not essential for the well being of the host (human or animal). **Penicillin**, for example, prevents susceptible bacteria from manufacturing a cell wall that is required for their survival but absent in animal cells.

By contrast, viruses use the host's biochemical machinery to live and reproduce. Because of this intimate relationship, many drugs that are toxic to the virus also cause significant harm to the host. The challenge scientists face is finding those subtle differences that are unique to viruses.

One highly fruitful approach has involved studying the complex life cycle of viruses, from their attachment to and entry into the host's cells, to their replication within the cells, to their release to infect new cells. Antiviral drugs have been developed that interfere with specific steps in this sequence.

PIONEER AGAINST VIRUSES. Acyclovir (also spelled *aciclovir*) prevents the virus from manufacturing DNA by interacting with two enzymes that are unique to these viruses. Just as penicillin started the antibiotic revolution, acyclovir was the first successful antiviral drug. It is effective against both the herpes simplex virus (HSV) and the varicella-zoster virus (VZV). HSV causes cold sores on the lips, conjunctivitis, and genital sores, whereas VZV can cause shingles and chickenpox. Acyclovir (Zovirax) reduces the time of healing of uncomfortable symptoms associated with these disorders.

Several important differences exist between antibiotics and antiviral drugs. Antibiotics are generally effective against multiple types of bacteria. By contrast, there are no all-purpose antiviral drugs, and existing drugs only act against a limited number of viruses. Antibiotics produce authentic cures of bacterial infections, while antiviral drugs only prevent viral reproduction and suppression of symptoms. When the drug is stopped, the virus returns, as does the disorder. Better antiviral drugs are vitally needed.

SEE ALSO Food and Drug Administration (1906), Salvarsan (1910), Penicillin (1928), AZT/Retrovir (1987).

Herpes simplex virus (HSV) particles consist of DNA genetic material covered by a protein coat (capsid), which is wrapped in a lipid layer, or envelope. Projections on the surface of the HSV particle bind to receptors on the white blood cell to create an opening through which the virus enters the cell.

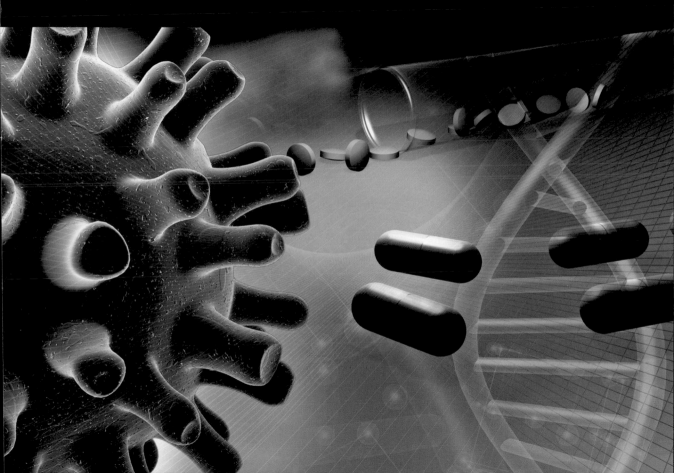

Biologic Drugs

Biologic drugs have revolutionized the treatment of an increasing array of medical conditions that have failed to respond adequately to traditional drugs. These include cancers, rheumatoid arthritis, and conditions affecting the skin, heart, and nervous system.

Now that we know more about the molecular basis of health and disease and have gained greater expertise in biotechnology, the development of biologic drugs has accelerated, complementing and, in some cases, replacing traditional drugs. These biologics can be identical to or can very closely resemble natural hormones, such as **human insulin**—the first biologic drug to appear in 1982—or **growth hormone**. Other biologics are monoclonal antibodies, stimulating or enhancing our body's immune system to zero in and block selective substances in the body or attack specific cell types, such as tumors.

Unlike biologics, traditional drugs are generally small molecules produced by chemical reactions, with a specific chemical structure. The active ingredient in approved generic equivalents must be identical to the original traditional drug. Moreover, the generic must be bioequivalent—that is, it must act in the body in the same way and to the same extent as the reference drug, as well as being freely interchanged with it.

By contrast, biologics are large and complex molecules produced by approaches involving recombinant DNA technology. Unlike traditional drugs, the composition of biologics and the effects they produce may differ significantly based on how they are prepared, even when there are only subtle differences in their preparation. Moreover, the final product is too complex to be characterized by existing analytical methods to determine whether it is chemically identical to the original.

Because biologics are so expensive, the development and approval of far less costly generic biologics have been subject to long and heated debate. In the United States, legislation was enacted in 2010 that enables the **FDA** to grant expedited approval to biosimilars—biologics that closely resemble but are not necessarily identical to the original product—but draft guidelines have yet to be finalized. Since 2001, the European Medicines Agency has had procedures for biosimilar approval, with the requirement that they produce the same effects and can be interchanged with the original.

SEE ALSO Food and Drug Administration (1906), Human Insulin (1982), Growth Hormone (1985), Herceptin (1998), Enbrel, Remicide, and Humira (1998), Iressa and Erbitux (2003), Avastin (2004), Lucentis (2006).

The twenty-first century has witnessed a distinct shift in the source of new drugs from plants and chemicals to biologic drugs. Biologic drugs are virtually identical to natural substances produced in our bodies. By applying recombinant DNA technology, it has become possible to produce virtually unlimited supplies of these highly specific and potent drugs. Because these drugs alter the fundamental causes of medical disorders, they offer more than mere symptomatic relief.

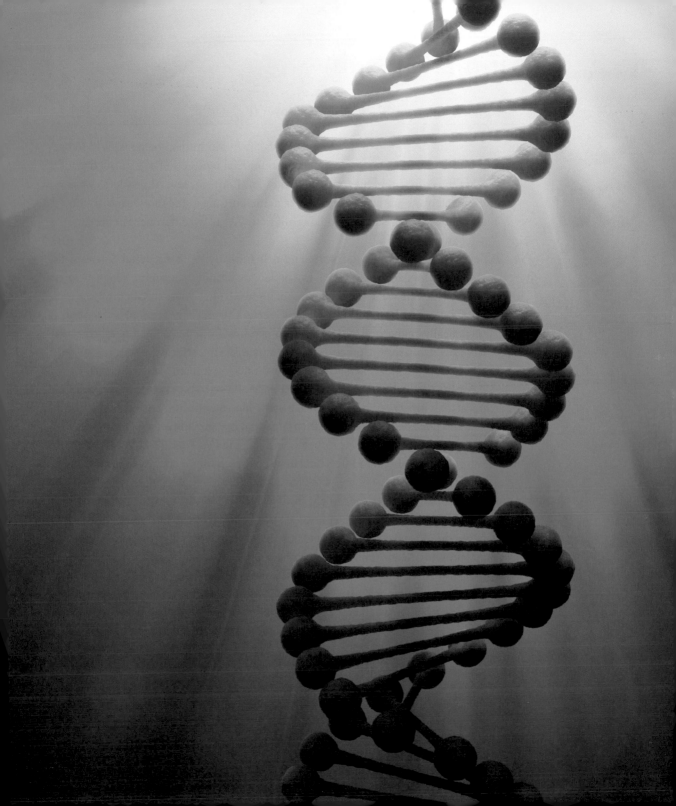

Human Insulin

Frederick Sanger (b. 1918), **Herbert Boyer** (b. 1936)

In 1922, **insulin** was shown to successfully treat diabetes in human patients. Within one year, Eli Lilly and Company began the first commercial production of a purified insulin extract from the pancreas of pigs (porcine) and beef. Early on, several problems were recognized: Scientists predicted a shortage of animal organs in the foreseeable future, and allergy and adverse reactions would result from the subtle differences between human and animal insulin.

A GIANT STEP FOR GENETIC ENGINEERING. In the early 1950s, Frederick Sanger, at the National Institute for Medical Research in London, determined the amino acid structure of insulin, for which he was awarded the first of his two Nobel Prizes in Chemistry in 1958. In 1977, Herbert Boyer of Genentech (Genetic Engineering Technology) produced the first genetically engineered, biosynthetic human insulin in the laboratory, which was licensed to Lilly. Utilizing the process of recombinant DNA technology, Boyer produced the insulin by inserting the genetic code for human insulin into an everyday bacteria. Maintaining the production of insulin to meet the world's needs ceased to be a problem.

Clinical trials in 1981–1982 established that the biosynthetic human and animal-derived insulins possessed comparable effectiveness but that the human insulin was not less likely to cause allergic reactions. Nevertheless, in 1982, the **Food and Drug Administration** and British authorities approved Lilly's human insulin, Humulin—the first approved drug developed by biotechnology but only a modest advance for medical science.

When insulin is injected too rapidly, the diabetic's blood sugar drops precipitously. Early signs of hypoglycemia may be missed, causing the diabetic to lose consciousness and perhaps even die. This has been a particular problem for patients switching from animal insulin to Humulin. More than 95 percent of insulin users in most parts of the world use biosynthetic human insulin, with the remainder using the porcine-derived type.

Biotech drugs—used to treat a variety of disorders including cancers, blood and clotting disorders, multiple sclerosis, cystic fibrosis, and growth deficiency—are among the most exciting new arrivals in medicine. And they all started with human insulin.

SEE ALSO Food and Drug Administration (1906), Insulin (1921), Orinase (1957), Glucophage (1958), Biologic Drugs (1982), Avandia (2010).

This illustration shows a ball-and-stick model of human insulin, which consists of two chains: one with thirty linked amino acids, the other with twenty-one.

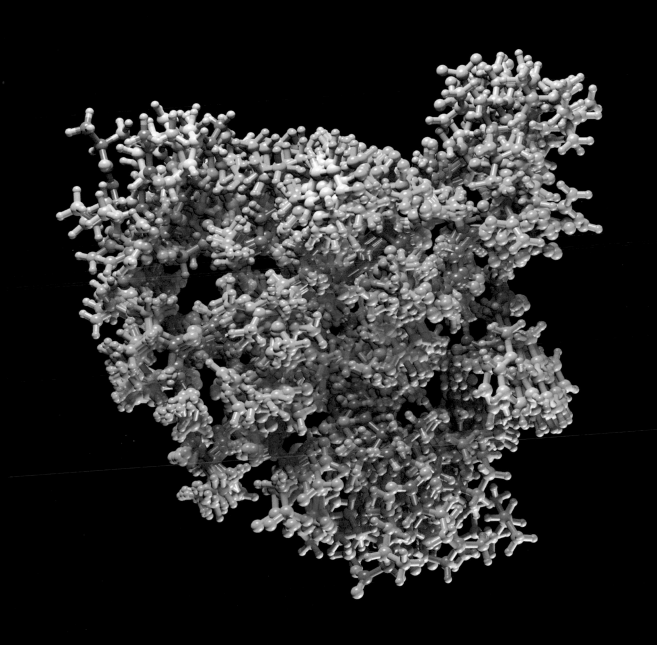

Accutane

Accutane is a highly significant drug for the treatment of severe acne vulgaris, in which the danger of scarring exists. Said to be the greatest advance in the treatment of acne, it often produces complete and long-lasting results after only a single fifteen- to twenty-week course of therapy, but because Accutane's use is associated with major adverse effects, it is only intended for use after other safer treatments have failed.

Acne, the most common skin disorder, results when sebum, an oily substance, is unable to pass through pores to the skin surface. The pores become clogged, infected with bacteria, and inflamed, producing skin eruptions referred to as acne pimples. Severe cases can leave permanent scars.

Mild cases of acne are treated with drugs applied to the skin that either kill the bacteria or unclog the pores. Tretinoin (Retin-A), a derivative of vitamin A, has been used as a topical cream since 1971 for the treatment of acne. In 1982, Hoffman-LaRoche introduced isotretinoin (Accutane, Roaccutane), which is chemically related to tretinoin but far more effective when taken by mouth. It is thought to act, in part, by decreasing sebum secretion.

Accutane's success in the dermatology clinics and marketplace has been more recently counterbalanced by major liability claims. Roche removed Accutane from the American market in 2009, but no shortage of generic equivalents exist. Hundreds of lawsuits are now pending, alleging that Accutane causes Crohn's disease and ulcerative colitis. Since the 1980s, controversy has also existed linking its use to depression and suicide.

No controversy, however, exists about Accutane and pregnancy. Accutane is highly likely to cause a wide range of major birth defects, and, without exception, it should never be used during pregnancy. In 2006, the iPLEDGE program was initiated in the United States to prevent pregnant women from receiving Accutane. To obtain the drug, women must obtain two consecutive negative pregnancy tests and agree to use two forms of contraception when engaging in intercourse. Given the drug's undisputed toxicity to unborn babies, it is mind-boggling that this drug can be purchased online, with no prescription required!

SEE ALSO Thalidomide (1957).

Propionibacterium acnes is a normal inhabitant of healthy skin. Excess sebum production causes pore blockage and provides favorable conditions for the overgrowth of P. acnes, which secretes chemicals that form the acne lesion.

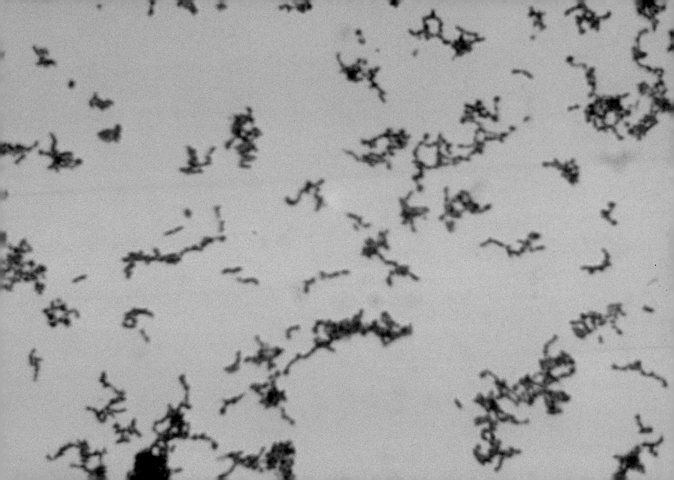

Cyclosporine/Ciclosporin

Hartmann F. Stähelin (b. 1925), Jean-François Borel (b. 1933)

Ancient Chinese and Roman myths tell of leg and heart transplants by healers and saints, but the first documented account dates back to the second century BCE, when an Indian surgeon transplanted skin to rebuild the nose of the recipient. The modern era of organ transplantation began in 1983, when cyclosporine became generally available. Surgeons had, at the time, mastered the basic techniques of transplant operations but were faced with the challenge of dealing with organ rejection, which can lead to transplant failure. Organ rejection results when the immune system of the recipient recognizes the transplanted organ as foreign and attacks it. The threat of such rejection is greatest during the early months following transplantation, although it can occur years later. Rejection involves T-cells and antibody mechanisms.

REJECTING ORGAN REJECTION. Cyclosporine (ciclosporin) acts in numerous and complex ways to suppress this immune response but primarily by interfering with T-cell function. Used to prevent rejection of kidney, liver, and heart transplants, the drug can be administered by intravenous injection (Sandimmune) or orally (Neoral). It is given before the operative procedure and then in progressively smaller doses for the lifetime of the transplanted organ. **Cortisone**-like steroids are often used with cyclosporine to suppress the inflammation associated with transplant rejection.

The most common and serious problem associated with the use of cyclosporine is kidney toxicity. Because this drug depresses the immune system, it makes the patient more susceptible to viral and bacterial infections and to developing certain cancers.

While there is no doubt that cyclosporine, the product of a fungus, was discovered in the Basel, Switzerland, laboratories of Sandoz (now Novartis), credit for its discovery has remained controversial. The primary contenders, both of whom participated in various stages of the development of this drug, are Hartmann F. Stähelin, a Swiss pharmacologist, and Jean-François Borel, a Belgian immunologist. Each of these researchers enjoys his own camp of supporters in the scientific community.

Thanks to cyclosporine and the newer immunosuppressants, organ transplantation has become relatively safe and routine. The greatest current challenge is the shortage of organs.

SEE ALSO Cortisone (1949).

To prevent rejection of a transplanted heart, kidney, or liver, cyclosporine is often prescribed for the rest of a patient's life. The legendary transplantation of a leg performed by Cosmas and Damian, twin brother physicians who were the patron saints of healers, is depicted in this fifteenth-century work.

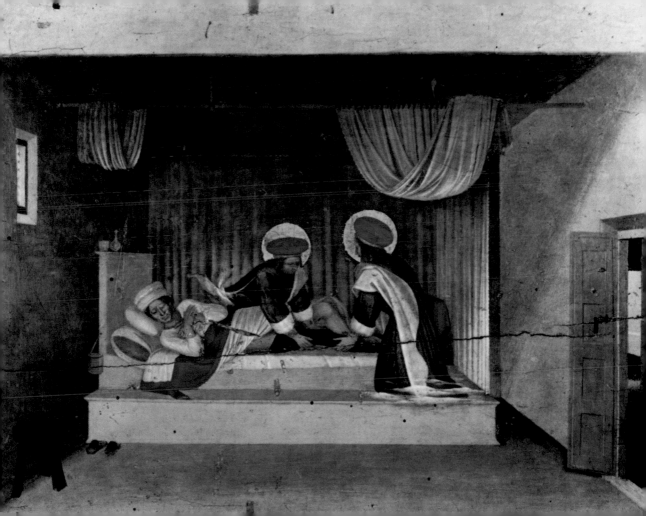

Propofol

Until recently, propofol was a drug known mainly by operating room personnel. In June 2009, propofol's name was on everybody's lips worldwide as the drug responsible for the death of the King of Pop, Michael Jackson.

Propofol is the most widely used preoperative anesthetic given by injection in the United States, replacing **thiopental**, which had reigned supreme for four decades. When injected intravenously, propofol is used to rapidly and gently induce anesthesia before the use of inhaled anesthetics, or it can be given alone by a continuous infusion to maintain anesthesia. Consciousness is lost in less than sixty seconds, and, unlike with thiopental, the patient recovers within minutes after the drug is discontinued and does not experience a hangover. This makes it a very valuable drug for outpatient (day-case) surgery.

Because propofol (Diprivan) can cause sudden and significant depression of breathing and a drop in blood pressure, it must always be used cautiously and in an operating room or facility in which breathing support is available immediately. When taken with **Valium**-related benzodiazepines, such as lorazepam (Ativan), the risk of respiratory depression is heightened.

After weaker sleep-producing drugs ceased to be effective, Michael Jackson's personal physician began giving him propofol for insomnia at the star's home every night for six weeks before his death. In the last days, additional drugs, including lorazepam, were given to facilitate his sleep. His death has been ruled a homicide, and his physician was convicted of involuntary manslaughter for failing to monitor the safe use of propofol, and he was sentenced to a four-year jail term.

The King of Pop was apparently not the only one addicted to propofol; other well-documented reports of abuse and addiction have appeared recently. These have primarily involved anesthesiologists and other operating room personnel who have easy access to the drug.

SEE ALSO Thiopental (1934), Valium (1963).

Propofol, a very commonly used, rapid-acting anesthetic, is administered via IV injection to induce anesthesia, or via IV infusion to maintain anesthesia. This drug should only be administered in a facility equipped to support heart and breathing complications. Michael Jackson, sadly, was not treated with propofol under these conditions.

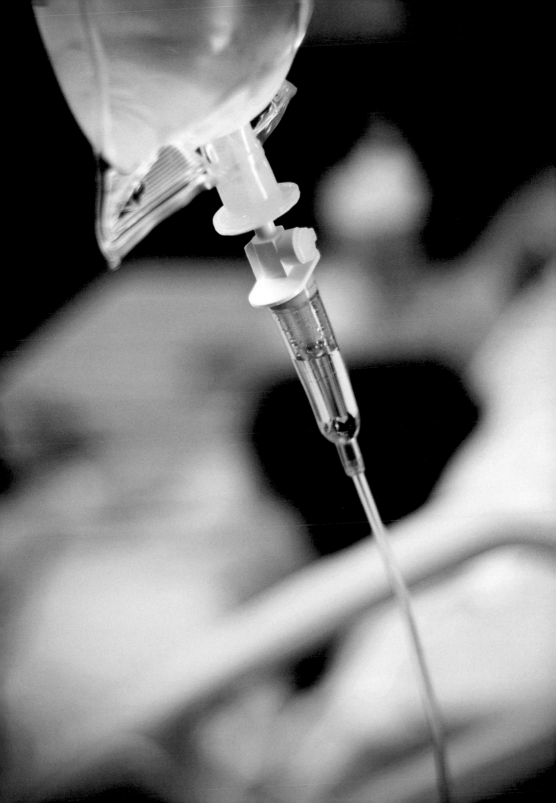

Growth Hormone

Growth hormone (GH) has only one approved medical use: the treatment of GH deficiencies in children and adults. Far greater public interest, however, has focused on its use to reverse the aging clock, to enhance athletic performance, and to breed livestock.

GH is produced by the pituitary gland, a pea-size structure located at the base of the brain. When obtained from human cadavers, pituitary supplies were understandably limited. However, since 1985, abundant supplies have been produced by recombinant DNA technology.

GH is needed for the normal growth of children and to maintain body fat, muscle, and bone in adults. Children with GH-deficiency typically receive six or seven injections each week for at least two years. Many children gain four inches the first year and three inches over the next two years, but not all respond satisfactorily.

Extravagant but scientifically unsubstantiated claims abound promoting the use of GH as an antiaging treatment. In a limited number of carefully controlled studies in healthy, elderly subjects, muscle mass increased and body fat decreased after administration of GH. However, no improvements were found in muscle strength, bone density, cholesterol levels, or other indexes associated with improved fitness.

The International Olympic Committee banned GH use in 1989. Nevertheless, there have been reports of athletes in power and endurance sports at the professional and amateur levels doping with this hormone. GH increases muscle mass and the speed at which injured tissue repairs itself, but there is no evidence that muscle strength is enhanced. Early studies are now underway to refine urine tests that can reliably differentiate between natural and injected GH.

Species-specific GH is commonly used to increase milk production by commercial dairy cows. However, its use to speed the rate of weight gain in cows—and, hence, beef's time to market—has provoked international furor. The United States and Canada favor its use, while the European Union has banned the importation of treated meats since 1988, based on concerns that hormonal residues in meat may increase the risk of cancer and promote the earlier onset of puberty in girls.

SEE ALSO Biologic Drugs (1982), Human Insulin (1982), Epoetin (1989), Antiaging Drugs (2020).

Just as inadequate secretion of GH in childhood leads to individuals of small stature, excessive secretion results in persons whose height is significantly above average. According to ancient scribes, Goliath's height was either 6' 9" (205.7 cm) or 9' 9" (297.2 cm). This David and Goliath fresco appears on a house wall in Regensburg in Bavaria, Germany.

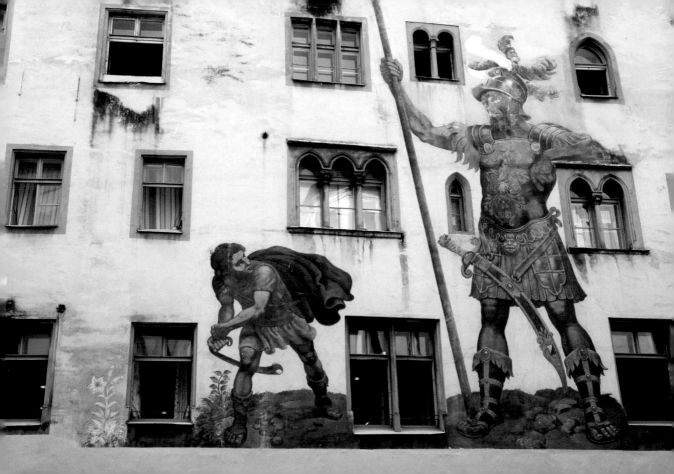

Crack Cocaine

The production, distribution, and sale of **cocaine** are illegal in most countries. Most illicit cocaine is produced in Colombia, with Bolivia and Peru as other major sources. The United States is the largest market for illicit cocaine, followed by Europe.

There are several forms of street cocaine, including the hydrochloride salt, "freebase" (pure), and crack cocaine, which differ in their physical properties and in the way they are taken. The hydrochloride salt can be dissolved in water and is either injected or snorted, whereas the freebase and crack forms are inhaled and absorbed into the blood through the nasal membranes.

Some users prefer to smoke cocaine. By using a highly volatile solvent, such as **ether**, users extract cocaine powder into freebase form, heat it over a fire, and inhale the fumes—an approach that is effective but very dangerous. When ether fumes are exposed to a flame, an explosion can result. In the mid-1980s, users discovered that when cocaine powder was dissolved in water, mixed with either ammonia or sodium bicarbonate (baking soda), boiled, and cooled, solid lumps or "rocks" of cocaine were produced; the resulting "crack cocaine" could be smoked. After inhalation, crack produces intense excitatory and euphoric effects within ten to fifteen seconds. Similar effects appear ten to fifteen minutes after snorting the drug.

Whereas the hydrochloride salt is expensive, crack is very easy to make, relatively cheap—and, hence, widely accessible. The use of crack assumed epidemic proportions in the 1980s. The U.S. Congress responded in 1986 by imposing minimum jail sentences of five years for both the possession of 500 grams (17.6 oz.) of cocaine powder or just 5 grams (.176 oz.) of crack. Over the years, many criminologists have pointed out that this sentencing disparity disproportionately affected blacks, who represent 80 percent of those convicted of crack possession, as opposed to users of powdered cocaine, who are predominately white. In 2010, the law was modified, increasing possession of crack to 28 grams (1 oz.) to trigger a minimum five-year jail sentence and reducing the illegal possession disparity from 100 to 1 to 18 to 1.

SEE ALSO Coca (1532), Ether (1846), Cocaine (1884), Methamphetamine (1944).

A sign posted in a tire repair shop in the Bywater section of New Orleans prohibits loitering, selling crack cocaine, and "cat selling" (prostitution). "NOPD [New Orleans Police Department] will be called."

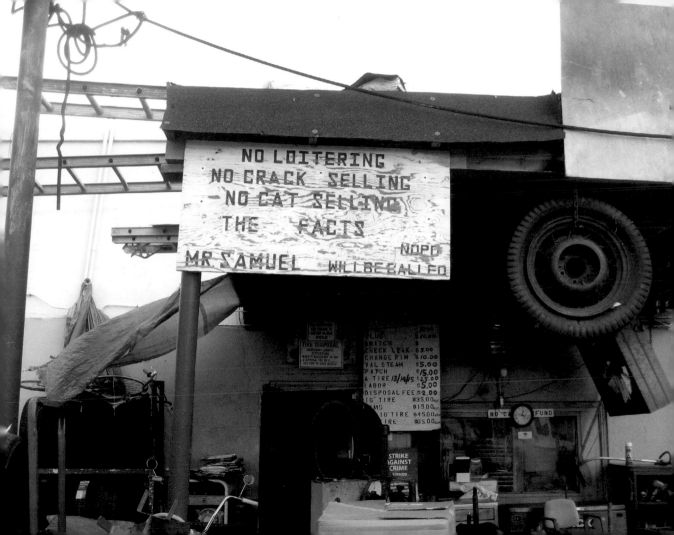

BuSpar

It's part of the human condition to worry about one's health, family, budget, or job. By contrast, generalized anxiety disorder (GAD) is intense worry that occurs frequently and often irrationally about many common day-to-day minor activities and events. GAD is common. In North America, some 3–5 percent of individuals over eighteen years of age experience GAD each year. BuSpar and the benzodiazepine **Valium** (diazepam) are often used to treat this problem.

BuSpar (buspirone), which gained FDA approval in 1986, doesn't chemically resemble the benzodiazepines. It does not have the same effects on sleep, muscle relaxation, or seizures, nor does it appear to cause a dependent state or produce its beneficial effects the way benzodiazepines do. The latter drugs interact with GABA (gamma-aminobutyric acid) receptors in the brain, while BuSpar acts on serotonin receptors. It is a very different drug.

Studies have compared BuSpar with Valium in GAD patients. Valium is highly effective in producing relief after only a few days. What's the problem with it, then? When used over an extended time, which is necessary to successfully treat GAD, Valium has the potential to be abused. BuSpar may not be as effective as Valium in GAD, but it is not sedating, neither is it subject to abuse when taken over many months. BuSpar is not recommended for relief of simple anxiety or panic reactions and must be taken for many weeks before its beneficial effects in GAD appear, however. Until it does work, Valium is sometimes given.

Some drugs interact with other drugs; BuSpar interacts with food. For example, the drug should not be taken with grapefruit juice, which contains chemicals that block liver enzymes that break down BuSpar (as well as statins and many other drugs), increasing its blood levels four-fold, which can result in adverse effects.

SEE ALSO Drug Receptors (1905), Phenobarbital (1912), Valium (1963), Xanax (1981).

There is no shortage of drugs, such as BuSpar, to relieve the stress and worry that people commonly experience in today's society. Drug benefits are relatively rapid but temporary, and a nondrug approach is usually required to produce long-lasting relief.

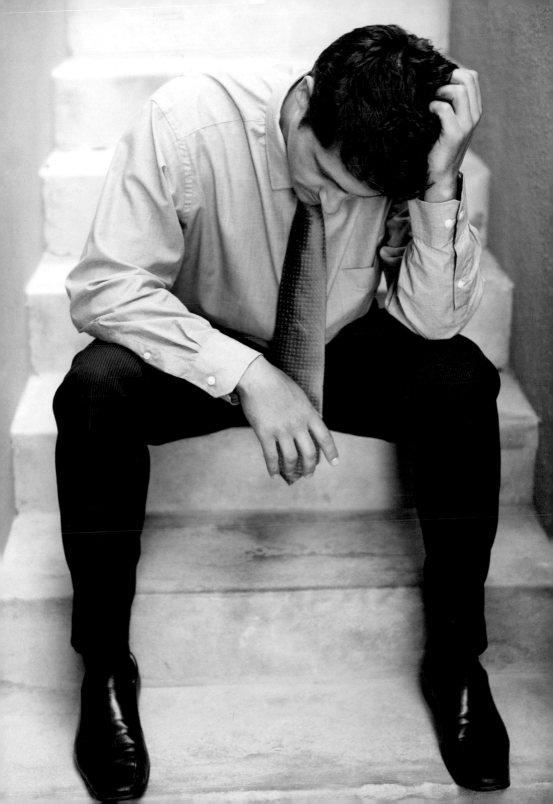

AZT/Retrovir

Jerome Horwitz (1937–2012), **Samuel Broder** (b. 1945), **Hiroaki Mitsuya** (b. 1950)

In 1981, a mysterious disease was sweeping through the gay population of San Francisco and New York. The disease, which devastated the immune system, was caused by the human immunodeficiency virus (HIV) and designated acquired immune deficiency syndrome (AIDS). Once this retroviral target had been identified, the search began for a drug treatment and led to the discovery of AZT (azidothymidine).

In 1964, Jerome Horwitz at the Karmanos Cancer Institute in Michigan initially synthesized AZT as a potential anti-leukemia drug, but it was proven ineffective. It was shown to be active against a retrovirus in the 1970s; but at this time, AIDS was unknown, and there was little interest in retroviruses. All this changed in the early 1980s, when AIDS patients were dying in droves around the world.

The National Cancer Institute (NCI) assumed responsibility for leading the government's efforts to find an AIDS treatment. To this end, the NCI's Samuel Broder conceived of an unusual partnership with the pharmaceutical industry. Companies could send potential compounds to the NCI, where they would be screened for anti-HIV activity. Burroughs Wellcome (now GlaxoSmithKline) had expertise in working with antiviral drugs such as **acyclovir**. In 1984, virologist Martha St. Clair and chemist Janet Rideout were instrumental in identifying and sending AZT to NCI, where Broder and Hiroaki Mitsuya more exhaustively examined it. Their positive laboratory findings were confirmed in AIDS patients at Duke University in 1985—news optimistically received by more than 10,000 AIDS patients. Clinical trials were initiated in January of the following year, and in an incredibly short fifteen months, the **Food and Drug Administration** approved AZT, which was renamed zidovudine and marketed as Retrovir.

This remarkable triumph of drug development and the NCI–Burroughs Wellcome partnership were marred by subsequent disputes over discovery credits, patent rights, and what was perceived to be an exorbitantly high price for the medication. AZT is now an integral component of a successful multidrug combination (**HAART**) used to both successfully treat AIDS and to prevent mother-to-child transmission of HIV during pregnancy and delivery.

SEE ALSO Food and Drug Administration (1906), Acyclovir (1982), HAART (1996), Viread (2011).

The human immunodeficiency virus (HIV), which causes AIDS, is surrounded by red blood cells. Anti-AIDS drugs have been developed to interfere with specific steps in the life cycle of the virus.

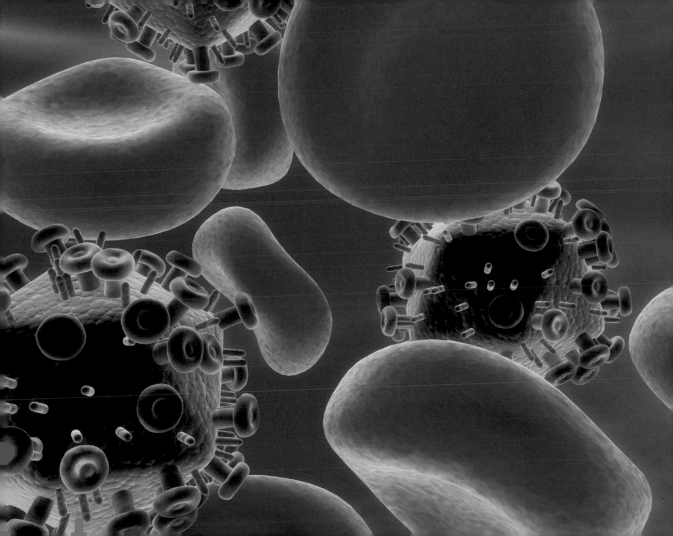

Cipro

Robert Koch (1843–1910)

Bacillus anthracis has long played a conspicuous role in science and warfare. During the 1870s, Robert Koch demonstrated that the microbe *B. anthracis* caused the disease anthrax. Moreover, Koch first noted that this microbe formed spores, permitting it to survive over extended periods under hostile environmental conditions. In 1937, Japanese researchers in occupied Manchuria tested aerosolized anthrax on prisoners and Chinese nationals. During World War II, British and American military scientists evaluated the feasibility of using bombs containing a *B. anthracis* spore payload, but these were never deployed in combat. Inexpensive, easy to produce, readily transportable and hidden, and very highly effective at low concentrations, anthrax is a preferred biological warfare weapon.

PROTECTION AGAINST BIOTERRORISM. In the fall of 2001, anthrax spores were used as a bioterrorist tool in the United States. After being exposed to spore-contaminated letters, twenty-two cases of inhaled and skin anthrax infections were reported, with five fatalities. (Anthrax is not spread from infected persons but rather from contact with or inhalation of anthrax spores.) Faced with a potential bioterrorist attack, some 10,000 persons in the eastern United States were offered the opportunity to take antibiotic therapy to prevent potentially fatal inhalation anthrax. Ciprofloxacin (Cipro) was one of a limited number of antibiotics recommended to protect exposed individuals.

Since its introduction by Bayer AG in 1987, Cipro has been one of several hundred brand names for ciprofloxacin, a member of the quinolone (or fluoroquinolone) class of antibiotics. These drugs have enjoyed great success, both medically and financially. More than twenty quinolones have been marketed worldwide—all bearing the family name *-floxacin* as a suffix—although some have been withdrawn.

Quinolones were initially intended for use as backup for the treatment of respiratory and urinary tract disorders when other antibiotics failed. However, notwithstanding their high cost, their activity against a very wide array of bacteria, relatively low toxicity compared with other antibiotics, and low-dosage frequency (taken one to two times a day), has led to their indiscriminate overprescribing, resulting in the development of bacterial resistance and the quinolone's diminished effectiveness.

SEE ALSO Tetracyclines (1948), Ampicillin (1961).

Cipro is highly effective for the treatment of anthrax (pictured), a potentially deadly infection. Because anthrax spores are easy to produce and effective at low concentrations, they are a choice bioterrorist weapon.

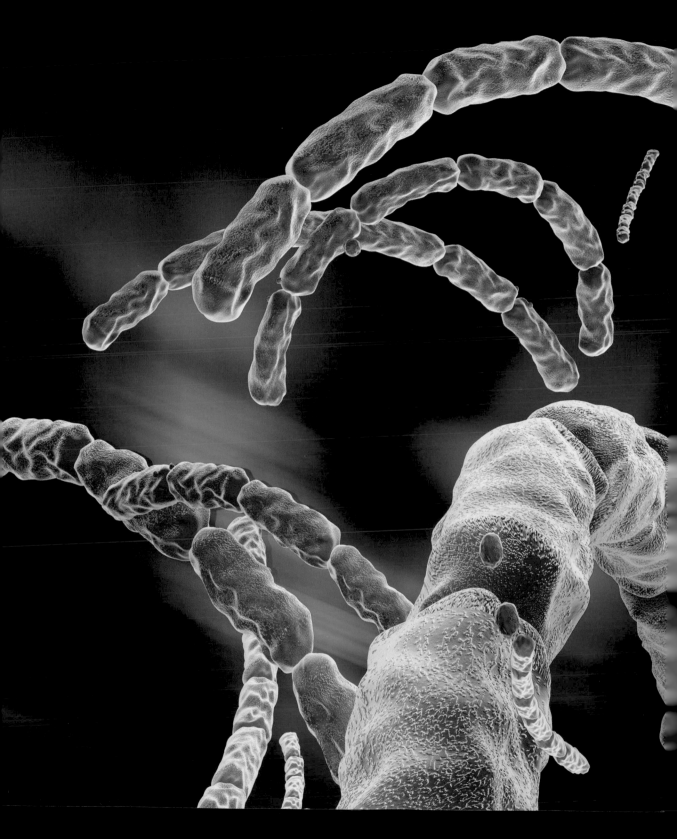

Mevacor

Lipitor (atovastatin), a statin, had sales of more than $12 billion in 2007, establishing it as the best-selling drug in history. Starting with Merck's introduction of Mevacor (lovostatin) in 1987, and now including more than six other similar drugs, the statins are the world's best-selling drugs, with annual sales of $40 billion. These are the most effective drugs currently available to reduce cholesterol.

Cholesterol is formed in the liver, and the statins block a critical step in their manufacture by inhibiting the enzyme HMG-CoA reductase. Statins also speed up the removal of cholesterol from the body. Both effects contribute to the 20–60 percent reduction of cholesterol blood levels seen after they are taken.

Who should receive statins? Elevated levels of cholesterol are a major risk factor for heart attack and stroke, leading causes of death in developed nations. By reducing LDL (bad) cholesterol levels, it's clear that these drugs prevent heart attack, stroke, and the risk of death by as much as 30–40 percent in individuals who have previously experienced a heart attack. In addition, people with increased risk factors for heart attacks, such as those with diabetes and high blood pressure, also benefit from these drugs, even if they have little or no elevation in cholesterol levels.

However, it is highly controversial whether the statins provide benefits to individuals with elevated cholesterol levels but who have not had a heart attack. The JUPITER study, funded by a pharmaceutical company (with vested interests in its positive findings) purported to show protection in this group, but these conclusions may have been biased. Moreover, consider the following: Experts agree that diet and exercise should be the first approach taken to lower elevated cholesterol levels. Failing that, should the statins be made freely available to everyone without a prescription? The answer differs depending on which side of the Atlantic you reside. The UK drug-regulatory agency voted yes in late 2004, while their U.S. counterparts rejected the same proposal months later, based on concern as to whether statins could be used safely in the absence of medical supervision.

SEE ALSO Diuril (1958), Captopril (1981).

Atherosclerosis is a condition in which the walls of an artery thicken because of a cholesterol build-up. This fatty plaque can narrow the vessel's diameter or rupture, causing a blood clot that blocks a blood vessel and increases the risk of heart attack or stroke. Mevacor, an inhibitor of cholesterol synthesis, is the world's all-time best-selling drug.

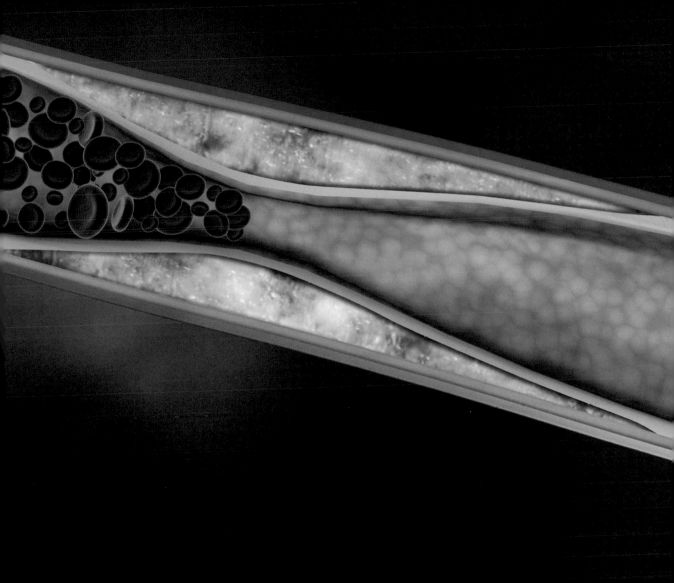

Prozac

Prozac and its half-dozen "band of brothers"—selective serotonin reuptake inhibitors (SSRIs)—are the most commonly prescribed class of antidepressants, in spite of questions regarding their effectiveness. However, there is no question that SSRIs cause fewer side effects and are safer when taken in overdose than the tricyclics.

During the 1970s and 1980s, the link between serotonin and depression became more convincing. Interest focused on the SSRIs, drugs that preferentially increase serotonin at mood-influencing sites in the brain. Prozac (fluoxetine), first approved in 1987 and marketed the following year, was later joined by Celexa, Lexapro, Luvox, Paxil, and Zoloft, plus a generous number of generic equivalents.

The approved medical uses of the SSRI differ somewhat around the world but often include anxiety and panic disorders, obsessive-compulsive disorders (think Lady Macbeth), and clinical depression. When used to treat severe depression, they start producing their beneficial effects in two to four weeks, which is comparable to the tricyclics. To reduce the risk of relapse, a common concern, antidepressants are generally taken for at least six months—and, often, for years—after recovery. Some 20–25 percent of individuals who abruptly stop taking these medications experience SSRI discontinuation (withdrawal) syndrome.

Notwithstanding their marketplace success, the use of SSRIs is embroiled in controversy. Some 30–40 percent of depressed patients receiving **placebos** improve, which complicates studies attempting to objectively demonstrate the effectiveness of SSRIs. Two critical meta-analyses of multiple studies appearing in 2008 and 2010 concluded that, when compared with placebos for the treatment of mild to moderate depression, SSRIs provided little or no benefit. SSRIs were, however, quite effective for treating severe depression. Regulatory agencies in the United States and United Kingdom have concluded that SSRIs can increase suicidal thoughts in children, adolescents, and young adults up to the age of twenty-four, although suicide attempts have not increased. This risk has not been shown for adults.

When Eli Lilly's patent for Prozac expired in 2001, they rebranded Prozac as Sarafem—same drug, different color capsule—at a much higher price than generic fluoxetine for "premenstrual dysphoric disorder."

SEE ALSO Placebos (1955), Tofranil and Elavil (1957), Monoamine Oxidase Inhibitors (1961).

The Professional Humorists' Club, a cartoon by Rea Irvin (1881–1972), appeared in Life *magazine in 1914. In the club's sitting room, various men exhibit sad, depressed, aggressive and angry moods. Irvin was* The New Yorker's *first art editor.*

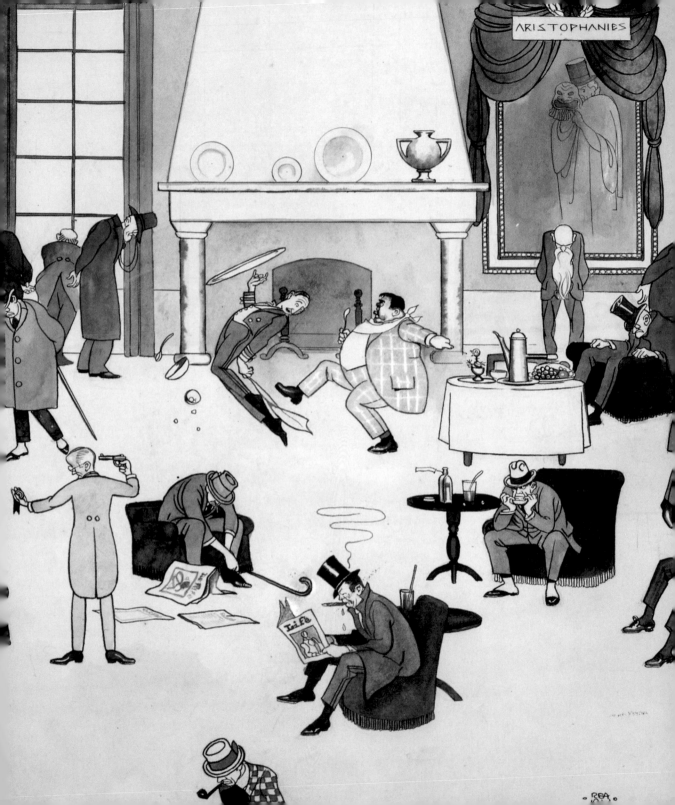

Ivermectin

One of the world's leading infectious causes of blindness is river blindness (onchocerciasis). Some 18 million people are infected with the disease-causing worm, which leaves 300,000 permanently blind and 500,000 suffering from visual impairment. Roughly 99 percent of all these cases occur in thirty countries in sub-Saharan Africa, with the remainder in Yemen and six Latin American countries.

The larva of the microscopic worm *Onchocerca volvulus* causes onchocerciasis, and the disease is spread by the multiple bites from infected blackflies that breed in fast-flowing rivers. Single oral doses of ivermectin (Mectizan, Stromectol), given at six- to twelve-month intervals, prevent the release of and kill the microfilariae (immature worms responsible for the disease), most likely by causing its paralysis. The drug also relieves the painful symptoms of onchocerciasis that affect the skin, and it prevents the disease from progressing to blindness. Ivermectin cannot kill the adult worm, however, neither can it reverse blindness once it has occurred. After the initial course of therapy, this generally well-tolerated drug is given at yearly intervals for ten to twenty years—the lifespan of the adult worm.

Since 1987, Merck, working with international aid organizations, has donated Mectizan. In 2008 alone, some 80 million people were treated, and thanks to this program, an estimated 600,000 cases of blindness have been prevented. There is hope that onchocerciasis will be eradicated in the coming years. However, in 2007, early signs of drug resistance were observed in the parasitic worm, and this could lead to a resurgence of the disease in communities previously thought to be brought under control.

Although the most dramatic effects have been seen in treating onchocerciasis, ivermectin is among the most broad-spectrum antiparasitic drugs for use in humans and animals. In humans, it is effective in treating threadworm and roundworm, as well as scabies and head lice. It is also given to dogs and cats to prevent heartworm and ear ticks.

SEE ALSO Praziquantel (1972), Artemisinin (1972).

The sculpture Gift of Sight *by R. T. Wallen depicts a boy helping an older man afflicted with river blindness. It is located in the World Bank's great atrium in Washington, D.C.*

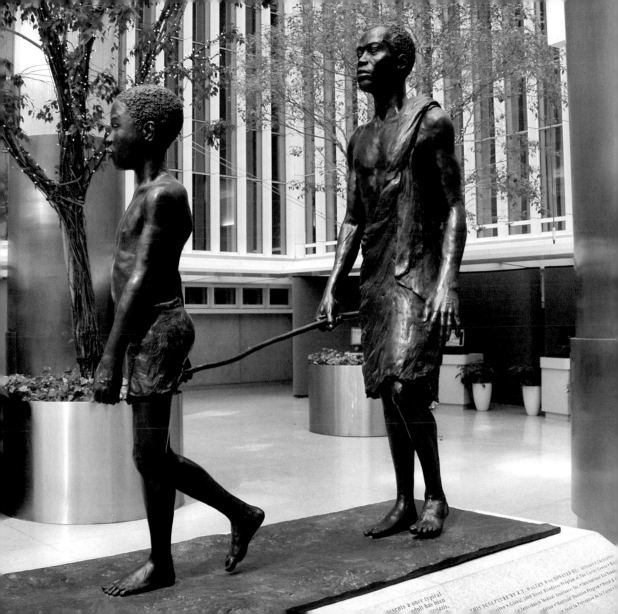

tPA

Désiré Collen (b. 1943)

A delicate balance exists between the ability of the body to control bleeding by forming a clot and the formation of a clot within blood vessels (thrombus) that can interfere with normal blood flow. Blocking blood flow in arteries that supply the heart can cause a myocardial infarction (MI), or heart attack. Similarly, in an ischemic stroke—the most common type of stroke—blood flow to the brain is blocked, markedly reducing the supply of oxygen and glucose and resulting in the death of brain tissue. In Western countries, heart attack and stroke are the leading causes of death, and stroke is second only to Alzheimer's disease as the most common cause of neurological damage.

Drugs can *prevent* clotting in blood vessels by decreasing clot formation (**warfarin**) or by interfering with the clumping of platelets (**aspirin, Plavix**). While these approaches are effective, ongoing heart attacks and strokes require the immediate restoration of blood flow to forestall long-lasting or permanent disability or even death. The odds of surviving after and recovering from a heart attack are greatly improved when blood flow returns within three hours of the time a heart attack begins. To limit the damage and disability associated with strokes, treatment should also begin within three hours of the first symptoms.

Thrombolytic drugs (clot-busters) are used to actively break up or dissolve existing blood clots that interfere with blood flow in the heart, brain, lungs (pulmonary embolism), or deep veins in the leg (deep-vein thrombosis). Normally, after an injury, a fibrin clot forms, plugging an injured blood vessel. Bleeding stops, the blood vessel is repaired, and the clot is dissolved by a natural thrombolytic chemical. This chemical— the enzyme tPA (tissue plasminogen activator)—plays an essential role in the biological process by promoting the conversion of inactive plasminogen to active plasmin, which breaks down the fibrin clot. The medical potential of natural tPA as a clot-buster drug was first recognized in 1980 by the Belgian physician-biochemist Désiré Collen.

Approved in some countries in 1987 for treating stroke and in the United States in 1996, commercial tPA (rtPA; Alteplase), manufactured by recombinant DNA technology, is the most effective and widely used thrombolytic drug.

SEE ALSO Aspirin (1899), Heparin (1916), Warfarin (1940), Biologic Drugs (1982), Plavix (1997), Pradaxa (2010).

A clot blocking the blood flow in the coronary artery is shown here. In an emergency, tPA can be used to dissolve the clot.

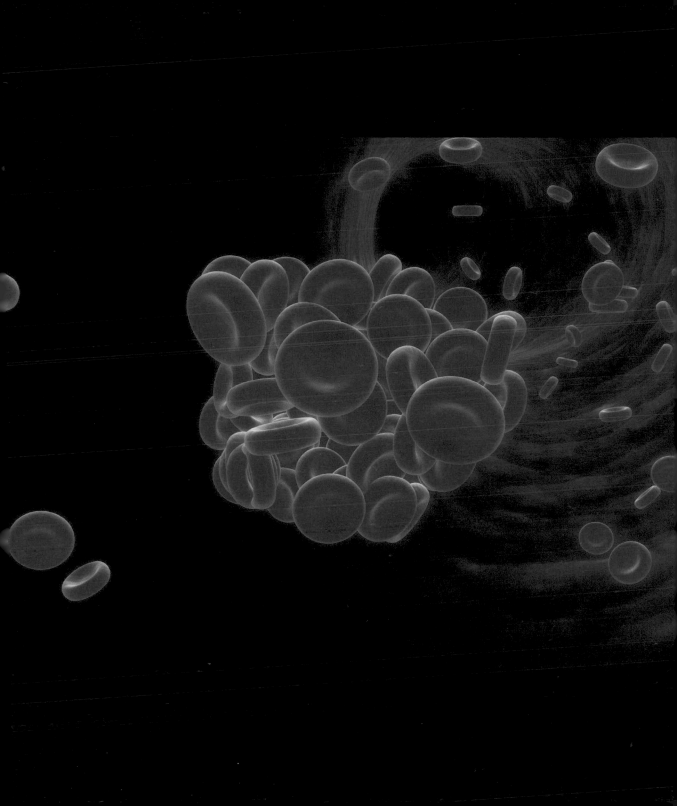

Rogaine

When it appeared on the market in 1979, minoxidil (Loniten) was considered by experts to be a major step forward in the treatment of high blood pressure. It was effective in the most severe cases and in patients who had failed to improve when taking other drugs. These benefits, however, were accompanied by a number of serious adverse effects, including the retention of fluids in the body and major heart problems.

While not dangerous, minoxidil's most interesting side effect, increased body hair growth, was cosmetically off-putting, in particular to women. This problem typically made its appearance within three to six weeks in four out of five patients taking the drug by mouth. Specifically, the body became blanketed with dark hair, starting on the face and progressing to the back, chest, arms, and legs.

Recognizing its commercial potential, Upjohn marketed minoxidil in a solution to be applied to the scalp in 1988. Called Rogaine in North America and Regaine in Europe and Asia, it was the first **Food and Drug Administration**-approved hair restoration product and is now available without a prescription.

Before running out and buying Rogaine and then immediately making an appointment for a haircut, read on: There are many causes of hair loss (alopecia), including medical conditions, hormonal disorders, stress, medications, cancer chemotherapy, and exposure to workplace chemicals. The most common type, androgenic alopecia, is seen in 95 percent of all instances of hair loss and occurs in genetically predisposed individuals.

Rogaine is only useful for androgenic alopecia. It is most effective in restoring hair on the crown of the head in slowly progressing (and not extensive) male- and female-pattern baldness. Past studies revealed that one-quarter of men experienced at least moderate hair growth, and one-third, only minimal growth. However, only one-fifth of women experienced moderate hair growth or better. Early signs of improvement take four months of treatment. Within several months after the medication is discontinued, new hair is lost.

In short, sadly, the cure for baldness has yet to be developed.

SEE ALSO Food and Drug Administration (1906), Diuril (1958), Captopril (1981), Proscar and Propecia (1992).

Rear view of a balding man. If Rogaine treatment proves successful, it might increase hair growth modestly on the crown of his head after four months of daily use.

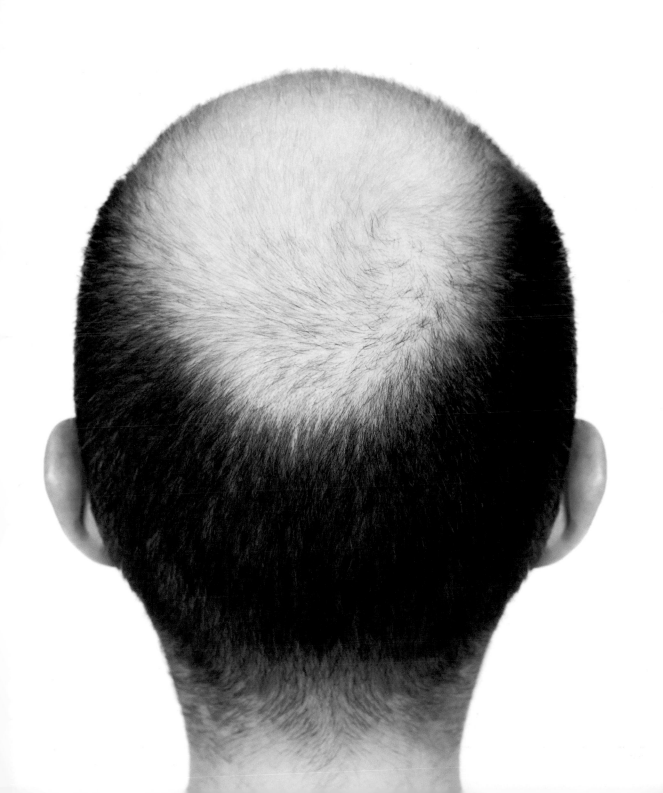

Mifepristone/RU-486

Drugs used for birth control can either prevent pregnancy or terminate pregnancy. These two groups of drugs act in different ways, and the ethical considerations and emotional responses regarding their use have generated varying degrees of controversy. Hormonal contraceptives prevent pregnancy by interfering with the release of the ovum or impairing the ability of the fertilized ovum to attach to the wall of the uterus. Although lower doses of mifepristone can prevent ovulation and be used as an emergency contraceptive (morning-after pill), it is primarily employed as an abortifacient to terminate an established pregnancy. It is the medical alternative to a surgical abortion.

Mifepristone was originally synthesized in 1981 by the French pharmaceutical company Roussel-Uclaf and assigned the designation RU-486. Marketed worldwide as Mifeprex and Mifegyne, it blocks the female hormone progesterone, which the body needs to maintain pregnancy. In 1988, it was approved in France for medical abortions. Many European countries approved its use during the 1990s, and the United States followed in 2000. To avoid antiabortion protests and boycotts in Europe and the United States, the rights to this drug have been commonly transferred to single-product (mifepristone) companies. In the United States, it can only be obtained directly from selected physicians.

In most countries, mifepristone is approved to terminate pregnancies of up to forty-nine days. It is taken in a dosing regimen with the prostaglandin-like drug misoprostol, which causes contractions of the uterus. Within twenty-four to seventy-two hours after drug treatment, uterine contractions occur, resulting in a miscarriage. Mifepristone is about 95 percent effective within two weeks.

Challenges to its approval and use have focused on its safety, adverse effects, and the ethical and religious issues associated with terminating pregnancies by abortions, whether surgical or medical. Almost all women experience abdominal pain, cramping, and vaginal bleeding—sometimes severe—for nine to sixteen days. Unlike surgical abortions, medical abortions can be undertaken in the privacy of the woman's home.

SEE ALSO Estrone and Estrogen (1929), Progesterone and Progestin (1933), Enovid (1960), Plan B (1999).

All pregnancy tests work by detecting human chorionic gonadotropin (hCG), a hormone that is only present if a woman is pregnant. Although home pregnancy tests can be very accurate, a positive test (shown here) may occur when the woman is not pregnant.

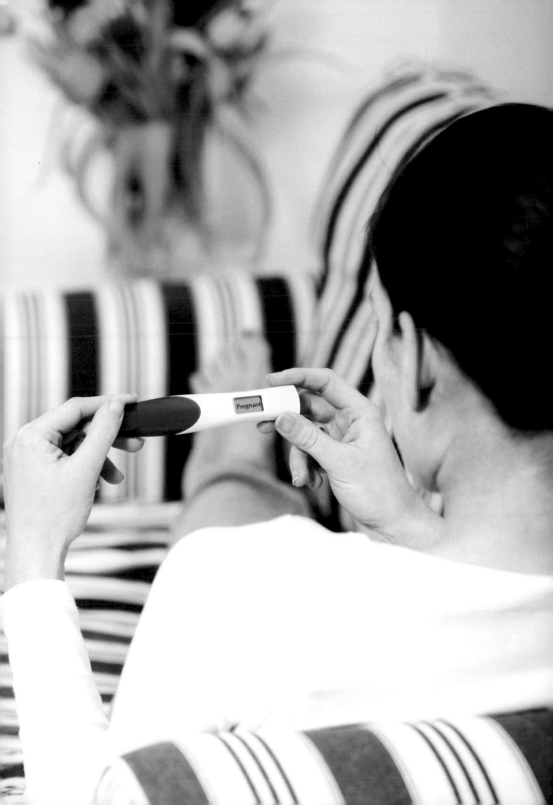

Prilosec

Robin Warren (b. 1937), **Barry Marshall** (b. 1951)

The search for relief from often highly distressful acid-related disorders accounts for the proton pump inhibitors (PPIs) being among the world's best-selling drugs. The PPIs are highly effective and generally safe drugs used for the healing of peptic ulcers and treatment of GERD and heartburn, which afflict half the adult population in Western countries on at least an occasional basis. In 1989, Prilosec (omeprazole), the first PPI, appeared.

Both the PPIs and the histamine H_2 receptor blockers, such as **Tagamet**, reduce the production of stomach acid, although they act in different ways. The PPIs, which reduce the production of gastric acid for longer periods, are more effective and overwhelmingly preferred. Their use is not without hazard, however. In 2010, it was reported that extended use of PPIs increased the risk of fractures involving the wrist, hips, and spine by 25 percent.

Antacids, Tagamet, and Prilosec all produce temporary relief of peptic ulcers although the symptoms return periodically. In 1981, Australian pathologist Robin Warren and physician Barry Marshall provided evidence that nondrug-induced stomach and intestinal ulcers were caused by a *Helicobacter pylori* infection. This bacterial infection is thought to be responsible for 80–90 percent of all such cases. For their work, Warren and Marshall received the 2005 Nobel Prize in Physiology or Medicine. It is now standard treatment to combine an acid-reducing drug with an antibiotic to cure this bacterial infection and prevent a recurrence of the ulcer.

Considering the sales potential of the PPIs, it should not be surprising that their manufacturers have been extremely resourceful in their marketing strategies. Depending on the country where they are sold, some of these drugs require a prescription, while others may be obtained with or without a prescription. Consider another marketing approach: With the expiration of AstraZeneca's patent on Prilosec in 2002, and with far less expensive generic equivalents on the horizon, the company introduced and very aggressively and successfully marketed Nexium to physicians and the public. Nexium is virtually identical to Prilosec, no more effective, not available generically, and far more expensive.

SEE ALSO Flagyl (1959), Tagamet (1976).

This highly magnified micrograph of gastritis (inflammation of the stomach lining) shows an infection of bacteria Helicobacter pylori.

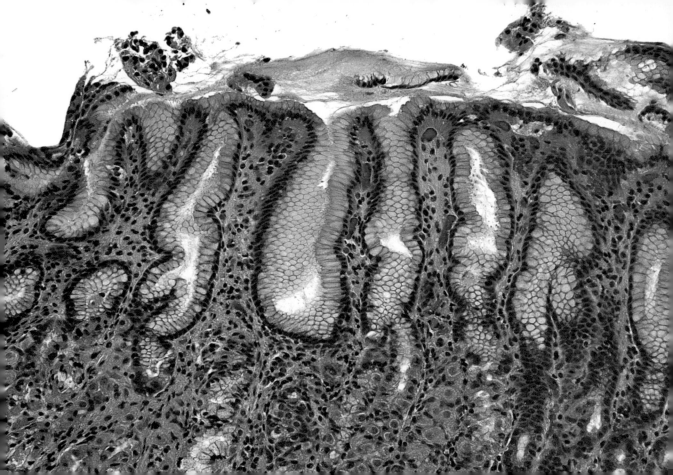

Clozapine

All medicine-taking involves balancing potential benefits vs. real and possible risks. When drugs are used to treat life-threatening or major medical conditions, the willingness of patients to assume these risks becomes greater. Clozapine is an excellent example of a drug that is often effective for the treatment of schizophrenia in many patients who have failed to respond to other drugs. This same drug, however, can cause a potentially fatal blood disorder.

From the start, clozapine was different. It was synthesized in the early 1960s and found to have promising antischizophrenic effects. Unlike **chlorpromazine** (Thorazine) and all similar "typical" antipsychotic drugs then available, it did not cause tremors and rigidity, so-called extrapyramidal symptoms (EPS) that resemble Parkinson's disease. Clozapine was the charter member of the "atypical" second-generation antipsychotic drug class.

Clozapine was first marketed in Europe in 1972, but three years later, it was withdrawn after causing agranulocytosis—a severe lack of infection-fighting white blood cells—and deaths in a number of patients. During the first months of treatment, agranulocytosis develops in 1 percent of clozapine-taking individuals—a risk that decreases over time. With the hindsight appreciation that it was effective when other drugs were not, clozapine (Clozaril) returned to the American and European markets in 1989. However, its use is accompanied by the caveat that blood tests must be conducted at very regular, specified intervals. These tests add considerably to the total cost of therapy.

Clozapine is arguably the most effective of all antischizophrenic drugs, but because of its potential dangers, its use has been greatly restricted. The drug is primarily given to "antipsychotic-resistant patients"—those 30–40 percent of individuals with chronic schizophrenia who are poorly controlled with other antipsychotic drugs. It is also approved for use in schizophrenics who are at high risk of suicidal behavior.

The effectiveness of clozapine has led to the development of newer second-generation drugs (such as **Zyprexa**) that are perhaps not as effective but are safer than clozapine. They are thought to produce their antischizophrenic effects by blocking both serotonin and dopamine receptors in the brain.

SEE ALSO Chlorpromazine (1952), Haldol (1958), Zyprexa (1996).

Don Quixote—the hero of what many authorities consider the greatest of all novels—suffered from delusions and hallucinations, which are classical symptoms of schizophrenia. But what would the world of literature be, had he been successfully treated with clozapine?

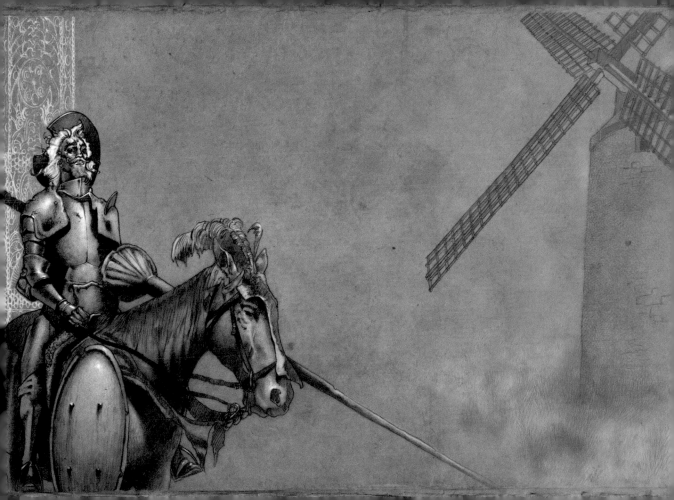

Epoetin

There have been no shortage of reports that competitors in the Tour de France and other high-visibility professional cycling events have been illicitly using an anti-anemia drug, EPO (epoetin alpha), to enhance their performance. When the margin of victory is measured in hundredths of a second, drug effects can provide the edge. However, EPO's primary use is for medical treatment.

Red blood cells (erythrocytes) carry oxygen from the lungs to the cells, where oxygen is used to produce energy. When erythrocyte levels are low (anemia), the blood carries less oxygen, resulting in weakness and fatigue. The hormone erythropoietin stimulates bone marrow to produce erythrocytes. When erythrocyte levels drop as the result of anemia or a shortage of oxygen supply, as might occur in high altitudes, erythropoietin output jumps, triggering an outpouring of erythrocytes into the blood.

Epoetin alpha (Epogen, Procrit) is a protein identical to human erythropoietin that is produced by DNA technology. This biologic drug is used to treat anemia in patients with kidney failure who are currently receiving or awaiting renal dialysis. It can be used to manage drug-induced anemias, such as those caused by **AZT** (zidovudine, Retrovir) in AIDS patients or by certain anticancer drugs. It is also used before and after surgeries to decrease the number of blood transfusions.

In 2012, a growing body of evidence revealed that manufacturer claims that these anemia drugs increased the survival or enhanced "life satisfaction and happiness" of kidney-dialysis patients were grossly exaggerated and that the risks of cancer and stroke were minimized.

"Blood-doping"—the use of red blood cell transfusions to increase blood's oxygen-carrying capacity—has long been used by some athletes in such endurance events as cycling and long-distance running. EPO has been shown to increase oxygen consumption and the time until exhaustion occurs in such endurance events. Unlike other performance-enhancing drugs, there are no reliable EPO detection tests. Its use is not without danger, however. If red blood cell levels become too high, the blood becomes abnormally thick, putting an excessive strain on the heart and potentially resulting in heart failure.

SEE ALSO Ferrous Sulfate (1681), Biologic Drugs (1982), Growth Hormone (1985), AZT/Retrovir (1987).

French baron Pierre de Coubertin (1863–1937) was founder of the International Olympic Committee and father of the modern Olympic Games, the first of which were held in Athens in 1896. He believed that competing was more important than winning. By contrast, the legendary football coach Vince Lombardi famously said, "Winning is not everything, it's the only thing."

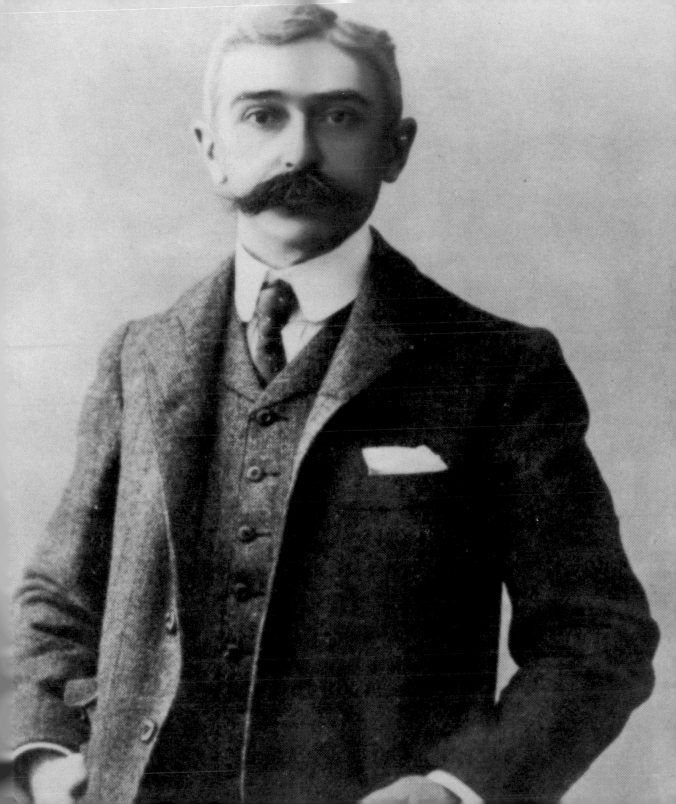

Botox

Jean Carruthers (b. 1949), **Alastair Carruthers** (b. 1945)

FROM FOOD POISON TO WRINKLE REMOVER. Botulinum toxin has undergone a number of reincarnations over the years, from a contaminant in improperly prepared foods, to a laboratory research tool to probe nerve-muscle communication, to a drug to treat problems involving eyes, muscles, and excessive sweating to, most famously, a drug that combats wrinkles for cosmetic purposes.

Food botulism, a rather rare but serious condition, is associated with improperly processed canned or preserved foods. During the nineteenth century, the problem was shown to be caused by a nerve poison produced by the bacterium *Clostridium botulinum*. Botulinum toxin, among the most poisonous of all substances, causes death by paralyzing the breathing muscles. It does this by preventing the release of the neurotransmitter acetylcholine from nerve endings responsible for activating muscles. Military laboratories have taken a keen interest in the toxin because of its potential in biological warfare.

During the 1980s, ophthalmologists employed it successfully to treat "crossed eyes" (strabismus) and "uncontrollable blinking" (blepharospasm), and the **Food and Drug Administration** approved it for these conditions in 1989. Some years later, it was found of value to control spasms of the neck and shoulders (cervical dystonia) and excessive underarm sweating.

During the course of injecting Botox for eye disorders in 1987, Vancouver ophthalmologist Jean Carruthers and her dermatologist husband Alastair accidentally noted that it relaxed the muscles and softened the frown lines between the eyebrows (glabellar lines), which gives the face an angry or tired look. The Carruthers never patented nor cashed in on their billion-dollar discovery, but Allergan, the Botox patent holder, did. Botox Cosmetic (botulinum toxin type A or onabotulinumtoxin A) was approved for this use in 2002. In addition, it is commonly used without the FDA endorsement, to reduce wrinkles on the forehead, lips, and neck, as well as to reduce crow's feet. The benefits are temporary, and repeat injections are needed every four months, at a cost of between $400 and $1,000 per treatment session, to retain or regain that youthful appearance. Expenses notwithstanding, Botox injections are the most commonly performed non-surgical medical procedure.

SEE ALSO Curare (1850), Neurotransmitters (1920), Food and Drug Administration (1906), Off-Label Drug Use (1962).

Botox injections are perhaps the most popular minimally invasive cosmetic procedures. In 2010, about 5.4 million injections were administered to men and women.

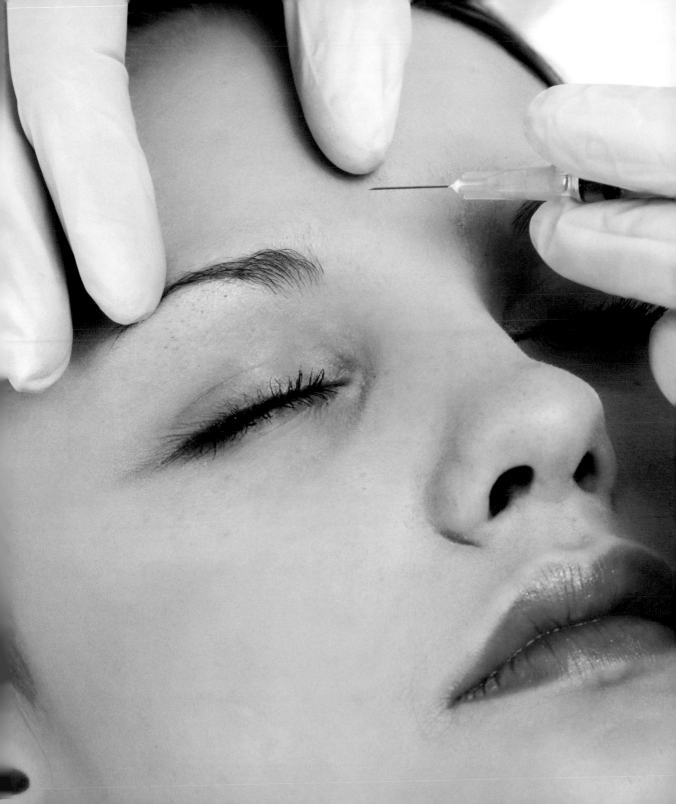

Imitrex

Patrick P. A. Humphrey (b. 1946)

Imagine a pulsating headache, usually on one side of the head, that persists for hours or days on end and that is accompanied by nausea, vomiting, and extreme sensitivity to light and sound. These symptoms often describe a migraine headache that affects some 30 million Americans. Affecting women three times more often than men, these headaches were previously attributed to a widening of the cranial blood vessels in the brain, but recent evidence suggests that these changes may be triggered by alterations in neuronal activity.

Serotonin is a **neurotransmitter** that controls many diverse brain functions, including mood, sleep, sexual behavior, and the widening and constricting of blood vessels. During the 1970s, Patrick Humphrey at Glaxo in England found that injections of serotonin alleviated migraine pain but, because of its actions at multiple serotonin receptor sites, produced many undesirable effects. His efforts led to the identification of a previously undiscovered serotonin receptor subtype that is primarily (but not exclusively) located in cranial blood vessels. Humphrey's next step was to develop a drug that acted on this serotonin receptor subtype to cause constriction of blood vessels that were distended during a migraine attack.

This drug was sumatriptan (Imitrex), approved for use in the United States in 1991. It is highly effective in terminating a migraine in some 70 percent of patients after being injected under the skin, taken by mouth, or used as a nasal spray. The triptans, of which Imitrex was the first of some half-dozen, have almost entirely displaced ergotamine, used since the 1920s but which caused many side effects. Triptans, however, are not effective for preventing the onset of a migraine attack.

Imitrex selectively constricts cranial blood vessels, but *selective* is not the same as *specific*. The same serotonin receptor subtype in the brain is also present in the coronary arteries that supply blood to the heart muscle. Imitrex can cause constriction of the coronary artery, which, in individuals with or at risk of heart disease, has led to heart attacks—sometimes with a fatal outcome.

SEE ALSO Drug Receptors (1905), Neurotransmitters (1920), Ergotamine and Ergonovine (1925).

Alice's Adventures in Wonderland, *was written by Lewis Carroll (Charles Lutwidge Dodgson) and illustrated by Charles Robinson. It has been suggested that the migraine aura (visual hallucinations) Carroll experienced may have served as an inspiration for his* Alice *books. If true, would Alice have existed if Carroll took Imitrex?*

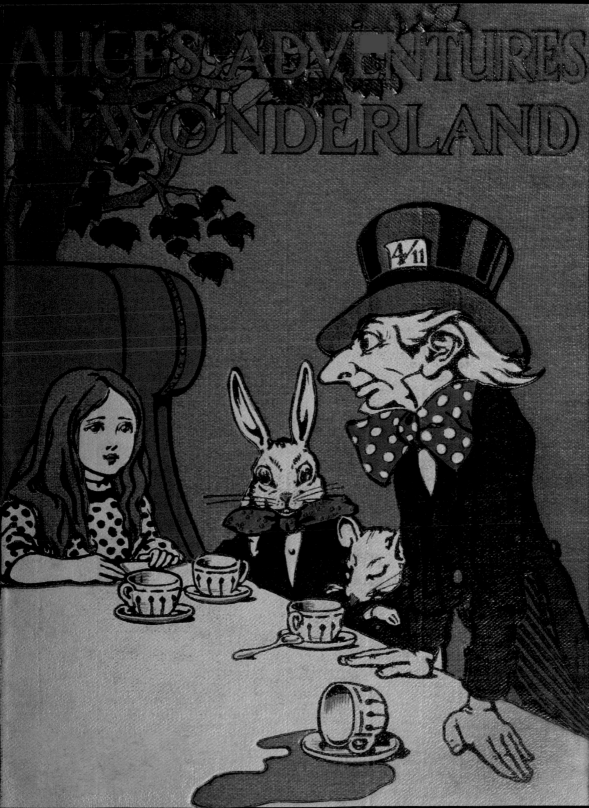

Nicotine Replacement Therapy

Scientific evidence linking smoking and lung cancer did not appear until the 1950s, although the link was long suspected. Over the years, aggressive and generously funded efforts by the tobacco industry attempted to suppress, obfuscate, and manipulate the research findings associating smoking with cancer, cardiovascular disorder, and pulmonary disorders. Experts now agree that cigarette smoking is the single most preventable cause of death and disease and that it is "the most important public health issue of our time."

The vast majority of cigarette smokers recognize the health hazards of smoking, and some 80 percent would eagerly kick the habit if they could. However, smoking is among the most difficult addictions to wrest free of, with most ex-smokers returning to smoking multiple times before quitting for life.

Nicotine is the addictive chemical in tobacco products. Its absence among erstwhile quitters is responsible for such nicotine withdrawal effects as irritability, difficulty concentrating and sleeping, depression, and increased appetite leading to weight gain. These effects may persist for weeks. Smokers have learned that nicotine craving and withdrawal can be prevented or readily suppressed by smoking or by taking nicotine.

First available in 1991, nicotine replacement therapy (NRT) provides this source of nicotine as a gum, transdermal patch, nasal spray, or inhaler. Unlike the immediate but transient pleasurable effects experienced after each puff of a cigarette, with NRT products, nicotine levels in the body remain constant throughout the day. As there are no major differences in the relative effectiveness of any of these approaches, it's a matter of personal preference which method is selected. When used in conjunction with a smoking cessation program, the chances of quitting are doubled. Although this sounds impressive, after one year, only 20–25 percent of smokers have been reported to have successfully quit, and the results of studies conducted in 2012 have even questioned whether NRT produces any long-term benefits. Although all NRT approaches cause side effects, these effects are far less harmful to health than continued smoking. The search continues for a safe and effective smoking cessation product.

SEE ALSO Methadone (1947), Chantix/Champix (2006).

Nicotine replacement therapy is intended to substitute harmful sources of nicotine, such as cigarettes, with less harmful sources, such as nicotine gum. These replacement products reduce cigarette cravings and nicotine withdrawal effects.

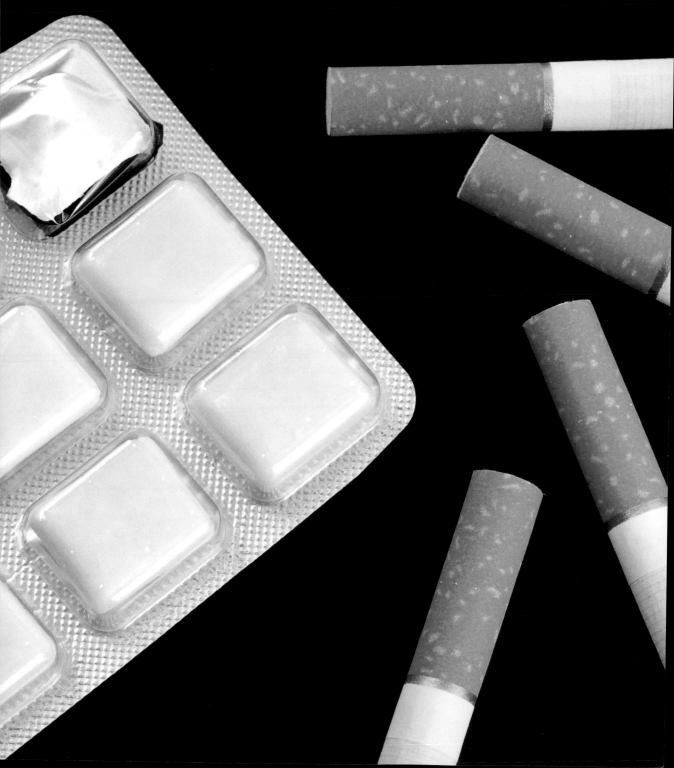

Neupogen

One of the great challenges patients receiving cancer chemotherapy and some anti-AIDS drugs face is their increased susceptibility to infections. Many of these drugs depress bone marrow, the site of blood-cell production. One of these blood cells is the neutrophil—the body's primary defense for fighting infections caused by bacteria and some fungi—which constitutes 50–70 percent of all white blood cells.

The production of white blood cells of the granulocyte type, of which the neutrophils are the most plentiful, is controlled by granulocyte colony-stimulating factor (G-CSF). Neupogen (filgrastim), a product of recombinant DNA technology, is produced in the bacterium *Escherichia coli* and differs only very slightly from human G-CSF. This biologic drug is used to treat neutropenia, an abnormally low level of neutrophils in the blood. The most common causes of neutropenia are some chemotherapy drugs or radiation used for cancer treatment—for which Neupogen was first approved in 1991—and **AZT**, an anti-AIDS drug. Neupogen is also given to stimulate granulocyte production in individuals either receiving or donating stem cells or after receiving a bone-marrow transplant.

Additionally, Neupogen is used to treat children and adults with severe chronic neutropenia. This rare, inherited condition is associated with a very pronounced reduction in neutrophils, causing the individual to experience very frequent and severe infections, with potentially life-threatening consequences. Gum disease, with a loss of permanent teeth, is also a common problem.

Neupogen provides yet another example of a potentially lifesaving drug that spares hospitalization and associated medical expenses—at a high personal cost. Neupogen speeds up the production of granulocytes that have been depressed, and within twenty-four hours after its injection, neutrophil levels increase. This reduces the incidence of infections and the need for intravenous antibiotics, necessitating fewer hospital admissions and shorter hospitalization periods when they occur. Unfortunately, these beneficial effects are transient, and the drug must be injected on a daily basis at an annual cost of $15,000–$20,000, which may not be covered by insurance.

SEE ALSO Amethopterin and Methotrexate (1947), Chloramphenicol (1949), Biologic Drugs (1982), AZT/Retrovir (1987).

A neutrophil (white blood cell) is defending the body by engulfing the invading anthrax bacteria.

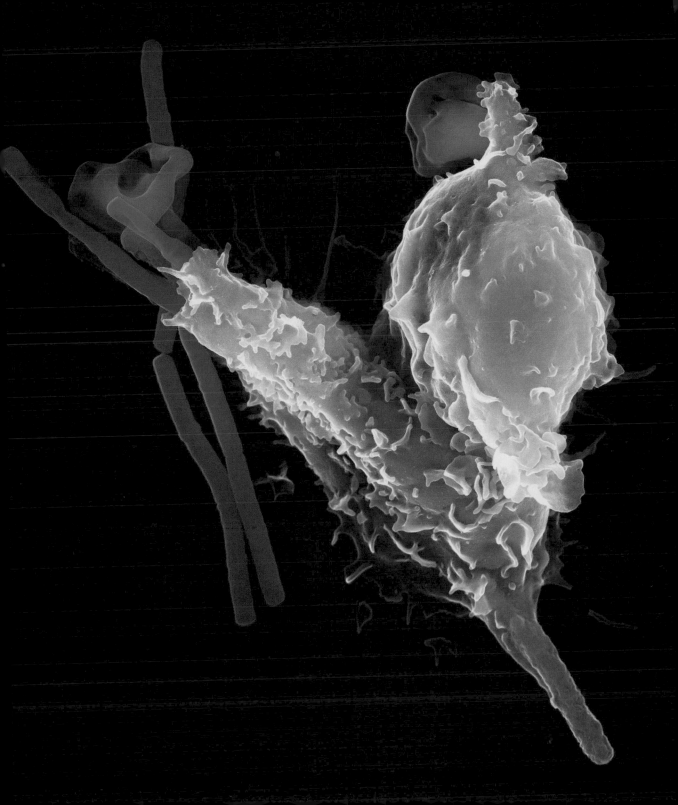

Proscar and Propecia

On the surface, you might very reasonably wonder what the prostate gland and hair have in common. The link is the hormone dihydrotestosterone (DHT), which is formed in the body from **testosterone**, the male hormone. DHT plays a critical role in the growth of the prostate gland and in causing male-pattern baldness—both problems of concern to aging males.

The drug finasteride blocks the enzyme responsible for the formation of DHT. Merck markets this same drug, taken only by men, as Proscar (1992) when used for prostate problems and as Propecia (1996), at a lower dose, for male-pattern baldness.

First, a little background: At the climax of male sexual stimulation, the ejaculate contains the prostate gland secretion that increases sperm movement and promotes egg fertilization by neutralizing fluids in the vagina. In young men, the prostate is walnut-size, but after age fifty, it begins to grow. This noncancerous enlargement is called benign prostatic hypertrophy, or BPH. As BPH progresses, it compresses the urethra—the tube draining urine from the bladder and out the body—decreasing how much can be urinated on each occasion and greatly increasing how often the urge to urinate occurs.

When taken over a six-month period, Proscar gradually shrinks the prostate gland and improves the symptoms of BPH, including increased urine flow. The drug also serves as a safer alternative to BPH surgery. However, Proscar's ability to prevent prostate cancer remains unclear.

High levels of DHT also cause hair follicles to shrink, leading to male-pattern baldness, which affects almost half of men by age fifty. Propecia restores hair growth and prevents further loss, primarily on the crown of the head. Have no fear: the hair will not grow to cover the eyes. The effects of Propecia are modest, with only about half the men showing what consumers would generally consider to be reasonable hair growth.

Both Proscar and Propecia must be taken indefinitely. Once their use is discontinued, the prostate resumes increasing in size and hair is, once again, lost.

SEE ALSO Testosterone (1935), Rogaine (1988) Flomax (1997).

Balding by the age of 23, Louis XIII (1601–1643) popularized wigs in the French court—a fashion that soon swept throughout Europe and remained in vogue for almost 200 years. Wigs were worn by women and men and viewed as symbols of wealth and status.

1992

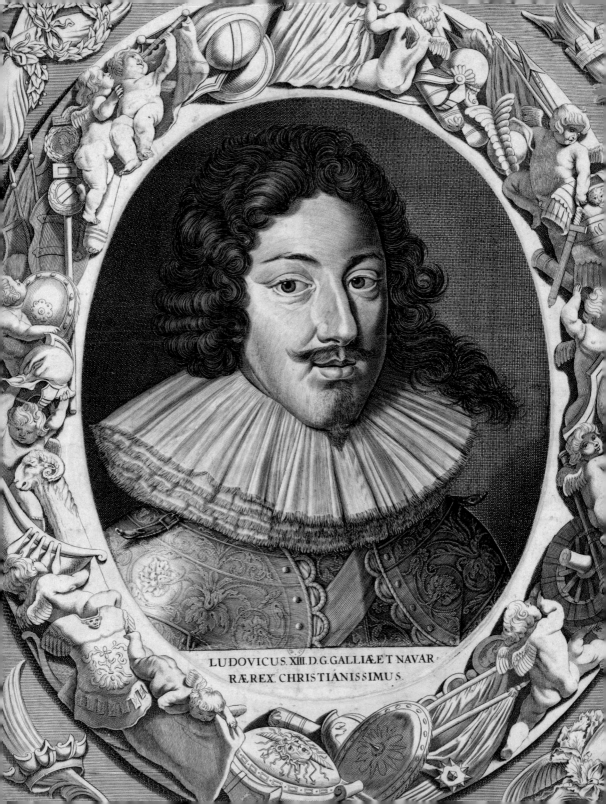

LUDOVICUS. XIII. D.G. GALLIÆ ET NAVAR
RÆ. REX. CHRISTIANISSIMUS.

Ambien

Normal sleep consists of two primary stages that cycle four to six times during the night: non-rapid eye movement (NREM) sleep—about 70–75 percent of total sleep—and rapid eye movement (REM) sleep, during which dreaming occurs. Hypnotics are a class of drugs taken to treat insomnia, a condition in which there is difficulty in falling asleep, staying asleep, or early morning awakening. The ideal hypnotic induces a state that resembles natural sleep and does not alter these phases. The **bromides**, barbiturates, and benzodiazepines all increase the amount of time spent in NREM sleep and decrease REM sleep. However, when the drugs are suddenly discontinued, the body attempts to catch up on lost REM time—a "REM rebound"—leading to excessive dreaming and sleep disturbances.

Two Z drugs, zolpidem (Ambien, 1992) and the newer zaleplon (Sonata, 1999), are distinct from benzodiazepines but act at the same benzodiazepine receptor that is involved with sleep. Both drugs shorten the time for sleep to occur, and Ambien increases the total sleep time. These drugs have several advantages over such sleep-promoting benzodiazepines as estazolam (ProSom), flurazepam (Dalmane), and triazolam (Halcion). The Z drugs do not appear to disrupt normal sleep patterns and cause minimal hangover residual drowsiness and depression the following day. Tolerance and physical dependence have been reported after the use of Ambien, however, so this drug is only recommended for short-term (less than four weeks) treatment of insomnia.

Instances of sleepwalking, in which individuals drive cars, cook, carry on complex conversations, or engage in sex, have been reported after taking Ambien and related drugs. U.S. Representative Patrick Kennedy (D-RI) crashed his car into a security barricade near the Capitol building at 2:45 a.m. in 2006 after taking two drugs: Phenergan, a heavily sedating drug being used for a stomach disorder, and Ambien. Shortly after this event, he admitted himself to a drug rehabilitation program to treat his addiction to prescription pain medications.

SEE ALSO Bromides (1857), Chloral Hydrate (1869), Paraldehyde (1882), Barbital (1903), Phenobarbital (1912), Nembutal and Seconal (1928), Librium (1960), Valium (1963).

The Office of War Information, operating from 1942–1945, assembled war news for domestic consumption and, using posters such as this one, endeavored to promote patriotism and increase worker productivity to support the war effort.

Federal Security Agency
U. S. PUBLIC HEALTH SERVICE

H. PRICE

Plenty of sleep

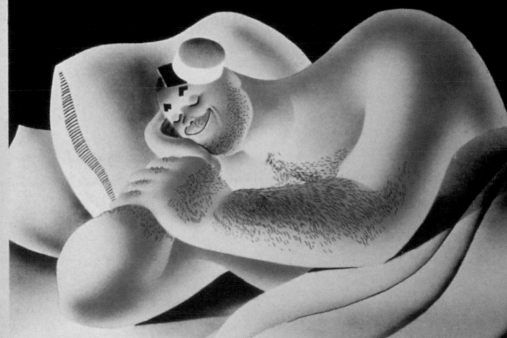

keeps him on the job

Cognex and Aricept

For many seniors citizens, the greatest fear is not heart disease, cancer, or stroke, but rather Alzheimer's disease (AD). AD is responsible for two-thirds of all cases of dementia, a slow and progressive decline in mental function leading to an impairment of memory, thinking, and reasoning. The risk of AD increases with age, but is not an inevitable consequence of aging. "Only" some 30 percent of people older than eighty-five are affected. Former president Ronald Reagan was formally diagnosed with AD at the age of eighty-three and became its public face when he notified the nation in 1994 that he was beginning "the journey that will lead me into the sunset of my life."

Although it may be suspected, proof of AD can only be established by postmortem examination of a brain with fragments of protein, clusters of dead and dying nerve cells surrounding a beta-amyloid protein fragment, and degenerated nerves. Among the most significant losses are those of cholinergic nerves, in which acetylcholine, a **neurotransmitter**, carries messages. Efforts have been directed toward increasing the brain concentration of acetylcholine, which would prevent its breakdown by blocking the enzyme cholinesterase.

Cognex (Tacrine), a cholinesterase inhibitor, has had a tumultuous history before and after its 1993 approval for the treatment of mild-to-moderate AD. Only 30 percent of patients benefit, and their benefits are modest and transient. At best, the drug slows the disease's progression and the loss of memory and cognitive function by months. It can cause severe abdominal pains, cramps, and, more important, liver toxicity. This, combined with the need to take Cognex four times per day, has led to its replacement by Aricept.

Aricept (donepezil), introduced in 1996, is thought to be more effective than Cognex for mild-to-severe AD. Taken only one to two times daily, it causes fewer side effects and no liver toxicity, but the search continues for drugs that prevent or stop the progression of AD and its associated cognitive decline.

SEE ALSO Physostigmine (1875), Neurotransmitters (1920), Anti-Alzheimer's Drugs (2014), Smart Drugs (2018), Antiaging Drugs (2020).

The official portrait of President Ronald Reagan was taken in 1981. Reagan, who served as president from 1981 to 1989, was formally diagnosed with Alzheimer's disease in 1994 and died ten years later. Since Reagan's diagnosis, his wife, Nancy Reagan, has been a public advocate for stem-cell research, which she believes could lead to a cure for AD.

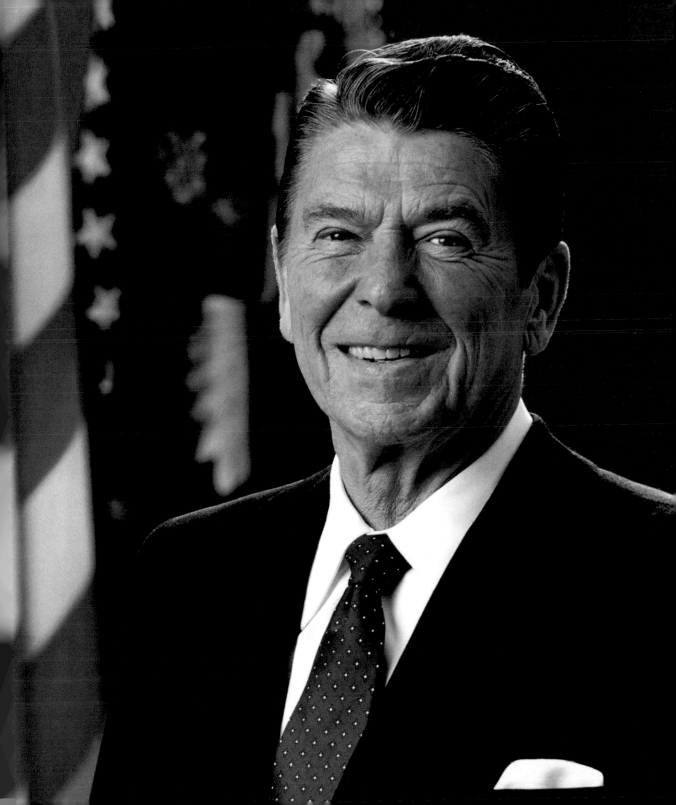

1993

Claritin

Benadryl and other earlier antihistamines developed during the 1940s and 1950s are very effective in treating allergies. However, if after taking these drugs you become drowsy during the daytime when trying to think clearly and drive attentively, is the relief worth it?

In 1986, the first non-sedating antihistamine, terfenadine (Seldane, Triludan), was brought to market. This newer, second-generation antihistamine did not cause drowsiness, because changes in its chemistry prevented it from entering the brain. Seldane was an effective drug, but because of its risk of causing a rare-but-life-threatening effect on heart rhythms, it was removed from the market in 1997.

During the intervening years, and after minor gun battles with the Food and Drug Administration (FDA), Claritin (loratadine) was approved in 1993. Four years later, the FDA modified its existing rules and permitted the **direct-to-consumer advertising** (DTCA) of prescription drugs. Among the first companies to take advantage of this change was Schering-Plough, which, in 1998, hired Joan Lunden—the former host of ABC TV's *Good Morning America*—to serve as spokesperson for a $40 million DTCA campaign for Claritin. Claritin sales rose 50 percent that year, raising $2.3 billion, and an additional 30 percent the following year. These ads ended when Claritin lost its patent protection in 2002, and generic equivalent drugs appeared. All was not lost for Schering-Plough, however: Claritin became available as a nonprescription drug that year.

What does it matter to the consumer if drugs, such as antihistamines, become available on a nonprescription basis? On the plus side, we can save time and money by avoiding a visit to their doctor and filling a prescription. On the minus side, there is no healthcare review of drug use, and insurance companies do not typically provide benefits for nonprescription drugs. Although Claritin and other second-generation antihistamines cause less drowsiness and are longer-acting, they are more expensive, and many experts do not believe that they work as well as the older first-generation drugs in treating allergies.

SEE ALSO Food and Drug Administration (1906), Neo-Antergan (1944), Benadryl (1946), Direct-to-Consumer Ads (1997).

Dust mites are among the most common causes of year-round allergies and asthma. These microscopic, eight-legged arachnids deposit waste products, which produce nasal symptoms of allergy or asthma when inhaled.

434

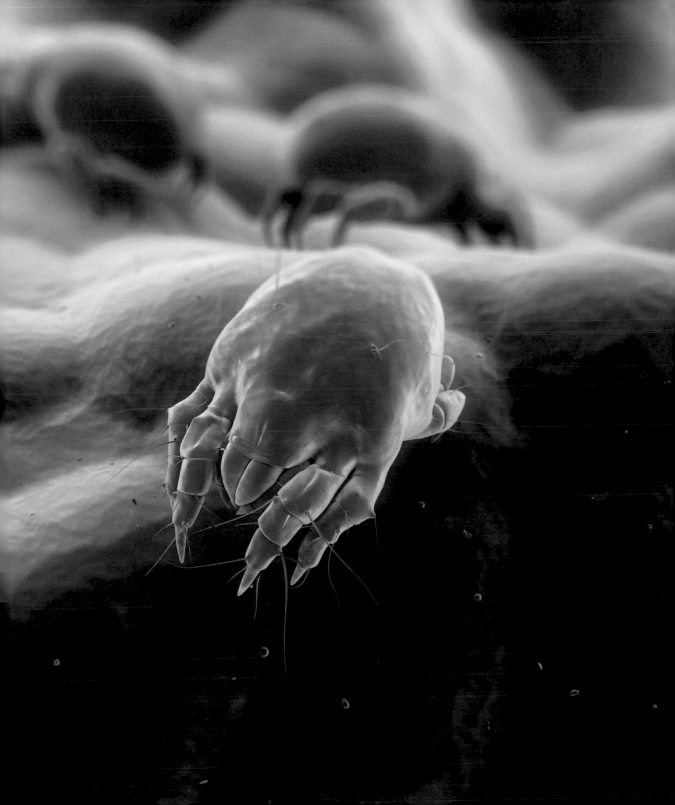

Ephedra/Ephedrine

Nagayoshi Nagai (1844–1929), **Ko Kuei Chen** (1898–1988)

When we think of traditional Chinese medicine, Ma Huang (*Ephedra sinica*) comes to mind. This drug, which may be the oldest medicine in continuous use, has been used in modern medicine; but more recently, it has been considered a potentially hazardous dietary supplement and a starting material for the manufacture of **methamphetamine**.

Teas prepared from the stems of *Ephedra sinica* date back to China some 5,000 years ago, when they were used to treat asthma, hay fever, and nasal congestion. In North America, Native Americans and Spaniards living in the southwestern United States used ephedra to treat sexually transmitted diseases.

Ephedra's active chemical, ephedrine, was isolated in the 1880s by the Japanese chemist Nagayoshi Nagai and was introduced into Western medicine in 1927 by the Chinese American pharmacologist Ko Kuei Chen. Ephedrine has had many uses over the years, including in the treatment of heart block and urinary incontinence; but most notably, it has been used to prevent asthmatic attacks.

Ephedra was in the twilight of its use as a medicine when it reappeared in 1994 in hundreds of dietary supplement products (as Metabolife 356), promoted for weight reduction and to enhance athletic performance. Ephedra alone or in combination with **caffeine** produces modest weight loss when taken over a period of four to six months. It is thought to act by speeding up the rate of metabolism. Evidence is lacking supporting the claim that ephedra, a stimulant banned in Olympic competition, enhances athletic performance.

Soon after its appearance, reports surfaced linking ephedra's use to heart attacks, strokes, seizures, and psychiatric disturbances. Unlike drugs, **dietary supplements** can be marketed in the United States without demonstrating that they are safe or effective. In 1997, the **Food and Drug Administration** began a decade-long successful effort to ban ephedra's sale, which was vigorously opposed by the supplement industry via congressional lobbying and in the courts. Public sentiment shifted to agree with the FDA in 2003, when Baltimore Orioles pitcher Steve Bechler died of heatstroke in which ephedra played a role.

SEE ALSO Epinephrine/Adrenaline (1901), Food and Drug Administration (1906), Methamphetamine (1944), Dietary Supplements (1994).

Traditional Mongolian Medicine (TMM) is based on the principles of Tibetan medicine and Tibetan Buddhism. Since the second half of the twentieth century, the practice of TMM has been revived, as has interest in indigenous medicinal plants. This Mongolian stamp (c. 1986) depicts Ephedra sinica *and is one in a series devoted to flowers.*

MONGOLIA

EPHEDRA SINICA

НАНГИАД ЗЭЭРГЭНЭ

40 ₵

МОНГОЛ ШУУДАН

1986

Dietary Supplements

As you peruse the shelves of your favorite pharmacy or health food store, you will find a group of products that closely resemble drugs but are not drugs. They contain one or a combination of vitamins, minerals, **herbs** or other botanicals, and amino acids intended to supplement the diet.

Many individuals worldwide report that they are using such dietary supplements (DS) as St. John's wort, echinacea, or black cohosh, as well as vitamins. The reasons why they use DS in addition to or instead of drugs are varied, but many consider them to be cheaper, more effective (they "restore health naturally, not with artificial chemicals"), and safer (which is not necessarily true).

The Dietary Supplement Health and Education Act (DSHEA), enacted in the United States in 1994, established the ground rules for DS, including how they differ from drugs and how the **Food and Drug Administration** views them. Drug products can claim to diagnose, cure, treat, or prevent disease. By contrast, the FDA considers DS to be foods that can claim to improve health by reducing the risk of disease. DS can also describe how the product benefits the organs or systems of the body (a "structure/function" claim) but cannot refer to a specific disease. It permits the claim that "calcium builds strong bones" but not that it can "prevent or treat osteoporosis."

Drugs must be proven to be safe and effective before the FDA grants them approval to be marketed. Manufacturers of DS are not required to submit such evidence or obtain approval to market their products. Unlike drugs, DS are not required to be standardized to avoid batch-to-batch variability and ensure reliability.

SOME WORK, SOME DON'T. Some DS have been found to be safe and effective, while others have not. Many more have never been adequately evaluated. The onus is on the FDA to remove unsafe products—a process that can take years, as was the case with ephedra.

SEE ALSO Herbs (c. 60,000 BCE), Pure Food and Drug Act (1906), Food and Drug Administration (1906), Kefauver-Harris Amendment (1962), Ephedra/Ephedrine (1994), Direct-to-Consumer Ads (1997).

Herbs are integral components of dietary supplements. Here, an herbal health market displays medicinal plant leaves.

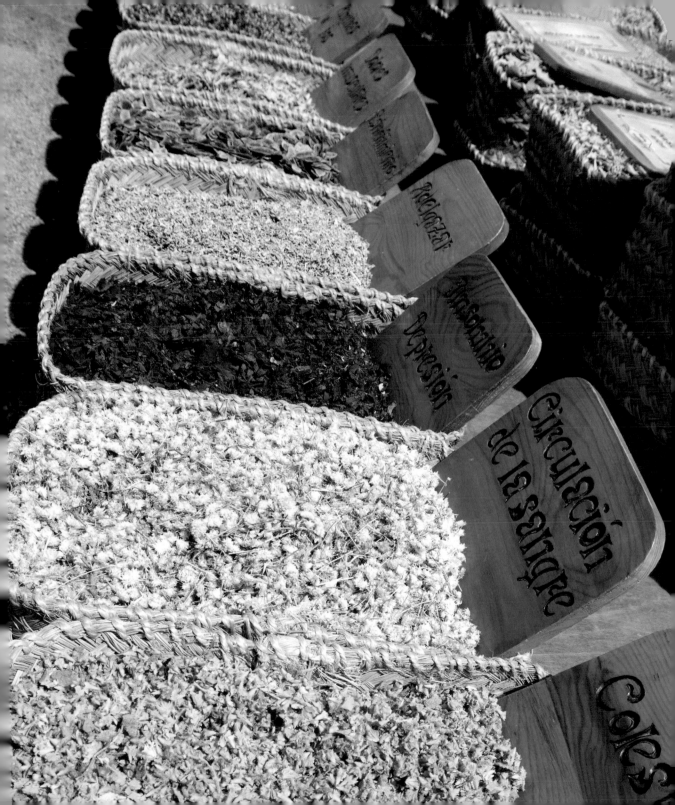

Fosamax

Suppose a drug is effective treating a long-term medical condition. How long is it prudent to continue taking it? When does the treatment cease to be helpful and begin to become risky? These are the puzzles facing physicians and their patients who are taking Fosamax and related biphosphonate drugs such as Actonel, Boniva, Reclast, and Atelvia for the treatment and prevention of osteoporosis.

Osteoporosis is a condition in which bone becomes less dense and at greater risk of fracturing. In developed countries, osteoporosis causes fractures in 30–50 percent of women and 15–30 percent of men older than fifty—fractures that may result from even minor traumatic events, like coughing or rolling over in bed. Since the late 1990s, highly effective drugs have been available for its treatment and prevention; Fosamax (alendronate), introduced by Merck in 1995, was the first drug of its kind.

Our bone mass normally builds up during our first thirty years, remains stable for the next twenty years, and then declines over the remainder of our lives. Osteoclasts are cells responsible for the resorption (breakdown) of old bone. In osteoporosis, Fosamax-like drugs decrease the number and activity of these osteoclasts, increasing bone-mass density (BMD) and reducing the risk of fractures by one-half. These drugs have been approved for the treatment and prevention of osteoporosis in post-menopausal women, but they have also been prescribed on a very long-term basis for healthy women, with no signs of osteoporosis or risks of fractures, with the hope of protecting their bones from fracturing later in life.

The routine use of Fosamax and other biphosphonates is now being questioned. These drugs do not appear to reduce the risk of fractures or to confer any real benefits in women who do not have osteoporosis. Far more troublesome are reports that they can cause a rare condition called osteonecrosis of the jaw (ONJ or jawbone death), as well as unusual thigh bone fractures and cancer of the esophagus. At this time, personal injury lawyers see a much clearer link between the use of these drugs and these rare conditions than does the general medical community.

SEE ALSO Evista (1997).

This x-ray depicts the spinal column of a male senior with osteoporosis. The most dangerous consequence of this condition is fracture—most commonly of the long bones and vertebrae. Multiple vertebral fractures (compression fractures) can lead to stooped posture, loss of height, chronic pain, and reduced mobility.

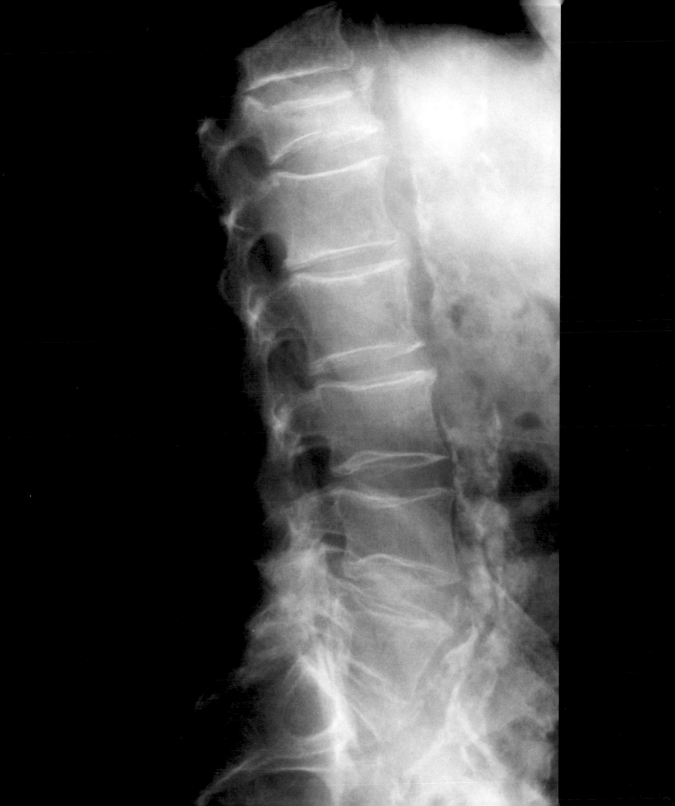

HAART

AZT was the first breakthrough in the treatment of AIDS (acquired immune deficiency syndrome), a failure in the immune system caused by HIV (human immunodeficiency virus). Over the years, other anti-AIDS drugs were discovered that work by mechanisms that differ from AZT, at other stages in the virus's life cycle. Additionally, such drugs could be taken in combination with AZT.

Although there are significant benefits associated with taking multiple anti-AIDS drugs, there are also many problems that rapidly multiply when three or four different drugs are taken each day. To work best, each drug must be taken at carefully specified times, and as might be anticipated, these times and their frequency differ for each drug. Moreover, these medicines cause a wide range of adverse effects, some of which are potentially serious. They can also interact with a bewildering array of other drugs, increasing potential toxicity or reducing effectiveness. To add to these various problems, the cost of many of these drugs is high. For most AIDS patients, multiple drugs are prohibitively expensive.

There are powerful benefits associated with using multiple drugs. Early on, it was recognized that HIV rapidly mutates and can transform itself from being drug vulnerable to drug resistant. However, the use of drugs in combination, which act in different ways, reduces the likelihood of the development of resistance. These combinations have been termed *highly active antiretroviral therapy*, or HAART, an approach that is recommended for all AIDS patients. A number of pharmaceutical manufacturers joined together, starting in 1996, to combine their individual drugs into single pills that can be taken twice daily. This reduces the likelihood that patients will skip doses, which fosters drug resistance.

FROM DEATH WARRANT TO CHRONIC DISEASE. In 2009, there were some 33 million individuals with HIV/AIDS worldwide—a total that has stabilized in recent years. The number of annual deaths has declined to 2.1 million in 2007, thanks to the available drugs. HAART does not cure AIDS—it must be taken for a lifetime—but it has decreased AIDS-related deaths by 50–70 percent and has transformed AIDS from a death sentence to a chronic disease.

SEE ALSO AZT/Retrovir (1987), Viread (2011).

This scanning electron micrograph is of HIV budding (depicted in green) from a lymphocyte (white blood cell, shown in blue). Treatment of HIV/AIDS involves the combined use of multiple drugs (HAART) that interfere with different phases of the HIV virus life cycle.

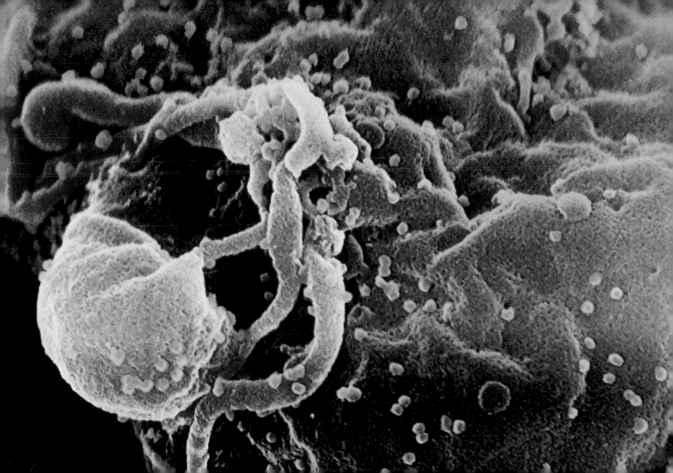

OxyContin

OxyContin is a classic case of a good drug gone bad. A highly effective drug for the relief of long-lasting pain, it has become among the most widely abused narcotics, sometimes with fatal consequences. Introduced to the American market in 1939, it was intended to be comparable to **morphine** in relieving pain when taken orally, but less likely to cause addiction. For many years oxycodone remained just one of many narcotics.

Oxycodone (5–10 mg) is now most often used with **aspirin** (a combination called Percodan) or **acetaminophen** (a combination called Percocet) to relieve moderate-to-moderately severe pain for a four-hour period, but some pains, such as those associated with cancer, may persist over extended periods or for the rest of a patient's life. In such cases, continuous pain relief is required around the clock. Recognizing this need, in 1996, Purdue Pharma introduced a specially formulated tablet that released oxycodone slowly over twelve hours. This was OxyContin. Purdue aggressively promoted OxyContin to physicians, claiming it caused only a modest high, had low abuse potential, and could be abruptly stopped without producing the withdrawal effects seen with other narcotics.

HILLBILLY HEROIN. OxyContin was an immediate success with physicians and patients alike and rapidly became a leading painkiller. Sales leaped six-fold between 1997 and 2005, and in 2008 sales were $2.5 billion in just the U.S. market. However, OxyContin also gained overnight popularity among addicts, who discovered that when the tablets were crushed, the entire contents of oxycodone were released at once. When injected or snorted, users experienced an immediate, intense high comparable to that of **heroin**. Its early popularity in rural Appalachia, later extending nationwide and internationally, led to its sobriquet, hillbilly heroin.

New nonmedical users of OxyContin numbered some half million in 2008. In 2010, a new plastic-coated tablet—said to be more resistant to being broken, crushed, or dissolved and injected—was introduced. Narcotic painkillers, including OxyContin, have been estimated to have been involved in 15,000 overdose deaths annually. Nevertheless, grossly misleading claims (misbranding) and advertising about the safety and abuse potential of OxyContin led the **Food and Drug Administration** to impose a $634 million fine against Purdue in 2007.

SEE ALSO Morphine (1806), Heroin (1898), Aspirin (1899), Food and Drug Administration (1906), Acetaminophen/Paracetamol (1953).

OxyContin and other opioids are used to control severe postoperative pain, as might be experienced after a hip replacement. In this image, the hip joint on the left has been replaced with a metal prosthesis.

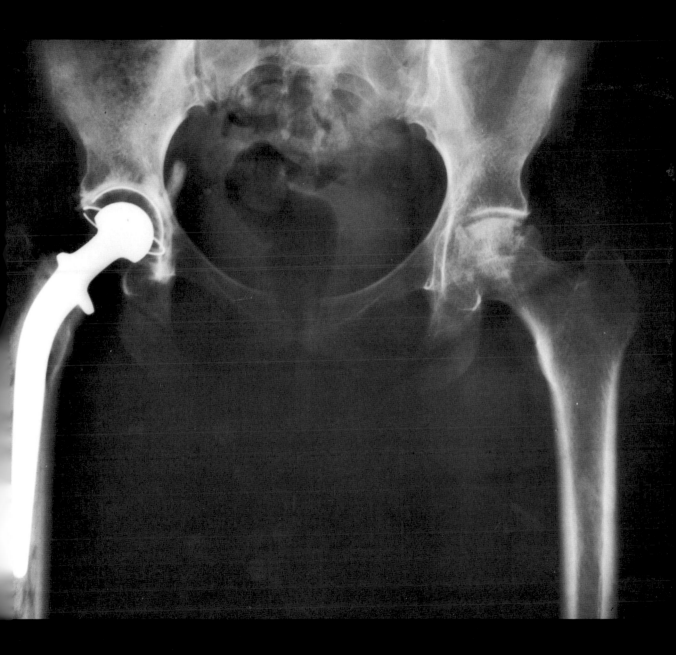

Zyprexa

When **clozapine** hit the market in 1989, it was clearly different from the older antipsychotic drugs such as **chlorpromazine** (Thorazine). It didn't cause tremors and rigidity, the so-called extrapyramidal symptoms (EPS) that resemble Parkinson's disease. However, **clozapine** (Clozaril) had a problem: It increased the risk of causing a potentially fatal blood disorder, agranulocytosis. Zyprexa (olanzapine), which appeared in 1996, resembled clozapine (no EPS) but without the blood problems. Perhaps overly simplistically, we now refer to the older chlorpromazine-like drugs as "typical" or first-generation antipyschotics, and the newer clozapine-Zyprexa drugs as "atypical" or second-generation antipsychotics.

The overwhelming majority of new antipsychotic drug prescriptions are written for such atypical drugs as Zyprexa, risperidone (Risperdal), and quetiapine (Seroquel). Many factors have contributed to their marketplace success, not the least of which have been aggressive promotional claims that these drugs not only cause fewer side effects but also are more effective than typical antipsychotics in controlling schizophrenia. These claims are largely based on drug company–financed studies. More objective clinical evidence from government-sponsored tests conducted in the United Kingdom and the United States have yielded conflicting results regarding their relative superiority. The jury remains out.

To varying degrees, the atypical antipsychotics—but, in particular, clozapine and Zyprexa—cause increased weight gain (sometimes very considerable) and potentially serious metabolic effects. These latter problems increase the risk of developing or worsening of existing diabetes, high blood pressure, and increased blood cholesterol levels associated with heart disease. Zyprexa's manufacturer has long sought to minimize these problems.

The distinction between typical vs. atypical antipsychotics is primarily based on their risk of causing EPS and their relative ability to block dopamine vs. dopamine-plus-serotonin subtypes of receptors in the brain. Beyond these, experts are not of single mind as to whether the claimed benefits and reduced risks are, in fact, different. There is a considerable cost differential between these antipsychotic drugs groups. Far less expensive generic equivalents are available for typical drugs, but only several atypical drugs, such as Clozaril and Zyprexa have generics. Are the differences in cost offset by their clinical benefits?

SEE ALSO Drug Receptors (1905), Neurotransmitters (1920), Chlorpromazine (1952), Clozapine (1989).

A faint, ghostlike figure appears in the distance, as might be imagined by a schizophrenic patient. Visual hallucinations are a symptom of schizophrenia, although they are not as common as auditory hallucinations.

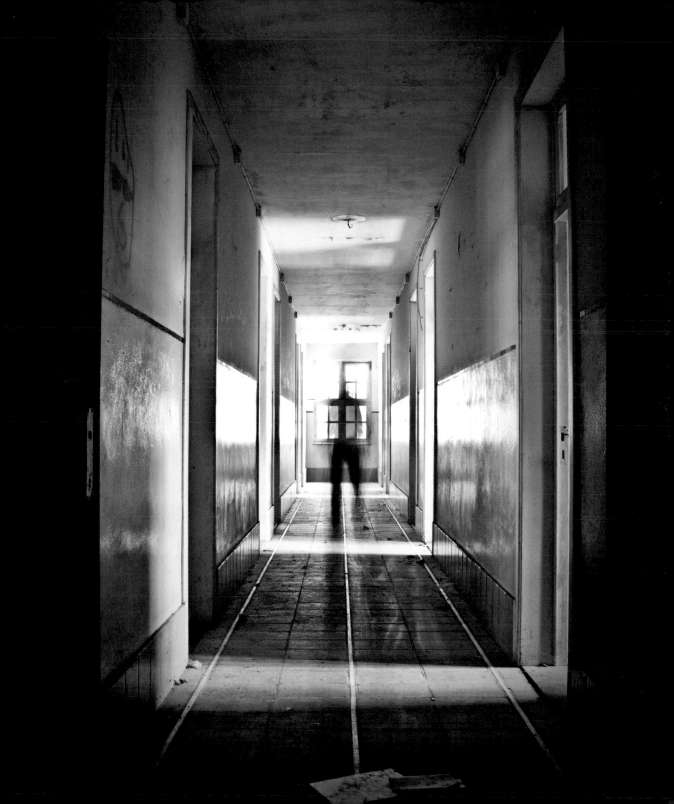

Plavix

Cardiovascular diseases are the leading cause of death in developed nations, and coronary artery disease (CAD), including heart attack, is the most common of these cardiovascular diseases. The antecedents of CAD are the buildup of cholesterol and other fatty materials in the walls of the coronary arteries that provide oxygen-rich blood to the heart. This buildup forms an atherosclerotic plaque, which promotes clot formation, potentially blocking blood flow—sometimes with a fatal outcome.

Nondrug measures slowing the progression of CAD include diet, exercise, and smoking cessation. Drug approaches include reducing cholesterol levels and interfering with the clumping of blood platelets. **Aspirin** and Plavix are the most commonly used oral anti-platelet drugs. These drugs vary in how they prevent platelets from clumping and show modest differences in their effectiveness, but they have a daily cost differential of pennies vs. dollars.

Neither drug breaks up existing clots. When taken immediately after a heart attack, aspirin reduces the risk of another heart attack or the death of heart tissue. Used on a chronic basis, aspirin prevents heart attack and stroke in individuals with a history of cardiovascular diseases, but its analogous benefits for those with no cardiovascular problems remain unclear. Its use for one to six months is also recommended after stents are placed in the coronary arteries.

Plavix (clopidogrel), approved for use in 1997 and for many years the world's second-best-selling drug, has been approved for use to prevent heart attack and stroke only in patients at risk for these problems. Plavix has been shown to be slightly more effective than aspirin, and their combination provides greater protection than aspirin alone. However, this combination also places patients at a greater risk of internal bleeding.

Plavix is a pro-drug, which means that to exert its anti-platelet effects it must first be metabolized by a liver enzyme (CYP2C19) to its active form. Some 2–14 percent of Americans are "poor metabolizers" and may be unable to derive the maximum protective benefits from Plavix.

SEE ALSO Aspirin (1899), Heparin (1916), Warfarin (1940), Mevacor (1987), tPA (1987), Pradaxa (2010).

Plavix is a very widely prescribed drug used to prevent the clumping of blood platelets (star-shaped cells) circulating in blood vessels. By reducing the risk of clot formation, it lessens the potential for heart attack and stroke.

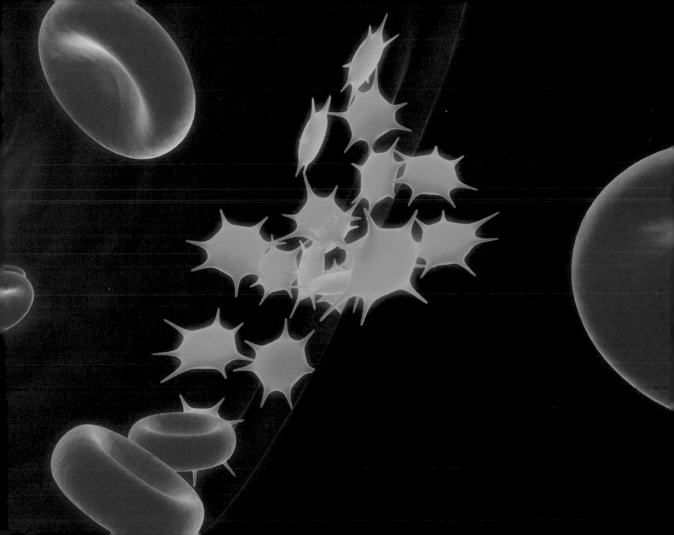

Direct-to-Consumer Ads

If you suffer from depression, asthma, an enlarged prostate, insomnia, high blood pressure, or elevated cholesterol levels, we have a prescription product for you! So proclaim the direct-to-consumer ads (DTCA) that flood television and print media. It was not always that way. Before 1997, information regarding your prescription drugs was restricted to healthcare professionals—primarily physicians. You were kept in the dark, and until relatively recently, the name of your prescription drug did not appear on its container.

That all changed in 1997, when the **Food and Drug Administration** authorized two types of DTCA: disease-awareness ads and product-claim ads. The first type discusses a medical condition but cannot refer to a drug name. It often points you to additional sources of information, which are usually drug manufacturers. Product-claim ads, the more common type, provide the drug's trade name and its medical use, along with a "brief summary" of the drug's benefits and risks. What are the upsides and downsides of these ads?

DCTA ads can improve patient awareness of their possible medical conditions and available drug treatments, as well as motivate patients to actively engage their healthcare provider for information. The ads can also alert patients about more effective medicines and significant adverse effects and risks associated with their drugs. However, some patients insist that the advertised medication is what they want prescribed. Broadcast ads accentuate the drug's benefits while minimizing the risks. Increased demands on physicians and pharmacists leave them little time to educate patients about misconceptions regarding the ads. When physicians acquiesce and prescribe newly introduced drugs, this can expose patients to uncommon but serious risks that only become obvious after large numbers of individuals have used the drug (e.g., **Vioxx**). Not surprisingly, DTCA almost exclusively promote products that enjoy patent protection and that are generally far more expensive than equally effective generic drugs, thus driving up healthcare costs.

Pharmaceutical manufacturers are spending some $4 billion a year on DTCA, and, obviously, they believe the money is well spent.

SEE ALSO Food and Drug Administration (1906), Celebrex and Vioxx (1998).

Prior to 1997, prescription drug-related information and ads in the United States were exclusively intended for healthcare professionals—in particular physicians, who were the drug prescribers. Since this time, prescription drug ads have been increasingly designed for the consumer. Such ads are only legally sanctioned in New Zealand and the United States.

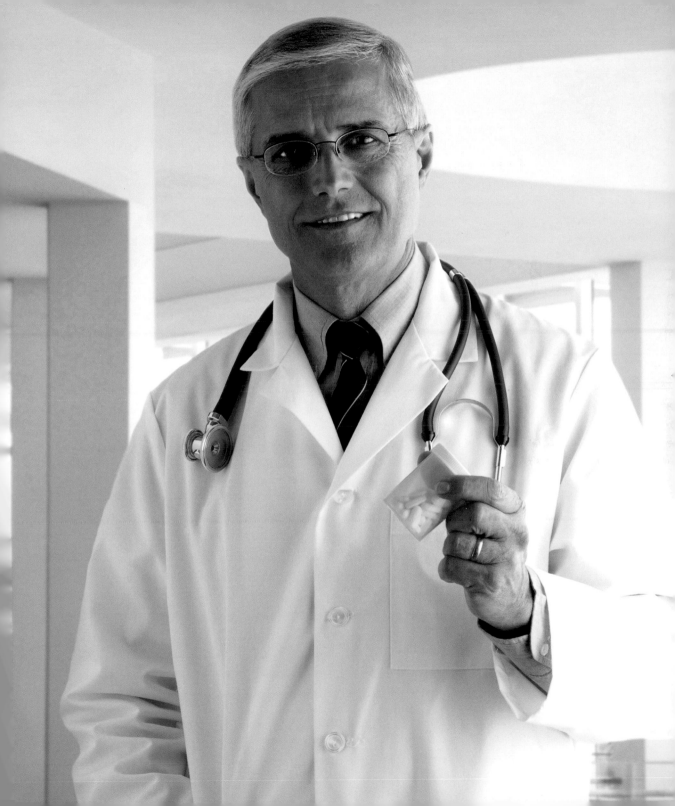

Synthroid

When two drugs are found to be bioequivalent, it indicates that they get into the bloodstream at the same rate and to the same extent and, therefore, are said to be interchangeable. At first glance, we might consider a discussion of bioequivalence to be rather esoteric and of primary interest to researchers and academics. However, in the case of Synthroid, interest in the subject sparked discussions on medical ethics, legal suppression of scientific results, conflicts of interest, scientist vs. scientist, and just plain bottom-line economics for the consumer.

Synthroid is the trade name for levothyroxine, a synthetic preparation of **thyroxine**, the principal hormone produced by the thyroid gland. Levothyroxine is the first choice for most patients who require replacement or supplementation of this hormone when their thyroid gland is operating sub-par. During the 1990s, Boots/Knoll sought to challenge generic manufacturers of levothyroxine, asserting that their products were not equivalent to Synthroid and should not be substituted for it.

Boots/Knoll commissioned a study in 1990 by Betty Dong at the University of California, San Francisco, anticipating the lack of equivalence. The results proved otherwise. The generic products were found to be bioequivalent to the far more expensive Synthroid, the second-best-selling drug in the United States, which enjoyed 85 percent of the market for levothyroxine. For six years, the manufacturer professionally attacked Dong's competence and successfully suppressed publication of these results by threatening legal action against her and the university. The results were eventually published in the *Journal of the American Medical Association* seven years after the study was completed. Class action lawsuits were brought against Knoll on behalf of patients who were overpaying for Synthroid, and the company rapidly agreed to settle for $98 million—a very small fraction of the company's profits during the delay.

This settlement did not end the Synthroid saga. In subsequent years, many clinical endocrinologists claimed that their patients were not responding to generic levothyroxine as they had to Synthroid and that the **Food and Drug Administration** criteria for bioequivalency were faulty. Nevertheless, the FDA remained resolute, and the generic products are now deemed bioequivalent.

SEE ALSO Food and Drug Administration (1906), Thyroxine (1914), Radioiodide (1946).

The thyroid, one of the largest endocrine glands, is located in the neck below the Adam's apple. Synthroid is a synthetic preparation of thyroxine, the primary hormone released from the thyroid gland.

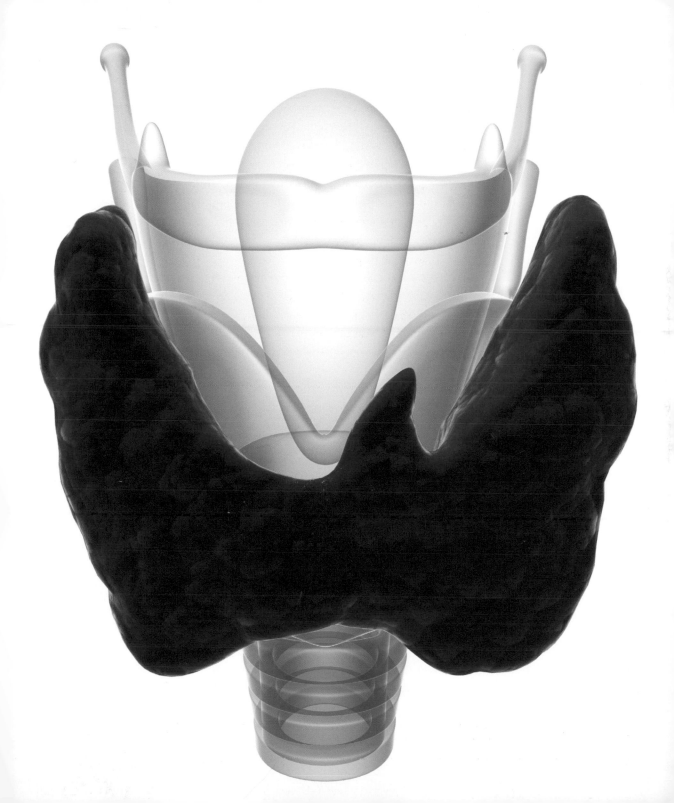

Evista

PROMOTING HEALTHY BONES AND BREASTS. In addition to its role as a female sex hormone, supporting the development of reproductive organs and secondary sex characteristics, **estrogen** also has a number of other metabolic effects. These include promoting the buildup of bone and affecting cholesterol levels.

Evista is like estrogen—it prevents bone loss and lowers LDL (bad) cholesterol— but it is also an anti-estrogen, blocking estrogen's growth-promoting effects on the breast and uterus. In 1997, Evista was marketed to treat osteoporosis and, more recently, to treat breast cancer.

Osteoporosis is a condition in which bone becomes less dense and more susceptible to fracturing, particularly at the hip. The World Health Organization ranks osteoporosis second only to cardiovascular disorders as a global healthcare problem. The highest risks of osteoporosis occur in the Scandinavian countries and the United States, with its frequency increasing in Asia, Latin America, and the Middle East. The highest incidence is seen among postmenopausal women and in both sexes over age sixty.

Bone is being continuously broken down and built up. Until the age of thirty, the balance favors buildup. Thereafter, a progressive breakdown of bone and a reduction in bone density and strength occur. Postmenopausal osteoporosis is caused by a lack of estrogen. Evista (raloxifene) slows the breakdown of bone and is used to prevent and treat osteoporosis in postmenopausal women.

Some 50–70 percent of patients with breast cancer have tumors that require estrogen for their growth. Evista, like **tamoxifen**, is an anti-estrogen that decreases the growth of cancer cells in such women with breast cancer. These drugs also prevent the development of breast cancer in women at high risk of developing the disease. Tamoxifen, like estrogen, stimulates the lining of the uterus and increases the danger of uterine cancer two- to three-fold. Evista, by contrast, has anti-estrogen effects on the uterus and does not appear to increase cancer likelihood.

SEE ALSO Estrone and Estrogen (1929), Tamoxifen (1973), Fosamax (1995), Herceptin (1998).

Bras are hung from a building along Broadway in New York City to promote breast cancer awareness.

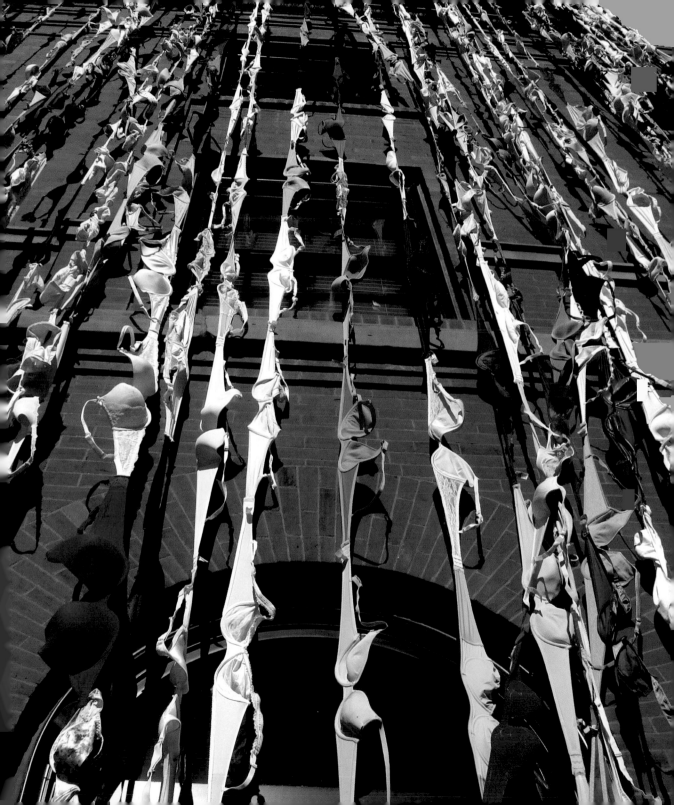

Flomax

It has been said that if you live long enough, you'll see everything. Similarly, if men live long enough, they'll develop benign prostatic hypertrophy (BPH). Characterized by an enlarged, noncancerous growth of the prostate gland, 90 percent of men older than eighty develop this condition.

The prostate gland lies under the bladder and surrounds the urethra, the tube through which urine exits from the body. The prostate's normal function is to produce a fluid in the semen that increases the lifespan of sperm. An enlarged prostate compresses the urethra, interfering with normal urination. Resulting problems include a weak urine stream and an inability to fully empty the bladder, resulting in the need to urinate multiple times during the day and night. Over-the-counter decongestants and antihistamines, common ingredients in cold remedies, can worsen these problems.

Two rather different drug approaches are used to treat this condition, but, unfortunately, neither produces a cure. Originally developed by the Tokyo-based Yamanouchi Pharmaceuticals, Flomax (tamsulosin) was approved for use in the United States in 1997. This drug is an alpha-1 adrenergic blocker that relaxes muscles in the bladder and prostate, increasing the flow of urine within two to three weeks after the drug is initiated. Other alpha-1 adrenergic blockers, such as prazosin (Minipress), have been used since the 1970s for the treatment of high blood pressure as well as for BPH. Unlike these drugs, which lower blood pressure by keeping small blood vessels dilated, Flomax has minimal effects on blood pressure.

By contrast, **Proscar** (finasteride) and Avodart (dutasteride) shrink the size of the prostate by preventing the synthesis of the hormone responsible for its growth. There is commonly a three to six month delay before symptoms improve. Saw palmetto, a traditional medicine of the Americas, is currently the most widely used herbal treatment for BPH. The mechanisms proposed for its effects on the prostate are similar to those of Proscar. Evidence supporting the effectiveness of saw palmetto for this condition is contradictory, although the balance may be slightly in its favor.

If drugs don't work, the final alternative is surgery. The most common procedure is transurethral resection of the prostate (TURP), in which part of the prostate is removed.

SEE ALSO Neurotransmitters (1920), Proscar and Propecia (1992), Dietary Supplements (1994).

Sufferers from benign prostatic hypertrophy can readily identify with this dripping faucet. Drugs like Flomax restore a full flow.

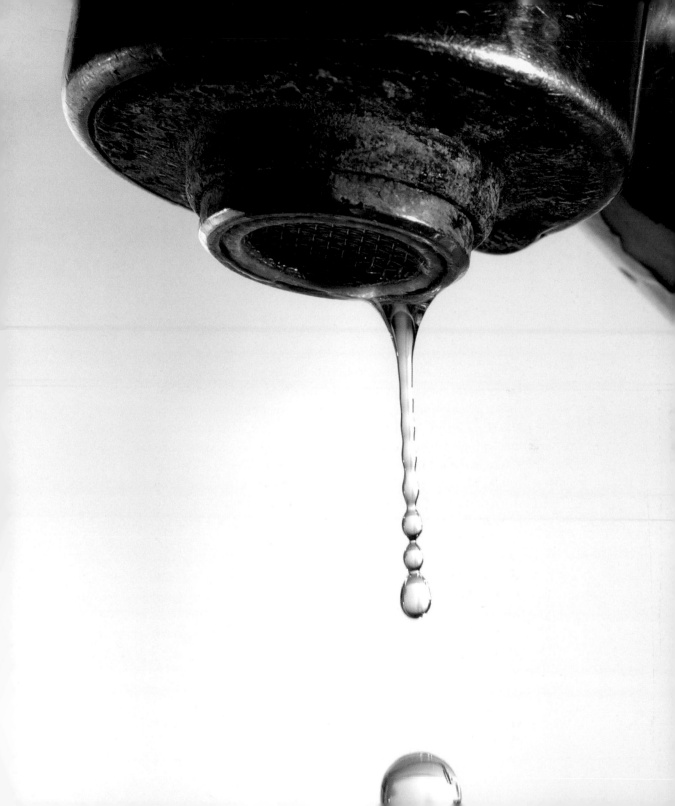

Celebrex and Vioxx

In 1970, **aspirin**'s myriad effects were attributed to its ability to inhibit the cyclooxygenases (COX), enzymes required for the synthesis of prostaglandins. The prostaglandins are a family of naturally occurring fatty acids that have a wide range of effects—some, desirable and protective; others, harmful.

The "good" prostaglandins, which require the COX-1 enzyme, protect the lining of the stomach from being eroded by stomach acids. By contrast, the COX-2 enzyme is involved in the synthesis of the "bad" prostaglandins that cause pain and the inflammatory response commonly in the joints. Aspirin, ibuprofen, and other nonsteroidal anti-inflammatory drugs (NSAIDs) inhibit both the COX-1 and COX-2 enzymes to a more-or-less equivalent degree, resulting in pain relief . . . at the risk of stomach ulcers.

Daniel Simmons, a chemistry professor at Brigham Young University, discovered the COX-2 enzyme in 1988. This led scientists to seek out drugs that that could selectively inhibit COX-2 while having little or no effect on COX-1. Pfizer's Celebrex and Merck's Vioxx, released in 1998 and 1999, met these objectives and were aggressively advertised in the United States in **direct-to-consumer ads** on television and in newspapers. These highly successful ads emphasized the drugs' pain-relieving effects for osteoarthritis, rheumatoid arthritis, and menstrual cramps, while causing fewer stomach ulcers. However, carefully controlled studies revealed that, while these drugs were effective, they were no better at relieving pain and inflammation and did not produce fewer adverse effects on the stomach than the older nonselective NSAIDs—drugs that could be purchased at a fraction of the price.

As early as 2001, reports appeared that linked the use of Vioxx to an increased risk of heart attack and stroke, with fatal outcomes reported in the thousands. In 2004, Merck voluntarily withdrew Vioxx from markets worldwide and is now defending individual and class-action lawsuits. Moreover, the drug company has been subject to scathing attacks in medical literature for withholding, manipulating, and misrepresenting data regarding the drug's safety. Great concern exists that similar risks may also exist with Celebrex, which continues to be marketed with other NSAIDs.

In other news, Pfizer settled a six-year lawsuit in 2012 that paid Brigham Young University $450 million in acknowledgment of its critical contribution leading to the development of Celebrex.

SEE ALSO Aspirin (1899), Acetaminophen/Paracetamol (1953), Direct-to-Consumer Ads (1997).

Osteoarthritis can affect any of the body's joints, including the spine, and occurs when the cartilage discs (shock absorbers) between the vertebrae degenerate. Celebrex and other NSAIDs relieve pain and reduce inflammation associated with osteoarthritis.

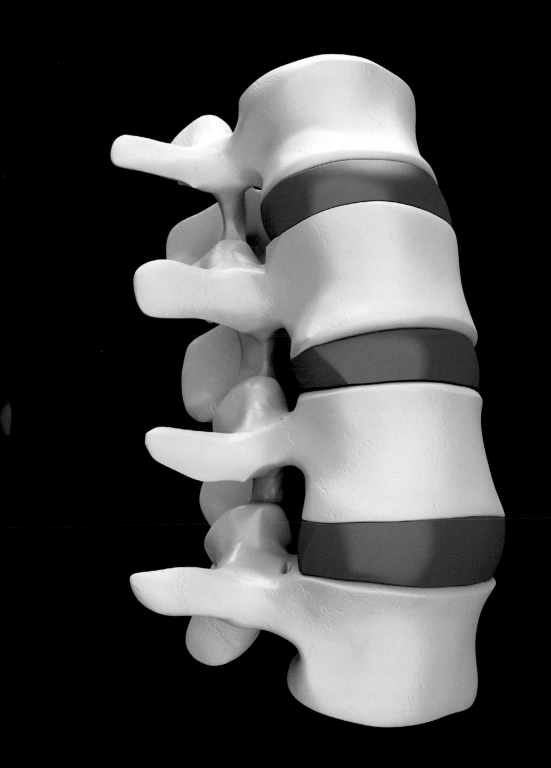

Viagra

Viagra ranks among the world's most familiar drug names and is synonymous with male sexual potency. It was among the first lifestyle drugs and subjects of **direct-to-consumer (DTC) ads** and medical condition awareness campaigns. In the process, it shined a light on impotence—long an unspoken, highly confidential medical condition.

Sidenafil (Viagra) was initially tested in the 1980s as a drug intended to treat high blood pressure and to promote blood flow to the heart muscle in angina. In clinical trials, however, its effect on angina was unimpressive, but an unanticipated side effect in comments by test subjects revealed a far more interesting and profitable possibility: Sidenafil produced erections, even in men who struggled with impotence. In 1998, Viagra became the first orally active drug approved in the United States for treating impotence, readily displacing the previous practice of drug injections into the penis. Viagra was highly effective (benefit in 70–80 percent of men), simple to take, and relatively safe. Within three years, Viagra had received regulatory approval in more than 110 countries and was being taken by 45 million men.

The traditional definition of impotence (now rebranded *erectile dysfunction*, or *ED*) was altered from the "persistent inability to initiate or maintain an erection" to the far more subjective "inability to sustain an erection suitable for satisfactory sexual performance." Pfizer launched DTC ads publicizing ED and Viagra—ads that featured former U.S. senator and 1996 presidential hopeful Bob Dole and the internationally acclaimed soccer superstar Pele. These efforts paid off handsomely: Viagra annual sales rapidly exceeded $1 billion.

Viagra was soon sharing the market with Cialis (vardenafil) and Levitra (tadenafil), which act faster and considerably longer. These drugs all act by a common and rather complex mechanism, causing the involuntary muscle in the penis to relax and increasing blood flow in blood vessels. To work, the male must first be sexually aroused—by whatever means. In the absence of such stimulation, the drugs fail to work. The search for a female Viagra have been unsuccessful to date, perhaps because of the especially complex nature of female desire, but hope is not yet lost.

SEE ALSO Mandrake (c. 200 BCE), Direct-to-Consumer Ads (1997), Female Viagra (2015).

The Kiss by Auguste Rodin is located near the Orangerie Museum in Paris. Since its introduction, Viagra has made satisfactory sexual relations possible for individuals with erectile dysfunction, but its benefits have not gone unnoticed by non-ED-afflicted males aspiring to achieve new romantic heights.

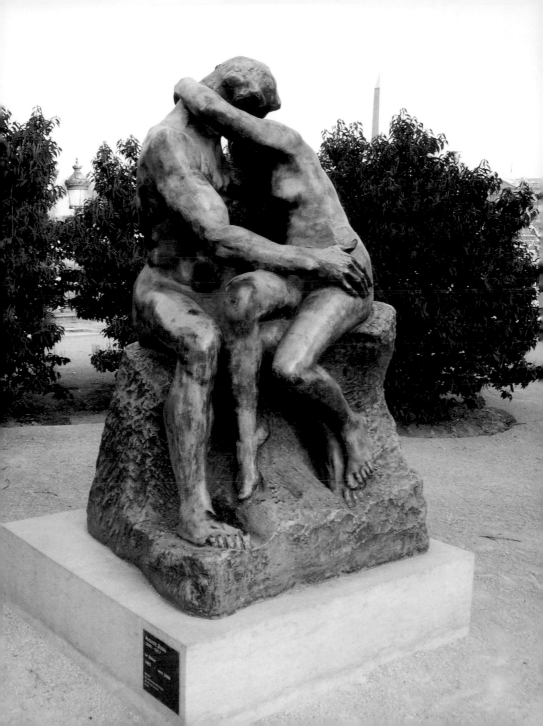

Herceptin

Dennis Slamon (b. 1946)

Breast cancer cells have a number of protein receptors that influence to what extent and how fast they grow, as well as what kinds of drugs are best used for their treatment. **Estrogen** receptors, for example, are present in 50–70 percent of breast cancer patients, and estrogen stimulates their growth. **Tamoxifen** is an anti-estrogen drug that blocks the estrogen receptor and prevents or slows the growth of the tumor.

Some 20–30 percent of breast cancers have an excess (over-expression) of the HER-2 gene that produces too many HER-2/*neu* receptors found on the surface of the tumor cell. Such tumors tend to be fast-growing and recurring. Herceptin (trastuzumab) is a monoclonal antibody that utilizes the body's immune defense system. It also acts, in part, by attaching to cells that contain HER-2/*neu* receptors and preventing the receptors from transmitting a signal that stimulates tumor growth.

A **biologic drug** marketed in 1998 by Genentech, Herceptin is only effective for the treatment of HER-2–positive tumor cells and can be used alone or in combination with other anticancer drugs for the treatment of metastatic cancers of the breast and stomach. Patients taking Herceptin have an increased survival rate, as well as a 30–50 percent reduction in the rate of relapses. However, these benefits come at the cost of heart failure in 2–7 percent of patients—a risk that increases significantly in individuals taking Herceptin with other anticancer drugs or who have a history of heart disease. More recently, Herceptin has been approved for the treatment of early-stage breast cancer.

Over a twelve-year period, Dennis Slamon, an American oncologist at Jonsson Comprehensive Cancer Center, University of California, Los Angeles, conducted laboratory and clinical research that led to the development of Herceptin. His discovery served as the basis for the 2008 made-for-television film *Living Proof*. The annual cost of Herceptin, between $50,000 and $100,000—and whether the drug's benefit justifies the cost—have been the subject of analysis and controversy.

SEE ALSO Drug Receptors (1905), Estrone and Estrogen (1929), Tamoxifen (1973), Biologic Drugs (1982), Evista (1997), Avastin (2004).

This ribbon model shows the antibody Herceptin Fab. These diagrams are three-dimensional schematic representations of the protein structure, showing its twisting and folding.

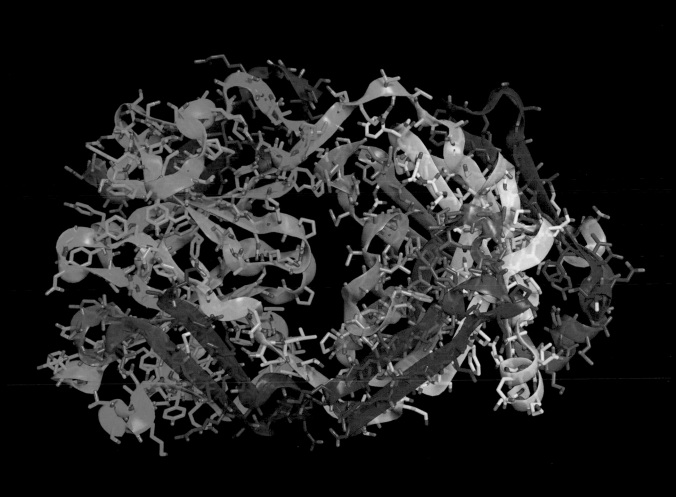

Enbrel, Remicade, and Humira

Ravinder N. Maini (b. 1937), **Marc Feldmann** (b. 1944)

Rheumatoid arthritis (RA) affects about 1 percent of the population worldwide and occurs in women about three times more often than in men. Symptoms of RA include inflammation, pain, and swelling of the hands and feet, often accompanied by destruction of the joints. Inflammation begins at the synovium—the membrane enclosing the joint cavity—progressing over several years to joint destruction.

Aspirin and related nonsteroidal anti-inflammatory drugs (NSAIDs), as well as **cortisone**-like drugs, reduce pain and inflammation without altering the progression of RA. By contrast, **methotrexate** and other DMARDs (disease-modifying anti-rheumatic drugs) slow the disease and delay joint deterioration. However, their mechanism of action is not clear.

During the 1980s and 1990s, Australian immunologist Marc Feldmann and Indian-born rheumatologist Ravinder N. Maini, working together at Imperial College School of Medicine, London, studied mechanisms underlying autoimmune diseases—in particular, RA. They found that tumor necrosis factor (TNF) was the most important chemical responsible for joint destruction. Attention was then directed toward developing **biologic drugs** that bind to and inactivate TNF.

The first such TNF-blockers were Enbrel (etanercept), Remicade (infliximab), and Humira (adalimumab), introduced between 1998 and 2002. These biologic-response modifying drugs are very highly effective for the treatment of moderate-to-severe RA, with more than 70 percent of patients showing an improvement in their symptoms (pain and swelling) within weeks after the start of therapy. They are even more effective when used in combination with methotrexate or another DMARD.

Because TNF-blockers are proteins, they are not active by mouth and must be injected. Remicade is injected intravenously generally at four- to eight-week intervals. As TNF plays a key role in the body's immune response against bacteria, the use of TNF-blockers increases the risk of severe infections, including tuberculosis.

Because joint destruction occurs within the first few years after symptoms appear, RA is now being treated more aggressively with DMARDs and TNF-blockers that slow the progression of the disease.

SEE ALSO Aspirin (1899), Amethopterin and Methotrexate (1947), Cortisone (1949), Biologic Drugs (1982).

This x-ray is typical of the hand of an individual experiencing rheumatoid arthritis—which, at the point shown, can no longer be reversed. Administering Enbrel and related disease-modifying anti-rheumatic drugs (DMARDs) at an earlier stage might have delayed the onset of joint deterioration and deformation.

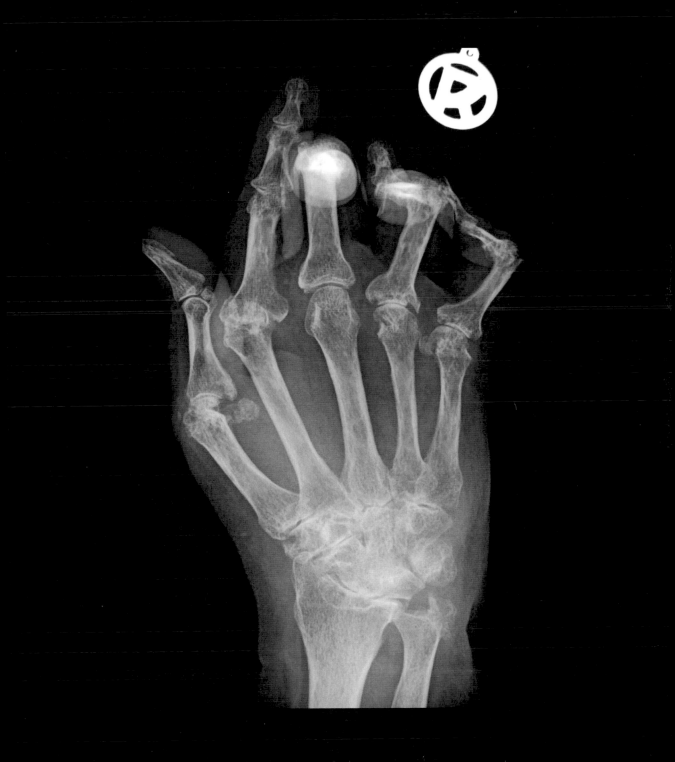

Plan B

Oral contraceptives (the Pill) are of two types: combination products, consisting of an **estrogen** and a progestin (**progesterone**-like drug), and the "mini-pill," containing only progestin. These products are taken once daily for twenty-one consecutive days, after which time menstruation begins. In the mid-1970s, studies showed that if high doses of either pill type were taken, breakthrough bleeding would occur. This led to the "morning-after pill."

The morning-after pills, emergency contraceptives (EC), are taken after sexual intercourse and are intended to prevent pregnancy resulting from a contraceptive failure, such as a broken condom, missed pills, the absence of any contraceptive, or sexual assault. The most widely used ECs are progestin-only (levonorgestrel) products, which are marketed in different parts of the world as Plan B, Levonelle, or NorLevo.

Plan B approval in the United States has been the subject of ethical concerns and political influences. Its effectiveness and safety are unquestioned: When taken within seventy-two hours of sexual intercourse, Plan B is 89 percent effective in preventing pregnancy. Nausea is the most common side effect. Most scientists believe that it works by preventing ovulation and fertilization of the ovum, rather than by preventing the fertilized ovum from attaching to the uterus. Unlike **mifepristone** (RU-486), it has no effect on established pregnancies; neither does it cause abortion.

In 1999, the **Food and Drug Administration** (FDA) approved Plan B as a prescription EC, intended only for occasional use. In 2003, an expert FDA advisory committee and FDA's own staff overwhelmingly recommended that it be made available without a prescription—a recommendation the FDA uncharacteristically rejected. Likely succumbing to political pressure from pro-life groups, the FDA argued that adolescents without medical supervision could not use Plan B safely, and that its use would lead to indiscriminate unprotected sex by teenagers. In 2009, a U.S. District Court called the FDA decision "arbitrary and capricious" and not based on good-faith reasoning. It ruled that Plan B be made available, without a prescription, to individuals older than seventeen. In 2010, the FDA approved—without political overtones—Ella. A drug only available by prescription, Ella is effective in preventing pregnancy up to five days after sexual intercourse.

SEE ALSO Food and Drug Administration (1906), Estrone and Estrogen (1929), Progesterone and Progestin (1933), Enovid (1960), Mifepristone (1988).

Conception may occur within hours of having sex, but the sperm-and-egg rendezvous is more common days later. It is generally believed that "morning-after pills" work by preventing or delaying ovulation, preventing fertilization, or by interrupting the fertilized egg from being implanted in the uterus.

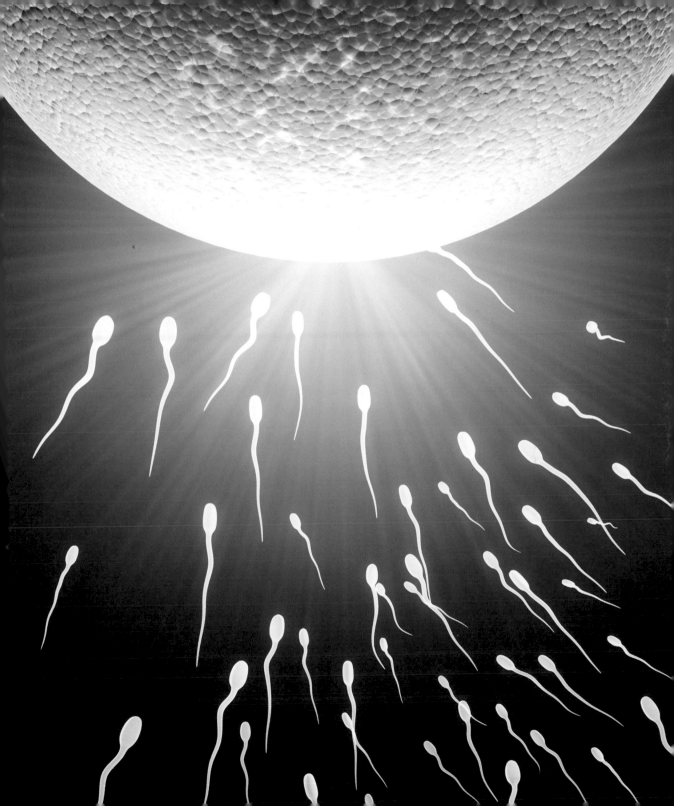

Gleevec/Glivec

Brian J. Druner (b. 1955), **Nicholas B. Lydon** (b. 1957), **Charles L. Sawyers** (b. 1959)

Gleevec or Glivec (outside the United States) represents a major advance in the treatment of cancer—a drug that *Time* magazine characterized as a "magic bullet" in a cover story in 2001, the year of its introduction. As of 2011, this drug has been found to be effective against eleven different types of cancer, including those affecting the blood, stomach, and digestive tract, several of which previously had poor survival rates. Of even greater significance for the future development of new anticancer drugs, Gleevec/Glivec (imatinib) is the first drug shown to act by zeroing in on a specific target associated with a certain cancer cell type.

In chronic myelocytic leukemia (CLM), normal white blood cells become cancerous. The survival rate with bone transplants and older drugs, such as interferon, was very low, and adverse effects were very high. With Gleevec/Glivec, the five-year overall survival rate is almost 90 percent, and side effects are relatively mild. CML, once a fatal disease, has been transformed into a treatable chronic disease.

The path for the discovery of Gleevec/Glivec was based on knowledge of the biology of CML and has provided a model for the development of other targeted therapies of cancer. By the 1980s, after several decades of research, it was known that all patients with CML had a chromosomal abnormality, dubbed the Philadelphia chromosome. Under normal conditions, the enzyme tyrosine hydroxylase signals cells to divide. Within the CML chromosome, however, are two genes that produced an abnormal tyrosine kinase protein that, when activated, signals an overproduction of white blood cells, resulting in CML.

During the 1990s, Brian Druner, an oncologist at the Oregon Health and Sciences University, Nicholas Lydon, formerly a biochemist at Novartis, and Charles Sawyers, a physician-scientist at the Memorial Sloan-Kettering Cancer Center, collaborated to find an inhibitor of tyrosine hydroxylase that was specific to CML. That compound was Gleevec/Glivec. As a result of their groundbreaking discovery, they were co-recipients of the 2009 Lasker-DeBakey Clinical Award, the "American Nobel Prize."

SEE ALSO Amethopterin and Methotrexate (1947).

Mary Lasker (1900–1994), who was instrumental in garnering federal financial support for the National Institutes of Health, was a driving force in increasing public awareness of disease and raising funds to support medical research. Since 1946, Lasker Awards (American Nobels) have been bestowed on individuals who have made major scientific contributions to treating and preventing human disease.

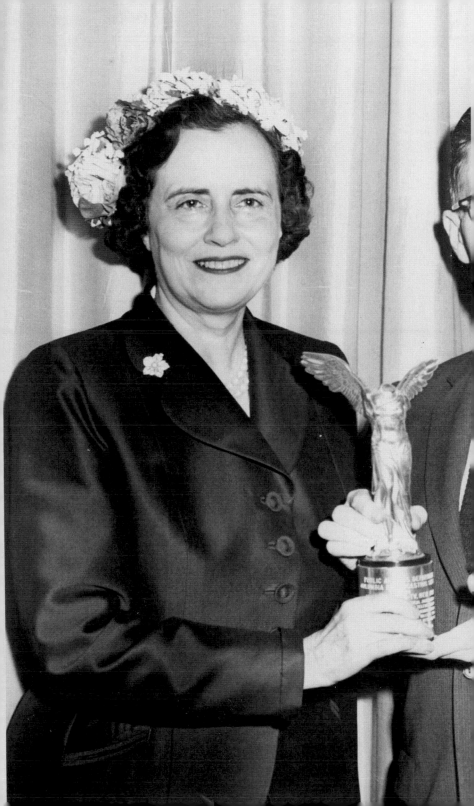

Iressa and Erbitux

Lung cancer is the leading cause of cancer deaths throughout the industrialized world, and colorectal cancer is not far behind. Untreated individuals with lung cancer survive an average of eight months, with a five-year survival rate of only 15 percent for treated patients. Similarly, only 9 percent of persons with advanced colorectal cancers that have spread (metastasized) survive five years beyond diagnosis. Depending upon the specific cancer type and stage of progression, surgery, radiation therapy, or drugs are the preferred treatment approaches.

Under ideal conditions, cancer chemotherapy (chemo) only kills cancer cells, while leaving normal cells untouched. Unfortunately, ideal conditions are not the reality. Existing chemo is, at best, more toxic to cancer cells, but all cells are damaged, leading to a wide range of side effects.

Biologic drugs, which include monoclonal antibodies, are designed to specifically target receptors located on the surface of cells that when over-activated can cause cancer. One of these is the epidermal growth factor receptor (EGFR), whose over-activity has been implicated in some cases of lung cancer and colorectal cancer. Approved for use in 2003 and 2004, Iressa (gefitinib) and Erbitux (cetuximab) block EGFR and are used for the treatment of lung cancer and colorectal cancer, respectively. Because of their serious side effects and questionable effectiveness, both drugs are often backups to other types of treatment.

Iressa is marketed in some sixty-six countries worldwide. In many countries in Europe and Asia, it has been approved for use alone as the first treatment for advanced cases of non-small-cell lung carcinoma (NSCLC). However, some clinical studies show that chemo-treated patients live longer than with Iressa. Thus, in the United States, Iressa has only been approved for individuals who have not benefited from chemotherapy.

Erbitux, when used with the chemo drug Camptosar (irinotecan), slows the growth of colon and rectal tumors. However, it does not improve the quality of life or increase the survival time of patients with advanced cases. Moreover, it has not been found to benefit patients whose colon cancer has not spread. The effectiveness of Erbitux remains to be shown in the clinics.

SEE ALSO Biologic Drugs (1982), Herceptin (1998).

The top of this image shows a microscopic view of excised lung cancer that has replaced normal lung tissue.

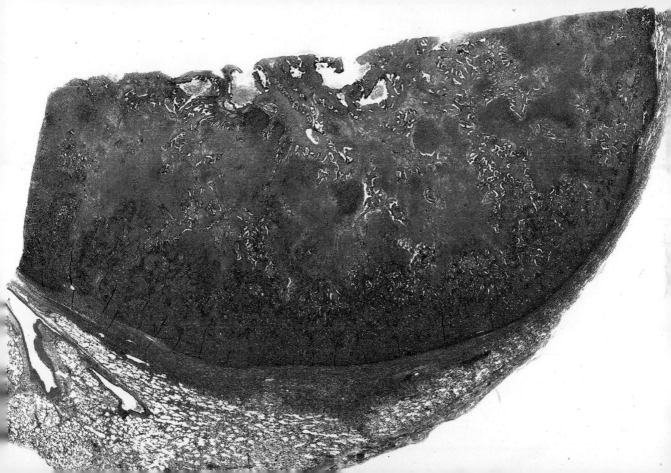

17P/Progesterone Injections and Gel

Some 12–13 percent of babies (500,000) in the United States and 5–9 percent in Europe are delivered before the thirty-seventh week of pregnancy and classified as premature or preterm. Prematurity is the leading cause of newborn mortality and illness in developed countries. Because their internal organs have not adequately developed, preemies are at greater risk for serious short-term and long-term complications, including cerebral palsy, for which prematurity is the leading single cause. Coupled with the parents' emotional distress are the medical expenses associated with extended periods of hospitalization, which can amount to many tens of thousands of dollars.

A 2003 federally funded study showed that injections of 17P (17-hydroxprogesterone caproate), given weekly starting no later than the twenty-first week of gestation, reduced the risk of preterm births in women who had had a prior spontaneous preterm birth. Not a new drug, 17P was approved for use in threatened miscarriages in 1956 and marketed and sold as Delalutin until 2000. After the 2003 results appeared, there was renewed interest in 17P, and compounding pharmacists specially prepared it for about $15 per injection or $300 for a full twenty-week course of treatment.

In February 2011, the **Food and Drug Administration** granted KV Pharmaceutical's application fast-track approval to exclusively market Makena (17P). This application had the enthusiastic support of numerous health groups, including the March of Dimes, which is dedicated to preventing premature births. Weeks later, the medical community was outraged when KV announced its intention to charge $1,500 per injection or $30,000 for a twenty-week treatment. Within a month, KV buckled slightly under the pressure and reduced its price to $690 per injection or $13,800 for twenty weeks—still almost fifty times more than the usual compounding pharmacist's price.

In 2011, news of another **progesterone** product appeared: a vaginal gel that, when applied daily during the second half of pregnancy, reduces premature births by one-half. Women in the study were those with a short cervix, a neck-like structure connecting the uterus and the vagina. The progesterone may act by keeping the cervix closed and the uterus inactive during pregnancy.

SEE ALSO Food and Drug Administration (1906), Progesterone and Progestin (1933), Diethylstilbestrol (1938).

The shorter the pregnancy, the greater the risk of infant morbidity and mortality. At twenty-four weeks, the infant has a 50 percent chance of survival. The premature infant faces multiple organ-system challenges, including problems in the development of the nervous system, cardiovascular complications, and very commonly, ailments affecting the respiratory system.

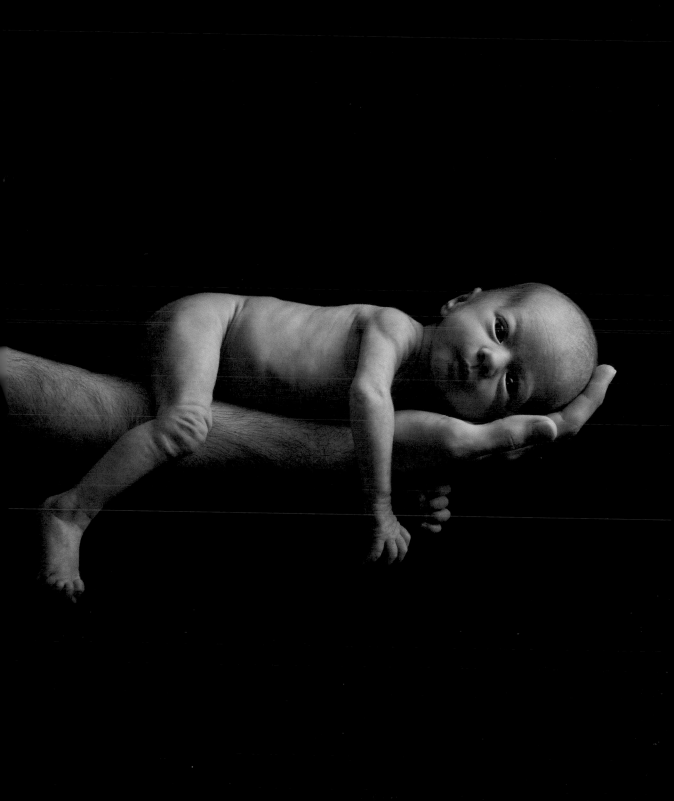

Resveratrol

The French diet is high in heart-unhealthy saturated fats, yet the French are reported to have a low incidence of heart disease. This so-called French Paradox was first brought to viewers' attention in a 1991 broadcast of *60 Minutes*, with the suggestion that an ingredient in wine, when consumed in moderation, protects the heart.

DID METHUSELAH DRINK RED WINE? Resveratrol, found in the skin of grapes and in red wine, is said to have health-promoting effects. This antioxidant is thought to protect the cells against free radicals, which damage cells, potentially shielding us from heart disease and cancer. Results of studies published in 2003 reported that resveratrol extended the lives of yeasts, worms, fruit flies, and short-lifespan fish. Mice fed a high-fat diet and treated with resveratrol had lower rates of obesity and diabetes, strong risk factors in heart disease. (To get a mouse-comparable dose of resveratrol, a human would have to consume 100 to1,000 bottles of red wine each day!) Other animal studies pointed to its anti-inflammatory and antidiabetic effects, its protection against brain plaque formation associated with Alzheimer's disease, and its reduction of skin cancer rates when applied to the skin.

After reading the promotional literature for resveratrol-containing **dietary supplements** found on the Internet, one reaches the inescapable conclusion that these same health benefits occur in humans. To date, we still anxiously await such positive findings. When taken as a pill, resveratrol is extensively broken down in the digestive tract and, after circulating in the blood and reaching the liver, is rapidly inactivated.

The pharmaceutical company Sirtris continues work on developing a synthetic resveratrol-like drug. This drug is theorized to work by activating SIRT1, a protein thought to extend the life of mice and, presumably, humans. For now, delay plans to celebrate your 120th birthday.

SEE ALSO Alcohol (c. 10,000 BCE), Dietary Supplements (1994), Antiaging Drugs (2020).

A number of studies suggest that, although red wine has a higher concentration of resveratrol than white wine, both wines, when consumed in moderation, produce comparable health benefits.

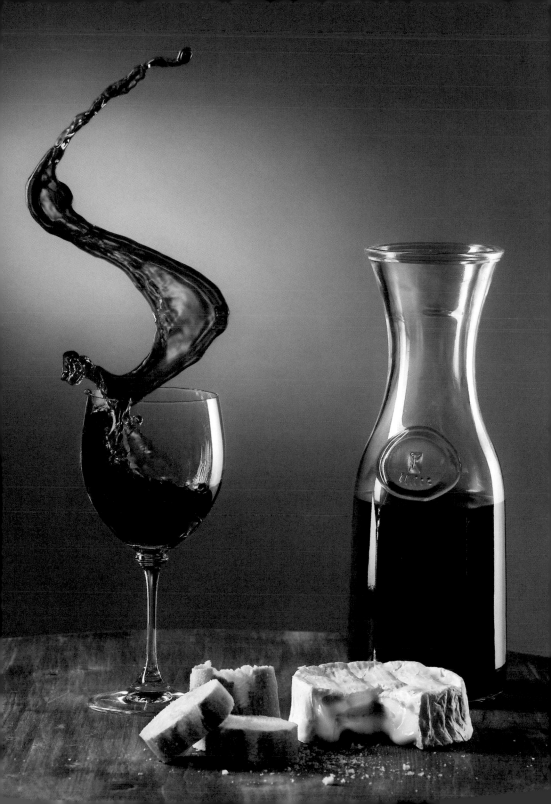

Avastin

Judah Folkman (1933–2008)

In 1971, Judah Folkman at Harvard Medical School proposed an original approach to the treatment of cancer, a concept that was dismissed by experts in the field for years. He theorized that, in order to grow and spread, tumor cells need a rich blood supply that provides them with adequate oxygen and nutrients, and that as the tumor increases in size, its requirements for blood supply become greater.

This increase in blood supply is accomplished by the influence of vascular endothelial growth factor (VEGF), which, when released, stimulates the formation of new blood vessels, a process called angiogenesis. Folkman proposed that inhibiting VEGF would prevent the growth of blood vessels surrounding the tumor, starving it and, thus, exerting an anticancer effect.

Avastin (bevacizumad), manufactured by Genentech, was the first angiogenesis inhibitor developed that works by this mechanism. A **biologic drug**, its large and complex molecules are produced by approaches involving recombinant DNA technology.

Since 2004, Avastin has become the world's best-selling anticancer drug, with annual sales of $6 billion in 2010. Used in combination with other antitumor drugs for the treatment of cancers of the colon, lung, kidney, and brain, Avastin was rapidly approved for the treatment of advanced breast cancer in the United States in 2008. To the dismay of many patients and their physicians, this approval was withdrawn in 2010, when the results of more detailed subsequent studies revealed that Avastin delayed tumor growth progression by only a few months, while subjecting patients to serious side effects. By contrast, the drug continues to be approved for use for advanced breast cancer in the European Union, based on the same information.

Because Avastin has been approved for marketing, physicians can continue to legally prescribe it on an **off-label** basis for breast cancer. However, insurance companies may no longer cover its $100,000 per year cost when prescribed for this condition. European drug regulatory authorities have, since 2010, permitted the manufacture of generic equivalents of Avastin and other biologic drugs (biosimilars).

SEE ALSO Off-Label Drug Use (1962), Biologic Drugs (1982), Herceptin (1998), Iressa and Erbitux (2003), Lucentis (2006).

To grow and spread, tumor cells need a generous supply of oxygen and nutrients, which are provided by a rich blood supply. Such increased growth of new blood vessels (vascularization) is seen here in the area of a uterine tumor. Avastin slows vascularization, producing its anticancer effects by starving the tumor.

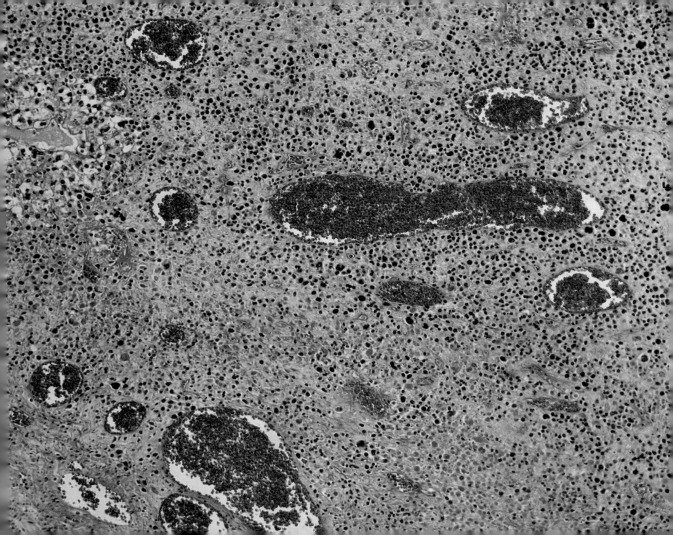

Gardasil

In 2006, Merck introduced a remarkable vaccine that prevented several types of human papillomavirus (HPV), which are responsible for causing 70 percent of cervical cancers and 90 percent of genital warts. Both are transmitted by sexual intercourse. The vaccine is not effective in treating these conditions but can prevent them when given in three injections over a six-month period. Hence, the manufacturer and governmental health agencies in the United States and Europe recommended that the vaccine be administered before adolescence, to girls as young as nine years of age, before they potentially become sexually active, and until twenty-six years of age. In 2009, approval was also given to market the vaccine for use in males aged nine years and over.

The vaccine's launch was initially accompanied by an apparent groundswell of political, medical, and public support, not only for its use but also for its mandatory administration in all eleven- and twelve-year-old girls as a condition for attending school. Texas governor Rick Perry was in the forefront of these discussions and, by executive order, in 2007 mandated vaccinations, bypassing the legislature. Months later, this action was overturned by his state legislature. In an effort to get state legislatures to pass such laws nationwide, Merck surreptitiously funded efforts by female state legislators but quickly terminated support after its involvement was disclosed.

GOOD MEDICINE, BAD POLITICS. Objections to mandatory vaccinations were soon voiced based on moral, political, financial, and health concerns. Socially conservative groups argued that the vaccine might encourage sexual activity in adolescent girls, who might think themselves now protected against sexually transmitted diseases. Some groups were opposed to all governmental mandates and interventions, regardless of how well intentioned. The series of shots cost around $360. Coverage by insurance companies is variable, and for many individuals, the out-of-pocket expense prohibitive.

Yet to be fully resolved are potential safety concerns associated with the vaccine and how long HPV protection lasts. Adverse reaction data and deaths have been subject to repeated analysis, and governmental health agencies in Europe and the United States have continued to conclude that Gardasil's health benefits outweigh any possible risks.

SEE ALSO Smallpox Vaccine (1796), Polio Vaccine (1954).

Out of the 150 to 200 types of HPV (pictured), 30 to 40 are transmitted through sexual contact, affecting about 80 percent of sexually active individuals. Most infections are temporary and cause no symptoms. In 5 to 10 percent of women, the infection persists and can progress to invasive cervical cancer over a 15- to 20-year period. Since the introduction of the Pap test in the 1940s, in which women are regularly screened, the death rate from cervical cancer has been reduced by 99 percent.

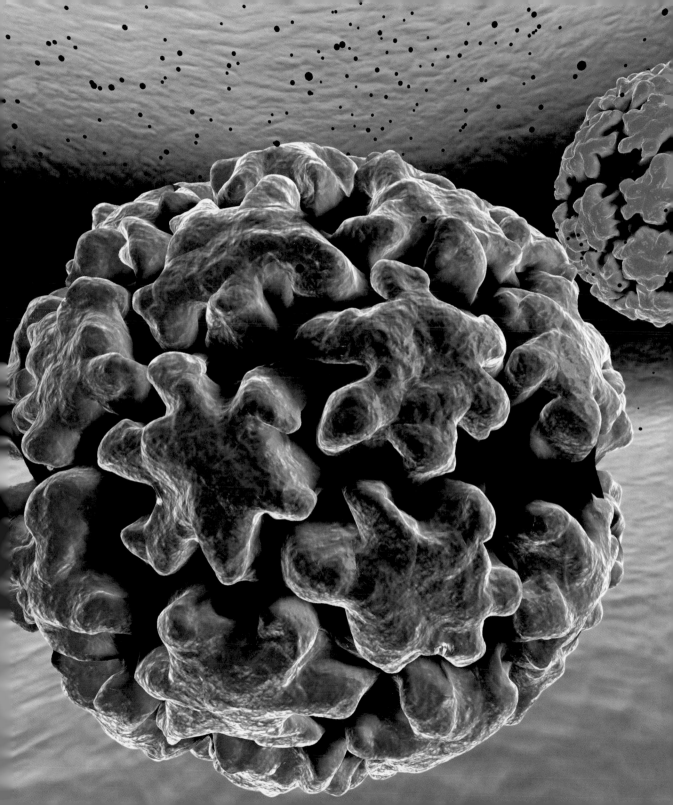

Chantix/Champix

The World Health Organization has estimated that by 2020, about 10 million people will die from smoking each year, 70 percent of whom reside in poor countries. In 2006, a long-awaited drug appeared on the market that was highly effective in promoting cessation of smoking, the world's leading cause of preventable death and disease.

Varenidine, marketed by Pfizer as Chantix in the United States and Champix in Canada, Europe, Japan, and other countries, was proclaimed by many to be a miracle drug that promoted smoking cessation, with no major safety concerns. This view was shared by international drug regulatory authorities, who very expeditiously approved its marketing. It was prescribed to more than 4 million persons in the United States within its first eighteen months.

Chantix/Champix works in two ways. Nicotine is the chemical in tobacco responsible for both its pleasurable effects as well as its potential to hook smokers. This drug acts on nicotine receptors in the brain to both block its pleasurable effects and to prevent the craving that occurs when the smoker attempts to quit.

It is not uncommon for individuals attempting to "kick the habit" to experience a depressed mood as they undergo nicotine withdrawal, and these changes in behavior were seen in many individuals who were taking Chantix/Champix, some of whom continued to smoke. Moreover, hundreds of individuals using this drug experienced suicidal thoughts. Highly aggressive and hostile behavior was exhibited, and the drug also worsened preexisting psychiatric illnesses and caused a recurrence of past behavioral problems. Consequently, drug labeling was revised in 2008 to include prominent and emphatic warnings of these potential psychiatric dangers. Moreover, the U.S. Federal Aviation Administration banned its use by pilots and air-traffic controllers.

Although still on the market, Pfizer's dreams of a multibillion-dollar drug have rapidly dissipated and been replaced by the vision of armies of lawyers pursuing personal injury lawsuits.

SEE ALSO Drug Receptors (1905), Neurotransmitters (1920), Methadone (1947), Nicotine Replacement Therapy (1991).

The neurotransmitter dopamine is thought to promote reward-seeking behaviors. Such activities, which may assume compulsive and addictive proportions, can include smoking, drinking, and pathological gambling, as well as drug taking, overeating, and having an overly active sex drive.

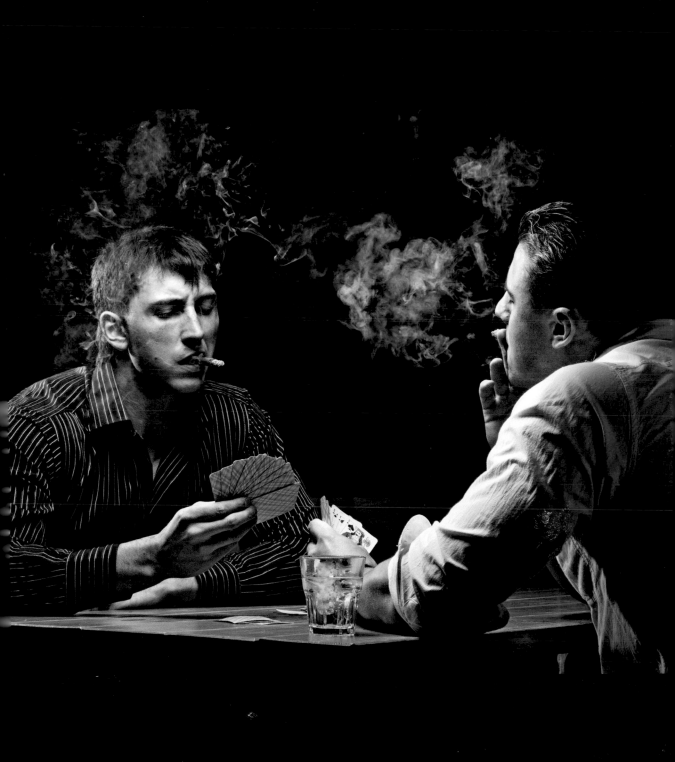

Lucentis

Age-related macular degeneration (AMD) is a major cause of blindness in individuals older than fifty-five. It is a progressive disease in which there is damage to the macula, the central area of the retina. A functioning macula is needed for sharp central vision required for reading and driving. Most cases of vision loss occur in individuals with advanced AMD, and almost all of these are associated with the wet form of AMD. In wet AMD, abnormal blood vessels grow under the macula, leaking fluid and blood, causing swelling and damage to the retina.

Introduced in 2006, Lucentis (ranibizumad) cannot cure AMD but can very effectively stop its progression by preventing the growth of new blood vessels by inhibiting vascular endothelial growth factor (VEGF). When injected directly into the eye at four-week intervals, this **biologic drug** stabilizes vision in 95 percent of patients and may, in some cases, be able to partially restore lost vision.

Genentech developed Lucentis specifically for the treatment of AMD. It is a fragment of the larger drug **Avastin** (bevacizumad), which is also a VEGF inhibitor and Genentech product. The smaller Lucentis molecule is thought to better penetrate the retina and stop the abnormal growth of blood vessels. Avastin is an anticancer drug that has been widely used around the world for AMD before and since the approval of Lucentis, with excellent results.

Why use Avastin instead of Lucentis? Lucentis costs forty times more than Avastin—$1,593 per dose vs. $42 per dose! Genentech's attempt to restrict the sale of Avastin for use in the eye has been largely unsuccessful and has generated considerable ill will among eye doctors.

In 2011, a large-scale, two-year National Eye Institute–funded study directly comparing the two drugs found that both drugs are just as effective in preventing AMD and improving vision, although Lucentis may cause slightly fewer side effects.

SEE ALSO Avastin (2004).

Hospital Corpsman Brian Long attempts to read a standard eye chart from twenty feet with the help of an optical refractor aboard the USS John F. Kennedy. Whereas infections are common causes of blindness in many developing countries, blindness is often attributed to age-related macular degeneration (AMD), which, in developed nations, can be treated with drugs like Lucentis if diagnosed early enough.

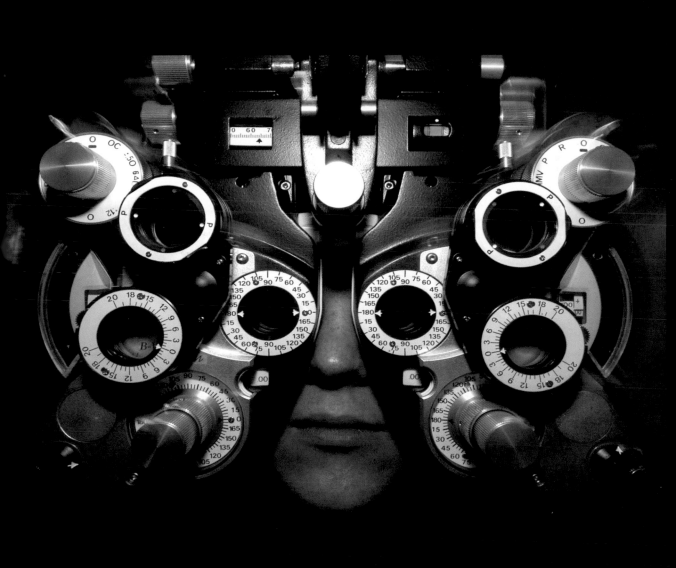

Avandia

Steven Nissen (b. 1948)

In 1999, Avandia and Actos were welcomed in the treatment of type 2 diabetes, by far the most common form of diabetes. Members of the glitazone class of oral antidiabetic drugs, Avandia and Actos work by increasing tissue sensitivity to insulin. Rezulin, the first member of the glitazone team, was effective but permanently benched in 2000 because it caused liver toxicity that was associated with several hundred deaths.

Avandia was aggressively marketed, becoming the best-selling drug for type 2 diabetes with sales of $3.2 billion in its high-water year of 2006. However, periodically over the years, in reports repeatedly dismissed by its manufacturer SmithKline Beecham (now GlaxoSmithKline, GSK), Avandia (rosiglitazone) use was linked to an increased risk of heart attack. However, these reports attracted national attention in 2007, when an article appeared in the prestigious *New England Journal of Medicine*. Cleveland Clinic cardiologist Steven Nissen provided evidence from GSK and **Food and Drug Administration** databases that Avandia increased the risk of heart attack and other cardiovascular problems by 43 percent. Avandia remained on the market but with additional warnings displayed on its label.

In 2010, uncovered documents revealed that GSK had withheld data and concealed information regarding concerns that Avandia caused heart problems. In fact, GSK had conducted a secret trial in 1999 comparing Avandia and Actos in terms of cardiovascular risks. Avandia fared poorly, and the results were never made public.

Most published independent studies in recent years have associated Avandia use to cardiovascular problems, and in September 2010, European and American drug regulators took action. The European Medicines Agency removed Avandia from the European market. In the United States, the drug will only be available to patients if their physicians attest that every other antidiabetic drug has been tried and that the patient is aware of its potential heart risks. Actos, marketed by the Japanese pharmaceutical company Takeda, does not appear to have heart or liver toxicity risks and remains the only unrestricted glitazone.

SEE ALSO Food and Drug Administration (1906), Insulin (1921), Orinase (1957), Glucophage (1958), Human Insulin (1982).

Diabetes is the leading cause of blindness in adults age 20 to 74. The three major eye problems experienced by the diabetic are glaucoma, retinopathy, and cataracts (shown here), which are associated with elevated blood-glucose levels. The results of some recent studies suggest that Avandia, while lowering blood glucose levels, may actually increase the risk of cataract development.

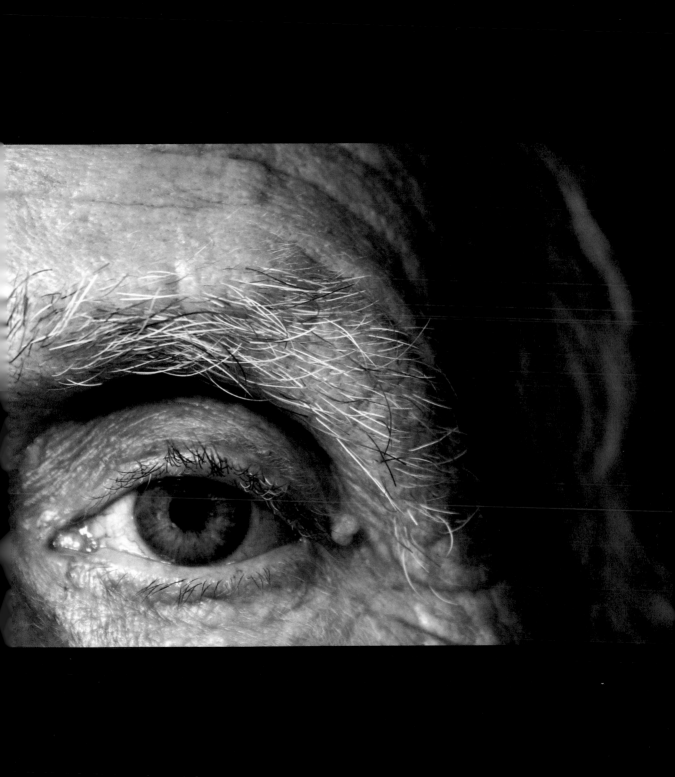

Provenge

Many old men die with prostate cancer, but most don't die because of it. However, some do. Traditional approaches for the treatment of advanced metastatic prostate cancer, in which the cancer has spread to other parts of the body and has failed to respond to hormone therapy, involve the use of chemotherapy (in which both cancer cells and normal cells are damaged or killed by anticancer chemicals), surgery, and radiation.

Provenge represents a new approach known as immunotherapy. The treatment is a vaccine but not a typical "preventive vaccine" such as those for measles, polio, or hepatitis. Rather, it's a "therapeutic vaccine" used after the cancer has been diagnosed. Said to be individualized for each patient, Provenge acts by mobilizing the patient's normal immunological response. White blood cells involved in the immune response are obtained from the patient's blood and sent to a laboratory, where they are mixed with a protein present on prostate cancer cells and an immune system booster. This mixture is then transfused back into the patient's body to specifically target the cancer cells. The patient receives three such treatments over a one-month period.

Seeking more evidence for its safety and effectiveness, the **Food and Drug Administration** rejected Dendeon Corporation's initial application to market Provenge (sipuleucel-T) in 2007. Their decision was greeted with white-hot protests, congressional lobbying, and even death threats by outraged prostate cancer patients, advocates, and investors.

WHAT IS FOUR MONTHS OF LIFE WORTH? The FDA was more amenable to the application in 2010. Common side effects are modest and include such flu-like symptoms as chills, fever, and fatigue. However, the benefits are also modest, extending median survival time from 21.7 months to 25.8 months. No change in the size or progression of the tumor growth is seen. The major question is whether the extra four months of life is worth the $93,000 cost of treatment. Your answer may depend upon whether you are the patient or family member who must pay for the treatment or whether you represent an insurance company or a governmental agency that will be picking up the tab.

SEE ALSO Food and Drug Administration (1906), Diethylstilbestrol (1938), Biologic Drugs (1982), Proscar and Propecia (1992), Flomax (1997).

This needle-core biopsy of the prostate gland shows the presence of prostate cancer. Whereas the cells at nine and ten o'clock are benign, a dense cluster of malignant prostate cells are present at two o'clock.

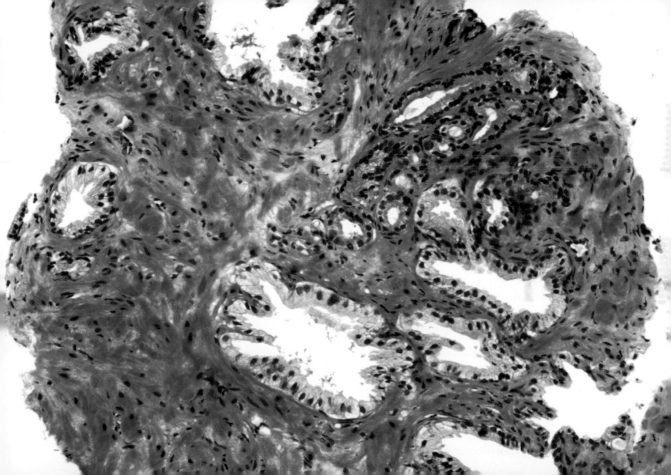

Gilenya

Multiple sclerosis (MS) is an autoimmune disease that has no known cause. White blood cells (lymphocytes) travel from lymph nodes to the brain and spinal cord, damaging the myelin sheath that surrounds and protects nerves. A reduction or blocking of messages between the brain and the body results. Symptoms vary greatly among individuals and include visual disturbances, muscle weakness, and problems with coordination and balance.

MS is highly unpredictable. Some patients exhibit a gradual but steady progression of the disease. More commonly, there are periods of remission lasting for months or years, alternating with relapses, or flare-ups, and a return of symptoms. Before the availability of Gilenya, **cortisone**-like steroids or interferon-beta (Avonex) relieved the MS symptoms and reduced the frequency or duration of relapses. However, these drugs failed to prevent the progression of MS and had many side effects.

In recent years, injectable drugs have appeared that decrease the frequency of MS relapses. These include Copaxone (glatiramer), approved in 1996, and Tysabri (natalizumad), a monoclonal antibody initially approved in 2004, withdrawn because of toxicity, and reintroduced in 2009. There is still no cure for MS.

BRAKING MS. Gilenya is a chemical modification of a natural immunosuppressant obtained from a fungus used as an eternal-youth product in traditional Chinese medicine. Between 2010 and 2011, Gilenya (fingolimod) was approved in North America, Europe, and Japan for the treatment of the relapsing form of MS. In clinical studies, Gilenya reduced the rate of relapses by one-half. The first oral drug to slow the progression of the disability associated with the disease and the frequency and severity of relapses, it is thought to act by preventing the release of lymphocytes.

Full assessment of the safety of Gilenya remains to be determined, but the drug is known to decrease heart rate, increase the susceptibility to infection, and cause swelling of the macula of the eye. The appearance of Gilenya has generated understandable enthusiasm among the 2.5 million MS patients worldwide. Time will tell whether it lives up to its potential.

SEE ALSO Cortisone (1949), Cyclosporine/Ciclosporin (1983).

In multiple sclerosis (MS), nerves lose patches of their myelin cover in a process called demyelinization. This photomicrograph shows a demyelinating MS lesion magnified tenfold.

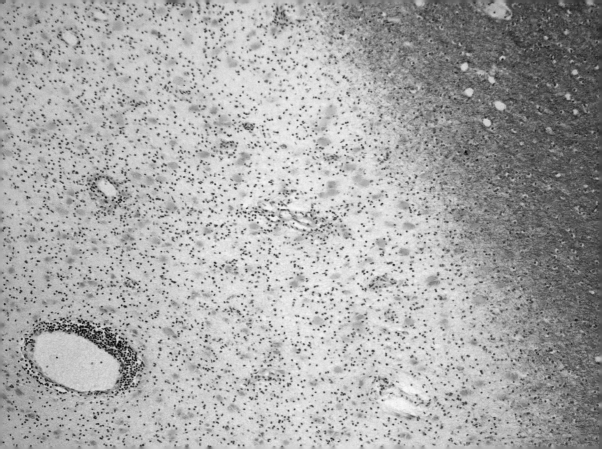

Prescription Drug Abuse

Michael Jackson was not the first celebrity to die as the result of a drug overdose. What caught our attention in 2009 was that legal prescription drugs—and not illicit substances—were responsible. Perhaps it should not have been surprising. While the use of **cocaine** and **methamphetamine** is decreasing, a sharp upswing in the abuse of prescription drugs has been occurring among teenagers and adults in the United States. In fact, the results of a 2010 study revealed a 400 percent increase in substance-abuse treatment admissions for prescription pain relievers between 1998 and 2008, which brings that number to more than 7 million current users, or 2.8 percent of the population.

The escalation in prescription drug abuse has been attributed to a number of factors. In addition to a greater supply and availability of drugs, the number of prescriptions written between 1997 and 2007 outstripped the increase in population by a factor of seven. More than half of these non-medical users identified their drug source to be a friend or relative who had an unused supply of drugs obtained from a physician to treat an authentic medical condition. One-fifth of prescription drug abusers "doctor shop," convincing physicians to write prescriptions that are not needed medically and identifying physicians known to freely write prescriptions on request. Still far easier is obtaining drugs through Internet sales, where few questions, with the exception of a credit card number, are asked.

Three groups of prescription drugs are most often abused. By far, the most common are painkillers such as Vicodin, **OxyContin**, Percodan, and hydrocodone, prescribed to relieve severe pain associated with trauma, an illness, or after an operation. Sedatives used to relieve anxiety or to promote sleep, including **Valium**, **Librium**, and **Xanax**, are also often abused. Stimulants such as **Ritalin**, Adderall, and Dexedrine (**amphetamine**)—prescribed for attention-deficit hyperactivity disorder (ADHD), weight loss, or narcolepsy—make up the third group.

These prescription drugs are perceived to be safer than street drugs because they are on the market and prescribed by doctors. In truth, they act in the brain in a similar manner to illicit drugs. Further, at the doses taken, and when used in combination with other drugs and **alcohol**, they become potentially dangerous—even lethal.

SEE ALSO Cocaine (1884), Amphetamine (1932), Methamphetamine (1944), Ritalin (1955), Librium (1960), Valium (1963), Xanax (1981), Propofol (1983), Ephedra/Ephedrine (1994), OxyContin (1996), Weight-Loss Drugs (2010), Smart Drugs (2018).

Users of prescription drugs mistakenly believe these drugs are safer than street drugs because they come from reputable manufacturers and are approved by the FDA. Drugs obtained from Internet sources are of inconsistent quality, are often counterfeit, and may contain ingredients and doses that are not safe or effective.

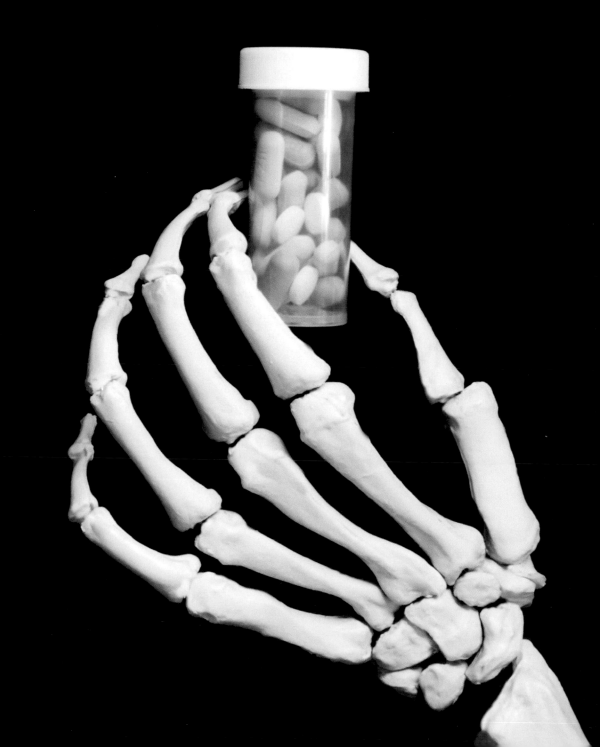

Weight-Loss Drugs

The developed world no longer has a monopoly on obesity. This is now an international problem facing almost all nations. The World Health Organization has projected that, by 2015, approximately 2.3 billion adults will be overweight and 400 million will be obese. Region-by-region, the percentage of obesity in 2005 was 3–4 percent in Japan and Korea, 7–10 percent in western Europe, 14 percent in Canada, 22–23 percent in Australia and the United Kingdom, and 30 percent in the United States, the developed world's leader.

Obesity is a leading preventable cause of death, increasing the risk of heart attack, high blood pressure and stroke, type 2 diabetes, and certain cancers. For many individuals seeking to lose weight, weight-loss drugs are a tempting shortcut. The challenge has been finding drugs that are both safe *and* effective.

Weight-loss drugs work in the following ways: (1) Decreasing the appetite by depressing the feeding center in the hypothalamus. **Amphetamine**-like drugs—the most widely used and approved for short-term use—act this way. (2) Interfering with the absorption of fats. Orlistat (Xenical, Alli) causes a very modest weight loss of 2–3 kilograms (4.4–6.6 lbs) after a year. (3) Increasing the body's rate of metabolism. **Dinitrophenol**, used in the 1930s, was highly effective at this but caused cataracts and severe toxicity.

Since the 1990s, approved drugs that were effective, such as Fen-phen, Redux, and Meridia, have been withdrawn because they increase the risk of heart attacks, strokes, and heart-valve problems. Acomplia (rimonabant) was approved in the European Union in 2006 and withdrawn three years later because its use was associated with depression and increased risk of suicide. In 2012, Qsymia (a combination of phentermine and topiramate) and Belviq (lorcaserin) were both approved for long-term use. Developing suitable drugs has proven to be an elusive challenge, with potential weight-loss products failing before approval or after marketing due to abuse potential, adverse effects, or questionable effectiveness. Time will tell whether these latest drugs effectively combat the rising tide of obesity.

SEE ALSO Amphetamine (1932), Dinitrophenol (1933).

The Portrait of a Gentleman (1630) is attributed to Charles Mellin. At 47 inches × 80 inches (121 cm × 203 cm), the size of this painting exceeds the size of the subject.

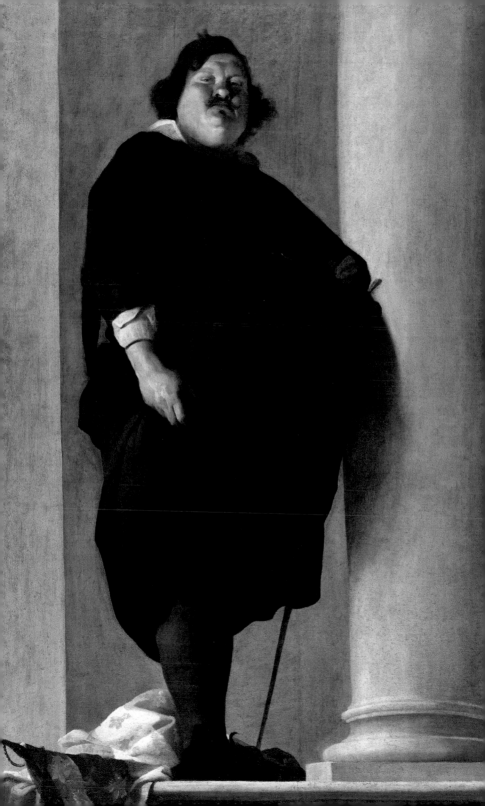

Pradaxa

Clot formation within blood vessels can be dangerous and life-threatening, a risk reduced with several types of drugs. **Aspirin** and **Plavix** prevent platelets from clumping to form a clot, while anticoagulants (blood thinners), such as **warfarin**, interfere with clotting factors in the blood. Warfarin produces its anticoagulant effects by blocking vitamin K, while newer drugs, such as Pradaxa, directly inhibit blood-clotting factors.

For more than six decades, warfarin has been preferred to prevent the formation of blood clots in the deep veins (deep-vein thrombosis, DVT), after hip or knee replacement surgery, and to prevent blood clots in patients with atrial fibrillation (AF), the most common heart-rhythm condition. AF is the major cause of stroke—one of the three leading causes of death in the developed world.

Warfarin (Coumadin), the most widely prescribed oral anticoagulant in North America, is highly effective but suffers from a number of limitations. For one, it interacts with many foods and commonly used drugs, leading to excessive anticoagulation and the risk of bleeding, or inadequate coagulation, with possible clot formation. Thus, the dose of warfarin must be carefully adjusted over days or weeks to fit the patient's unique needs, necessitating frequent blood testing (INR) and regular healthcare monitoring.

In 2010, the **Food and Drug Administration** approved Pradaxa (dabigatran), two years after its approval in Canada and Europe. Pradaxa reduces the risk of DVT and stroke in patients with AF by 35 percent more than warfarin does. Unlike warfarin, treatment with Pradaxa does not require blood monitoring to adjust dosage or dietary modifications, and it interacts with few drugs. However, these benefits come at a price. Well-documented cases of severe internal bleeding have occurred, and the risk of heart attacks is increased. More than 540 deaths were reported to have been associated with Pradaxa in 2011, leading all other drugs, including warfarin, which accounted for 72 deaths. This risk is greater in individuals older than seventy-five and those with impaired kidney function. Unlike warfarin, which has a specific antidote (vitamin K), no antidote is available to counteract the life-threatening bleeding caused by Pradaxa.

SEE ALSO Aspirin (1899), Warfarin (1940), Plavix (1997).

Prevention of clot formation with warfarin or Pradaxa after joint replacement surgery or for people with atrial fibrillation can be lifesaving. Physicians are now faced with a quandary, however: Use Pradaxa, a potentially dangerous but more effective and easier-to-administer drug, or use warfarin, a time-tested anticoagulant with a specific antidote that can reverse its blood-thinning effects?

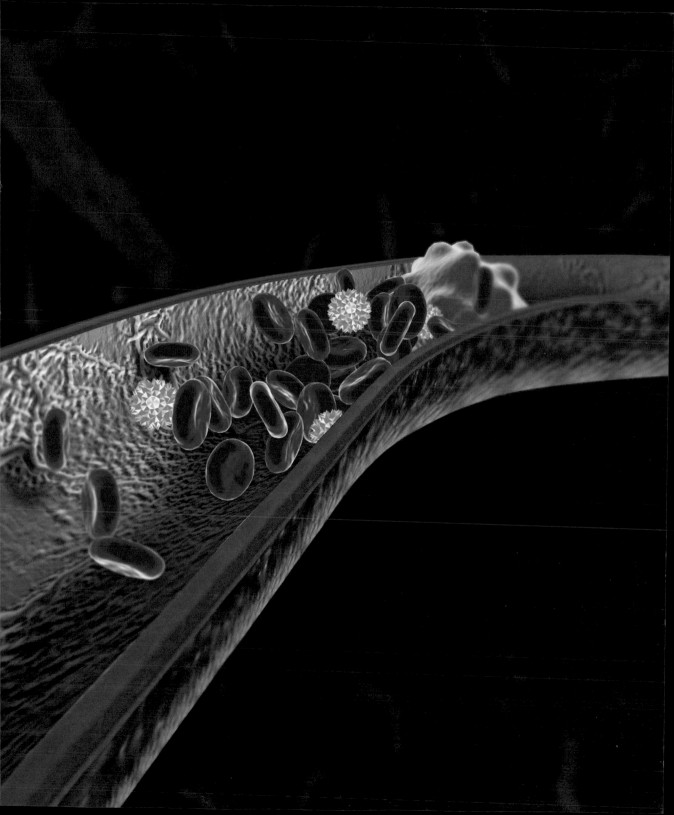

Viread

Some 33 million people worldwide are currently infected with the HIV virus, most of whom are sexually active and can spread the disease to uninfected, and often unsuspecting, partners. While drugs that treat HIV/AIDS are now available, it would be far preferable to prevent the disease from spreading to uninfected individuals. After fifteen years of unsuccessful efforts, preliminary results of two separate studies conducted in Africa in 2010 and 2011, using the Gilead Sciences anti-AIDS drug Viread (tenofovir) in a vaginal gel and pills, provide reason for optimism. Viread blocks reverse transcriptase, an enzyme the HIV virus requires for the synthesis of DNA. Without DNA, this virus cannot multiply.

In Africa, 60 percent of AIDS-infected individuals are women, virtually all of whom became infected through sexual interactions. For these women, preventing infection through abstinence, monogamous partners, or using condoms is beyond their control. Attempts have been made to develop a Viread vaginal gel that would allow them to reduce—although not necessarily eliminate—the need for the man's cooperation. This same gel has been reformulated to be applied to the rectum for use by men and women to protect them from the risk of HIV infection after anal sex.

In other studies, a daily dose of pills containing either one (Viread) or two anti-AIDS drugs (Truvada) reduced the risk of infection in uninfected heterosexual men and women and gay men by 63–73 percent. In this study, a greater rate of protection was seen in the more medication-compliant subjects.

Many questions and challenges remain before AIDS prevention becomes an established reality. These products must be used daily or hours before intercourse. Long-acting products that work for months or even years after administration on a single occasion—such as an AIDS vaccine—would obviously prove far more effective and ideal. Affordability of these expensive drugs has been, and remains, a major challenge. A Medicines Patent Pool was established in 2010 that permits generic pharmaceutical companies to copy patented AIDS drugs at a very low price for use in developing countries.

SEE ALSO Smallpox Vaccine (1796), Fluorides (1945), Polio Vaccine (1954), AZT/Retrovir (1987), HAART (1996).

This illustration shows the AIDS Memorial Quilt, first displayed on the National Mall in Washington, D.C., in 1987. Over two decades, the quilt expanded in size from 1,920 panels to more than 48,000 panels, becoming the largest community-art project in the world.

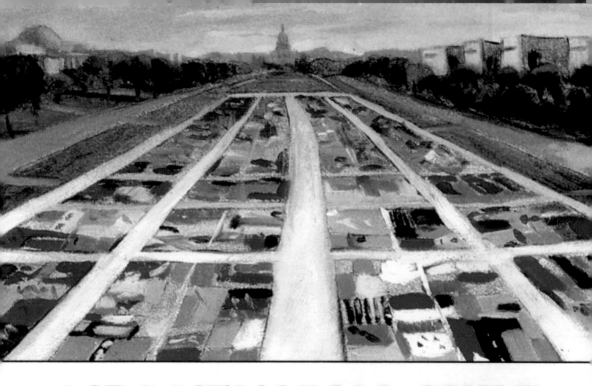

AIDS MEMORIAL QUILT

Victrelis and Incivek

Hepatitis C affects some 130–170 million people worldwide, including 3.2 million Americans, with 20 percent of the affected individuals developing cirrhosis of the liver and liver cancer. Worldwide, hepatitis C infections cause at least 250,000 deaths annually. Approved in 2011, experts view Merck's Victrelis (boceprevir) and Vertex's Incivek (telaprevir) to be the most dramatic advances in the treatment of hepatitis C in decades. These orally administered drugs double previous cure rates to 80 percent and shorten the drug treatment period by one-half, to as few as twenty-four weeks.

Hepatitis is an inflammation of the liver, the body's largest gland. The liver performs a number of complex functions involving digestion, nutrient and vitamin metabolism, synthesis of proteins required for blood clotting, removal of bacteria from the blood, and the metabolism and inactivation of foreign substances, such as drugs. Hepatitis has a number of causes, including infections by several types of virus, the most common of which are designated A, B, and C. They differ in their severity, mode of transmission, prevention, and treatment.

Hepatitis A is often mild and primarily spread by ingestion of fecal-contaminated food or water. Available vaccines are 95–100 percent effective in preventing this condition. Hepatitis B is more severe and is most commonly transmitted by sexual contact with an infected individual, by sharing contaminated needles, and during childbirth, when an infected pregnant woman transmits the virus to her baby. The hepatitis B vaccine—among the safest of vaccines—provides protection to more than 85 percent of individuals after the second dose.

Before the testing of blood supplies in 1992, millions of Americans became infected with hepatitis C after blood transfusions. Now, most individuals become newly infected after sharing contaminated needles, and they are unaware of their infection until years later, when symptoms of liver damage become evident. Earlier hepatitis C treatments with interferon and ribavirin acted by boosting the immune system. By contrast, Victrelis and Incivek block protease, an enzyme the hepatitis C virus requires in order to reproduce itself. Other protease inhibitors are integral components of drug cocktails (**HAART**) used to treat HIV/AIDS infections.

SEE ALSO Acyclovir (1982), AZT/Retrovir (1987), HAART (1996).

The liver, the body's largest internal organ, is highlighted in this illustration of the human abdominal cavity. The liver is a soft, pinkish-brown, triangular organ, normally weighing about 3.5 lbs. (1.6 kg).

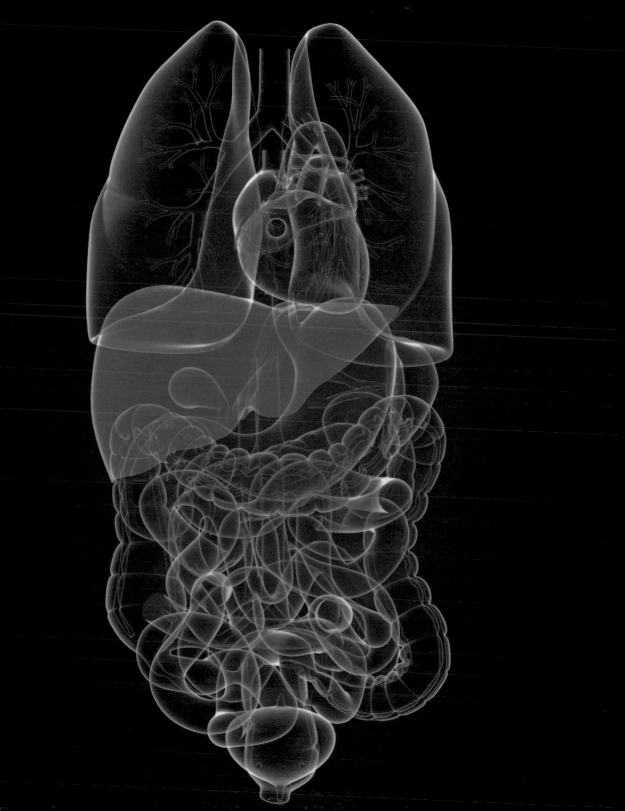

Benlysta

After almost a six-decade interval, a new drug, Benlysta, was approved for the treatment of lupus in 2011. This drug benefits only some of the 300,000 to 1.5 million patients in the United States, 90 percent of whom are women—and not necessarily those at greatest risk. In 1955, approved drugs included **cortisone**-like steroids and Plaquenil, the latter developed for the treatment of malaria. Benlysta is intended to be used in combination with these older drugs, ideally permitting a reduction in the dose of steroids, whose use is associated with severe side effects, and in the frequency of the periodic lupus symptoms.

Systemic lupus erythematosis (SLE or lupus) is a debilitating, serious, and potentially fatal autoimmune disease in which the body's antibodies attack its own connective tissues. Affected tissues include the joints, skin, kidneys, and brain. This chronic disease often has symptom-free periods that may continue for years. Symptoms (referred to as flare-ups) include swelling or pain in the joints, sensitivity to light, fever, chest pain, skin rashes, and fatigue.

Although Benlysta is perceived to be an advance in the treatment of lupus, and its approval by the **Food and Drug Administration** generated considerable enthusiasm in the lupus community, the drug appears to represent more of a step forward than a major breakthrough for treatment. Patients of African descent do not appear to derive benefit from Benlysta, and it was not evaluated in patients with severe forms of the disease. Moreover, only one out of eleven patients derives benefit after treatment.

Benlysta (belimumab) is a monoclonal antibody developed by Human Genome Sciences. It is the first class of drugs found to block the activity of BLyS or B-lymphocyte stimulator, which is thought to energize the production of autoantibodies that attack the body's own tissues. Notwithstanding Benlysta's modest benefits, it may lead to the development of more effective drugs that act in a similar manner.

SEE ALSO Food and Drug Administration (1906), Cortisone (1949), Biologic Drugs (1982).

The term lupus *(Latin for wolf) refers to the resemblance between facial lesions caused by the disease and a wolf's bite, as noted by twelfth-century Italian physician Rogerius. Recently, lupus has been called "the great imitator" because its symptoms can mimic other more common medical disorders. Benlysta represents an advance in the treatment of lupus but, regrettably, is only a modest step forward.*

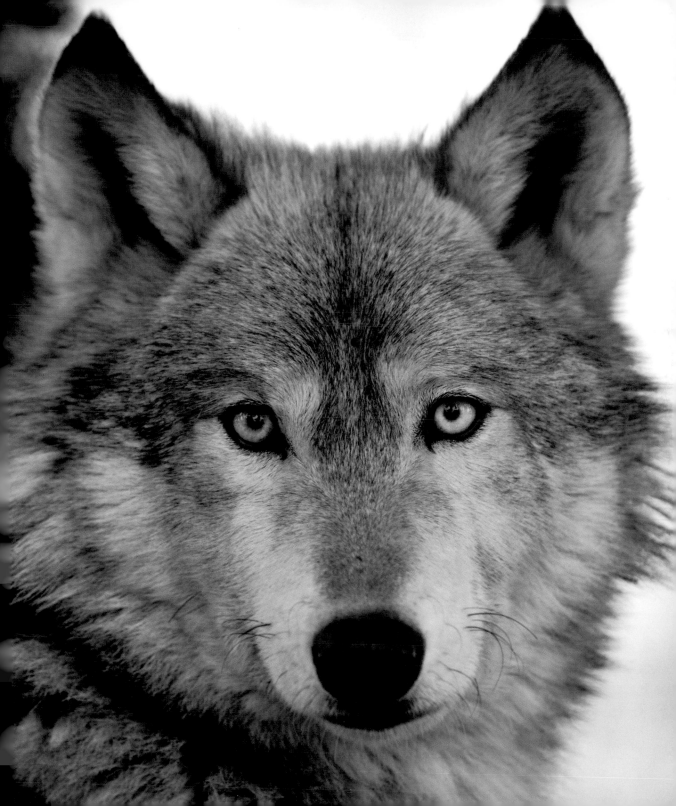

Broad-Spectrum Sunscreens

A suntan has long been a sign of social status. Historically, darker-skinned people were viewed as members of the lower class, while those with fair skin were perceived to be wealthy, with excessive time for leisure. After Coco Chanel returned from the French Riviera with a suntan in the 1920s, however, tanning became the vogue and remained so until the late 1970s, when the dangers of excessive exposure to the sun were recognized.

The greatest of these risks are skin cancers—now the most common of all cancers, accounting for 2–3 million new cases globally each year. Although less common than other skin cancers, melanoma is the most dangerous. Annually, it is responsible for some 130,000 new cases of skin cancer worldwide and three-quarters of all skin cancer deaths, numbering about 50,000. Incidence of skin cancer is expected to rise with depletion of the ozone layer and increased exposure to ultraviolet radiation (UVR).

UVR is divided into two major bands: UVA and UVB, the latter of which is responsible for burning and inducing skin cancer. More recently, it has been recognized that UVA exposure, which penetrates into deeper layers of skin, may not only increase the carcinogenic effects of UVB but may itself cause skin cancer, as well as premature skin aging.

Sunscreens have sun protection factor (SPF) ratings, which, to date, have only reflected protection against UVB. Under ideal sunscreen application conditions (rarely achieved in practice), SPF ratings of 15 block 93 percent of UVB, while SPF 30 ratings block 97 percent. Although UVA protection has not traditionally been considered in SPF, new rules effective in 2012 in the United States mandate that products claiming to be "broad spectrum" provide equal protection against UVB and UVA, and that only those with SPF 15 or higher can claim protection against skin cancer and premature skin aging.

Sunscreens, usually containing a mixture of ingredients, are of two major types: chemical sunscreens that absorb UVR transmission and thereby block its transmission to the skin, and physical sunscreens (e.g., zinc oxide and titanium dioxide), which act by reflecting and scattering UVR and protect against UVB and UVA. Regrettably, there is no international agreement regarding acceptable active ingredients in sunscreens and their concentrations.

Doris Kenyon (1897–1979) was a popular actress starring in some sixty silent and sound movies between 1915 and 1939. Kenyon's pale look was considered in vogue until the 1920s, when being tan became all the rage. The use of sunscreens is now a health issue and not a fashion statement.

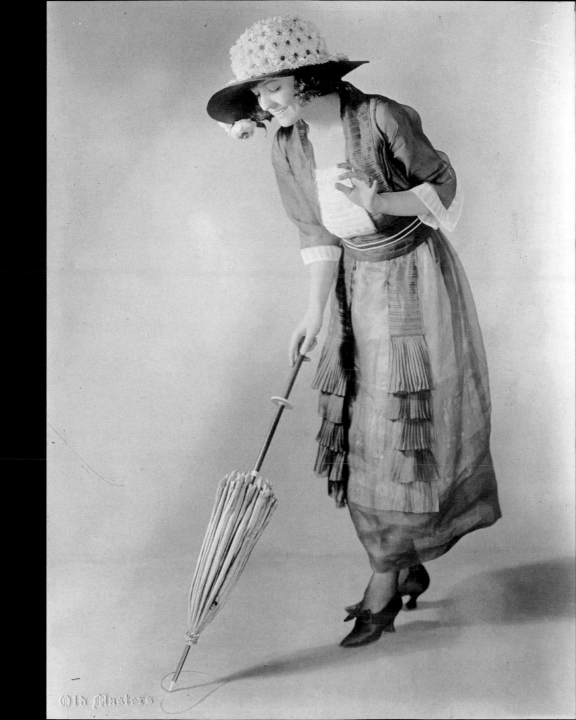

Kalydeco

Affecting 30,000 patients in the United States, cystic fibrosis (CF) is one of the most common inherited diseases leading to death among Caucasians. In CF, the body produces very thick, sticky mucus that clogs the lungs, allowing bacteria to collect and causing the patient to cough and wheeze. The flow of digestive enzymes from the pancreas that break down and absorb food is also impaired, causing nutritional problems. Patients are prone to respiratory tract infections, and, over time, they lose their ability to breathe. The average life expectancy of a CF patient is thirty-seven years.

After the CF gene was first identified in 1989, early attempts to use gene therapy by inserting the correct gene into the lungs proved unsuccessful. Of the more than 1,800 genetic mutations that can cause CF, about four percent of CF patients—1,200 individuals in the United States—were found to have a mutation in the G551D or CF transmembrane conductance regulator (CFTR) gene, which makes a protein that controls the movement of chloride and water into and out of cells. When this protein does not function normally, mucus thickens, damaging the lungs, digestive system, reproductive system, and other organs.

In 2012, Kalydeco (ivacaftor), developed by Vertex Pharmaceuticals and with the support of the Cystic Fibrosis Foundation, was approved for the treatment of CF in the United States and Europe for children older than six years. Described as a "medical breakthrough," Kalydeco represents one of the first drugs that corrects an underlying specific genetic defect rather than just providing symptomatic relief.

Referred to as a CFTR potentiator, Kalydeco works by helping the protein made by the defective gene to function better. Individuals receiving the drug by mouth exhibit significant and sustained improvement in lung function, and they also gain weight. On the downside, Kalydeco does not reverse permanent lung damage caused by CF. Also, priced at $294,000 for a year's supply, it is among the most expensive prescription drugs in the United States

Only those patients with a defective CFTR gene benefit from taking Kalydeco, but studies combining Kalydeco with a second drug are underway, with the goal of helping 90 percent of CF patients.

SEE ALSO Gene Therapy (2020).

The pancreas (pictured) secretes digestive enzymes into the duodenum that promote the absorption and digestion of fats and proteins. In CF, mucus blocks the pancreatic ducts, preventing these enzymes from reaching the intestines and causing malnutrition and weight loss. Children taking Kalydeco have been reported to gain weight.

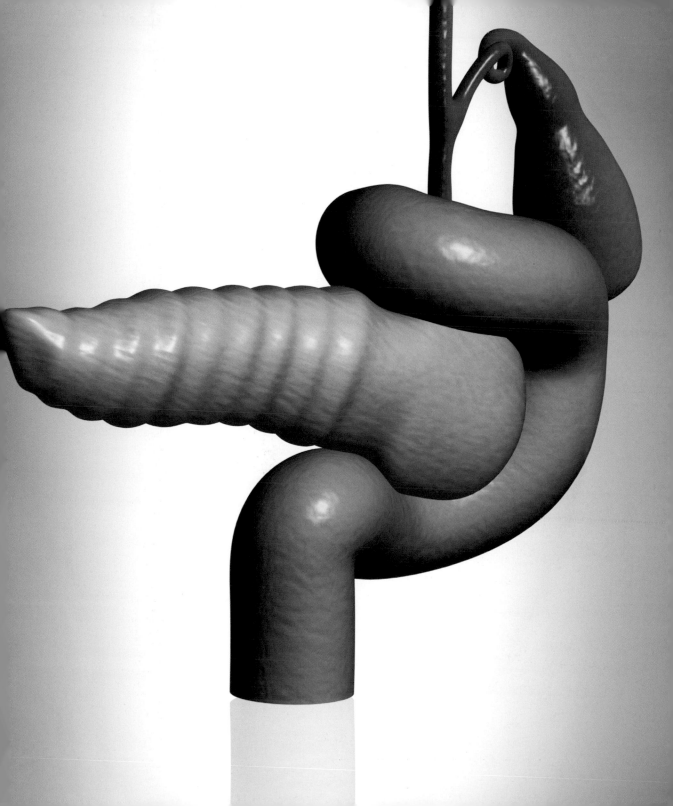

Anti-Alzheimer's Drugs

Alois Alzheimer (1864–1915)

As our population ages, so will the increased prevalence of Alzheimer's disease (AD), arguably the most terrifying consequence of aging, with the loss of memory and of the self. The World Health Organization estimates that four of every 1,000 people worldwide will have AD in 2015. Scientists are searching for causes, for ways to detect it earlier, and for drugs that will prevent, slow, and even reverse its progression.

In 1906, German psychiatrist-neuropathologist Alois Alzheimer accurately described a patient with progressive memory, language, and behavioral problems. Upon her death, he found changes in brain tissue—namely, the presence of twisted bands of fibers (neurofibrillary tangles) and dense deposits surrounding nerve cells (neuritic plaques). Six decades later, scientists recognized that a correlation existed between the mental decline and these specific brain changes, leading to the recognition that AD is a disease and not an inevitable consequence of aging.

These damaging brain changes begin long before—perhaps one or more decades before—memory loss or cognitive decline appears. Some scientists believe that when these cognitive signs become evident, the damage has been done, and it's too late for existing drugs to correct the underlying causes. Researchers are exploring simple and accurate diagnostic tests for AD before cognitive symptoms appear. PET scans of the brain, involving radioactive imaging, are able to detect plaques, and spinal taps can detect beta-amyloid, a protein that forms plaques. Still farther back in the disease process are genetic influences (such as the ApoE4 gene) that increase the risk of AD by hastening the accumulation of beta-amyloid.

If these diagnostic tests for early detection of AD prove reliable, ongoing debates will swirl in the medical community: How early should individuals with memory deficits be labeled with AD? More fundamentally, should such diagnostic tests even be conducted in routine medical practice, since AD is currently untreatable?

One active approach in anti-AD–drug development is looking at how to block gamma secretase, an enzyme that chops down a larger protein to form beta-amyloid. Clearly, other approaches are needed to combat this devastating disorder.

SEE ALSO Neurotransmitters (1920), Cognex and Aricept (1993), Smart Drugs (2018).

Two elderly men are playing Xiangqi or Chinese chess, one of the most popular board games in China. Some research suggests memory games may slow the progression of Alzheimer's disease.

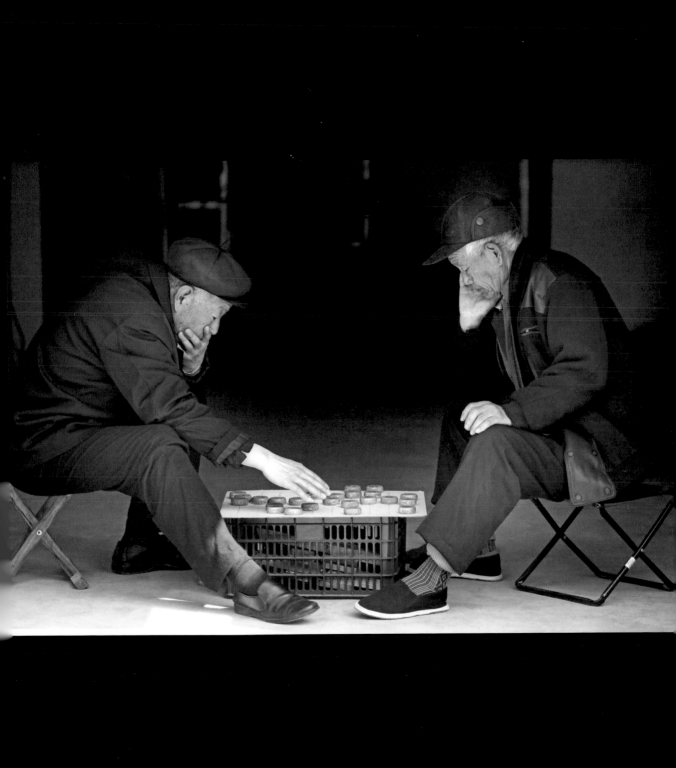

Female Viagra

The 1998 appearance of **Viagra** brought erectile dysfunction (impotence) out of the shadows and revolutionized its treatment. It was also a multibillion-dollar seller worldwide for Pfizer. What about women? Based on multiple reports, 29–43 percent of women experience low libido or hypoactive sexual desire disorder (HSDD), with personal distress, at some time in their life—hence, the need for a drug that increases female sexual desire. The use of Viagra seems obvious, but the premise has faltered based on the realization that the relationship between arousal and desire differs dramatically in men and women.

Arousal almost invariably leads to desire in men but not necessarily in women. Viagra increases blood flow to the genital area—a marker of sexual arousal—in both sexes. However, in women, the key linkage between arousal and desire is far more complex, and their critically sensitive "sex organ" appears to be the brain. Viagra does not work on the brain and, thus, does not increase female desire. Pfizer abandoned hopes of having a pink Viagra in 2004. What other approaches are there?

Although typically thought of as a male hormone, **testosterone** is secreted by the female ovaries and adrenal gland. Testosterone levels decrease with age—dramatically so after menopause—and hormonal deficiency may contribute to HSDD. Intrinsa, a testosterone-containing skin patch produced by Procter & Gamble, was approved for use in post-menopausal females in Canada in 2002 and in Europe in 2007, but the **Food and Drug Administration** rejected it. Their 2004 rejection was said not to be based on effectiveness but on concern regarding its long-term safety and potential for off-label use to increase muscle mass and strength.

By contrast, Boehringer Ingelheim exploited the "sex/brain/body" link in conceiving the development of its female libido-enhancing drug. Flibanserin, a non-hormone with complex effects on the brain's neurotransmitters, was reported by women to increase "sexually satisfying events," but in 2010, the FDA rejected it because it did not increase sexual desire during clinical studies.

A testosterone-like drug may yet prove to be the elusive female Viagra that increases sexual desire. Nevertheless, some doubt exists as to whether HSDD is an authentic medical disorder or merely a marketing gimmick to sell drugs.

SEE ALSO Mandrake (c. 200 BCE), Food and Drug Administration (1906), Neurotransmitters (1920), Testosterone (1935), Dianabol (1956), Off-Label Drug Use (1962), Viagra (1998).

Venus, the Roman goddess of love and beauty, is depicted in Botticelli's La nascita di Venere *(The Birth of Venus). This masterpiece was painted in 1486 and is now displayed in the Uffizi Gallery in Florence, Italy.*

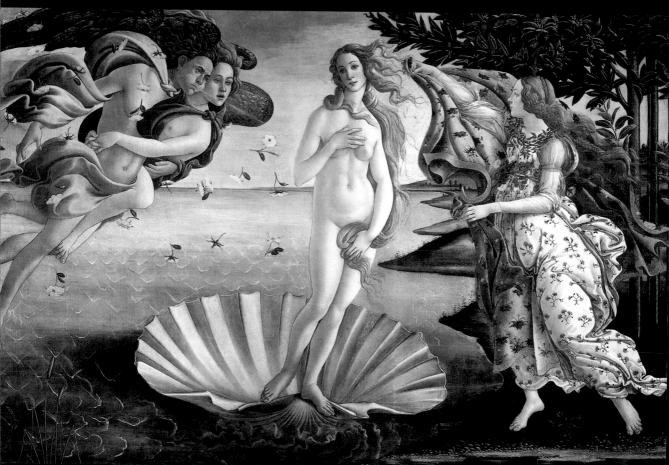

Smart Drugs

Move Over, Einstein and Mozart. If we believe ads appearing on websites or in print, we are but one pill, Power Bar, drink, or **dietary supplement** away from having a greater attention span or powers of concentration—perhaps even a greater memory, capacity to learn, ability to solve complex problems, and reasoning prowess. These "miraculous" products are variously called smart drugs, cognitive enhancers, and nootropics (from the Greek, "toward the mind").

Some purported smart drugs are nutrients and herbals available at health food stores. Others have been approved for use for Alzheimer's disease or Parkinson's disease but have never been shown to enhance memory. Currently, the most widely used smart drugs are stimulants, such as **Ritalin** (methylphenidate) and Adderall (**amphetamine** salts), which treat attention deficit-hyperactivity disorder (ADHD) or Provigil (modafinal), prescribed to counteract narcolepsy.

As many students and rising executives will attest, stimulants do promote alertness, decrease drowsiness, and increase concentration. However, evidence that such drugs enhance the user's ability to solve complex problems, write great books, compose symphonies, or make more rational long-term decisions is now absent.

In theory, how might the smart drugs of the future help the user achieve such wonders? Perhaps by increasing the supply of or efficiency in utilizing nutrients and oxygen in the brain. Increasing the synthesis, creating mimics, or improving the effectiveness of **neurotransmitters**, hormones, or other essential brain chemicals required for memory might work. Still others might facilitate the flow of information between nerves or enhance the utilization of memory stores. Some of these drugs may be of benefit in the treatment of Alzheimer's disease, and perhaps some anti-Alzheimer's drugs will enhance normal memory.

Assuming such drugs were safe, effective, and available, who could get them, and would their selective availability be good or bad for society at large? Would using smart drugs in school or on the job provide an unfair advantage, or would they be more like tutors that maximize mental abilities? As we learn more about brain function and its chemistry, such drugs appear to be on the not-so-distant horizon.

SEE ALSO Neurotransmitters (1920), Amphetamine (1932), Ritalin (1955), Dietary Supplements (1994).

This spherical fused gyroscope comes close to achieving perfection, differing from a perfect sphere by no more than 40 atoms. Used in NASA's Gravity Probe B experiment in 2004, it tested and confirmed two key predictions from Einstein's 1916 general theory of relativity. Einstein, synonymous with genius, is refracted in the background image.

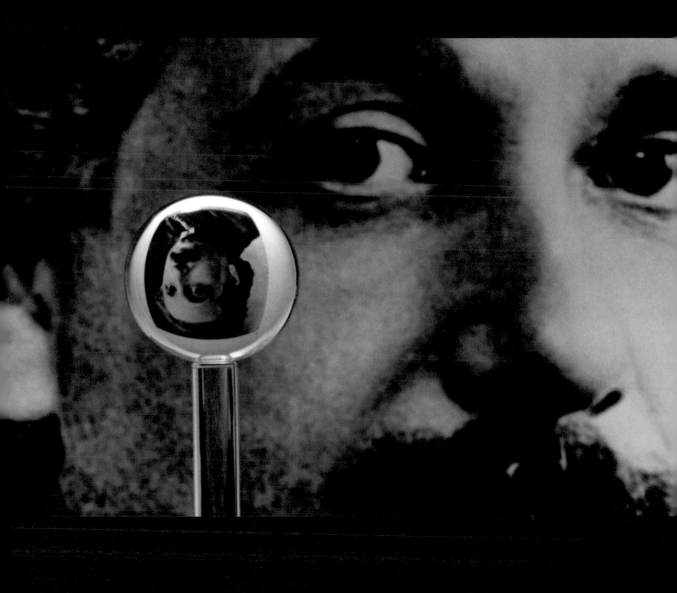

Antiaging Drugs

We have long sought to arrest, eliminate, or even reverse aging evidenced by the deterioration of our organs, sensory systems, and minds. Antiaging strategies have varied from subsisting on a low-calorie diet of fresh fruits and vegetables, to moving to Shangri-La, to imbibing from the Fountain of Youth. More immediate and tangible are the pills, vitamins, hormones, and creams being promoted, with extravagant and largely unsubstantiated claims of benefit.

What doesn't work? Three of the most widely promoted antiaging products are the hormones **testosterone**, DHEA, and human **growth hormone** (GH). Whereas administering testosterone improves the physical and psychological state of men with low testosterone levels, its benefit in older and healthy men has not been established, and it may potentially cause harm. Similarly, no benefits occur after elderly people have taken DHEA (dehydroepiandrosterone), which is converted to testosterone in the body. Although GH is medically used to stimulate growth, its safety and effectiveness as an antiaging product have yet to be established in appropriately controlled studies.

Some of us are content with merely concealing the outward appearance of aging by using anti-wrinkle products, such as **Botox**. Alternatively, a wide assortment of creams and lotions contain alpha-hydroxy acids (AHAs) that cause the top dead layer of skin to peel and be replaced by new layers of smooth skin. Their most distinguishing characteristic is their extremely high price.

What may work? **Resveratrol**, obtained from the skin of grapes, was found in some studies, but not others, to extend the lifespan of yeast, worms, flies, and mice. By exploring how it may act at a molecular level, a compound with a similar action— perhaps activating a specific life-extending protein—may be of benefit in humans.

However, perhaps more important than living many more years is our ability to remain in good health until our days end. For the moment, only a healthy diet, abstinence from smoking, and exercise appear to ward off the ravages of advancing age.

SEE ALSO Testosterone (1935), Growth Hormone (1985), Botox (1989), Dietary Supplements (1994), Resveratrol (2003).

Der Jungbrunnen *(also referred to as* Fons Juventutis, *or "Fountain of Youth," 1546), an oil painting by Lucas Cranach the Elder, currently hangs at the Gemäldegalerie in Berlin. Note the elderly women entering the fountain on the left and emerging as youthful beauties on the right.*

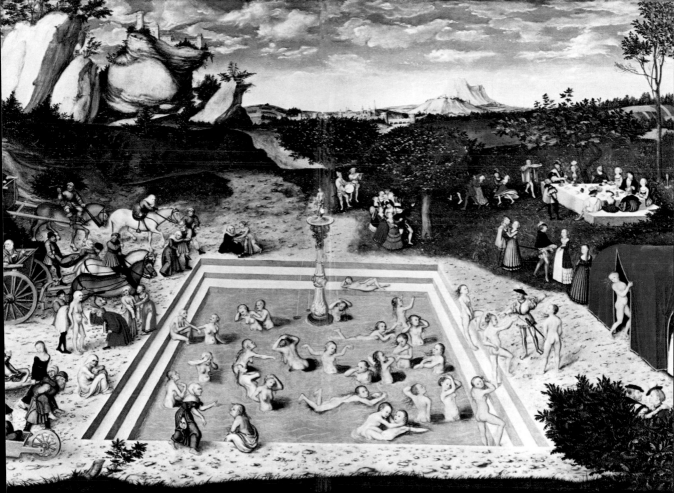

Gene Therapy

In 1972, Theodore Friedmann and Richard Roblin published what many consider to be the first in-depth consideration of the use of gene therapy for the treatment of human genetic diseases. Since the early 1990s, gene therapy has been hyped as a game-changing medical treatment, but after being plagued by an almost unbroken series of failures—including a subject's death in 1999—all clinical therapy trials in the United States were suspended for a number of years. Then in 2011, gene therapy was successfully used to treat the first well-known genetic disease, hemophilia B, a disorder caused by a defect in the gene for clotting Factor IX. This treatment success, involving six patients, has reinvigorated hope for a technique first conceptualized in 1972 and attempted in a human subject in 1990. The genetic defect was carried by Queen Victoria and was passed to her male descendants, who married into the royal houses of Europe.

The most common approach in gene therapy involves introduction of a normal gene into the genome to replace a missing or defective gene responsible for causing or preventing a disease. The gene carrier (vector) is usually a virus that transports the therapeutic gene to its target cells in the patient. Once delivered to its target, the therapeutic gene enters the cell's interior and begins producing a protein that restores the cell's function to normal.

To be successful, gene therapy must overcome a number of challenges. Once delivered to the intended cells and then activated, the therapeutic gene must be stable and long-lived in order to provide long-lasting benefits. As a foreign substance, the virus must evade attack by the immune system—a problem that limits repeated treatments. Also, once inside the patient, the viral vector must not restore its capacity to cause disease.

Gene therapy remains an experimental approach to prevent or treat disease. For the foreseeable future, until essential challenges are overcome, it appears unlikely to replace drugs. The best candidates for gene therapy are those disorders caused by a defective single gene, such as hemophilia, cystic fibrosis, sickle cell anemia, and Tay-Sachs disease. Far more challenging will be such multi-gene disorders as heart disease, high cholesterol, diabetes, cancers, and Alzheimer's disease.

SEE ALSO Biologic Drugs (1982), Kalydeco (2012).

The Romanovs were the ruling family in Russia in the late nineteenth and early twentieth centuries—a reign that abruptly ended in 1918 when Tsar Nicholas, his wife Alexandra, and their children were murdered during the Bolshevik revolution. Their only son, Prince Alexei, was prone to excessive bleeding, attributed to hemophilia caused by a defective gene passed down from his great-grandmother, Britain's Queen Victoria.

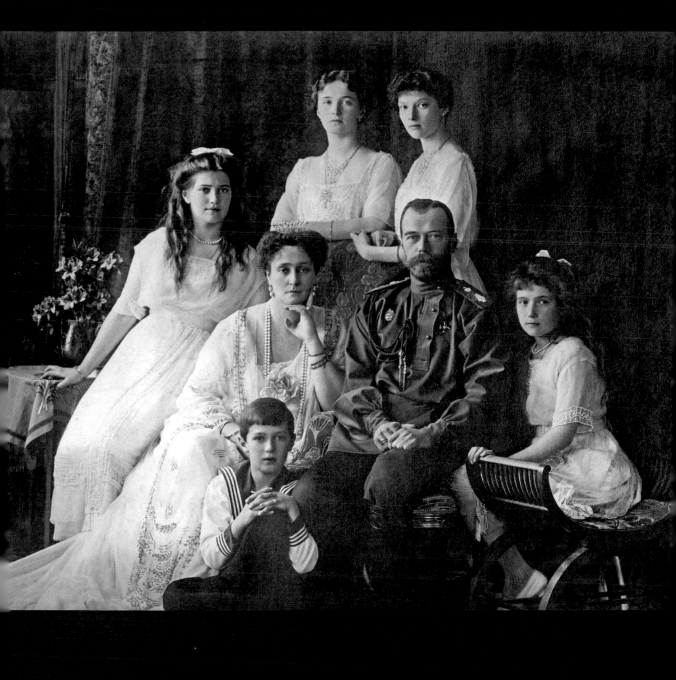

Further Reading

The following list contains some of the many sources I've used to write this book. It is also intended to provide you with more in-depth information on the drugs I've discussed. A number of Internet sources are ongoing and reliable, offering detailed and up-to-date information on most of the drugs that continue to play a role in modern medicine. These include: the Centers for Disease Control and Prevention (*www.cdc.gov*); Mayo Clinic (*mayoclinic.com/health/drug-information/DrugHerbindex*); Medline Plus (*www.nlm.nih.gov/medlineplus/druginformation.html*); and PubMed Health (*www.ncbi.nlm.nih.gov/pubmedhealth/s/drugs_and_supplements*). The compilation of the best or most significant drugs is highly subjective. I welcome your comments about any significant or interesting drug that might be included in future editions of this book at mcgeraldweb@gmail.com.

General Reading and Sources

Brecher, E. M., and Editors of Consumer Reports, *Licit & Illicit Drugs: The Consumer Union Report on Narcotics, Stimulants, Depressants, Inhalants, Hallucinogens, and Marijuana—Including Caffeine, Nicotine, and Alcohol.* Boston: Little, Brown, 1972. [Brecher, 1972]

Brunton, L. L., Lazo, J. S., Parker, K.L., eds., *Goodman and Gilman's The Pharmacological Basis of Therapeutics*, New York: McGraw-Hill, 2006. [Bruton, Lazo, 2006]

DiPalma, J. R., ed., *Drill's Pharmacology in Medicine*, New York: McGraw-Hill, 1971. [DiPalma, 1971]

Drill, V. A., *Pharmacology in Medicine*, New York: McGraw-Hill, 1954. [Drill, 1954]

Emsley, J., *Elements of Murder*, New York: Oxford University Press, 2005.

Gerald, M. C., *Pharmacology: An Introduction to Drugs*, Englewood Cliffs, NJ: Prentice-Hall, 1981.

Goodman, L. S., Gilman, A., *The Pharmacological Basis of Therapeutics*, New York: Macmillan, 1955. [Goodman, Gilman, 1955]

Hart, C. L., Ksir, C., *Drugs, Society and Human Behavior*, New York: McGraw-Hill, 2012.

Osol, A., Farrar, G. E., Pratt, R., eds., *The Dispensary of the United States of America*, Philadelphia: Lippincott, 1960. [Osol, Farrar, 1960]

Sneader, W., *Drug Discovery: A History*, West Sussex, England: John Wiley, 2005.

Sollmann, T., *A Manual of Pharmacology*, Philadelphia: W.B. Saunders, 1942. [Sollmann, 1942]

Tyler, V. E., Brady, L. R., Robbers, J. E., *Pharmacognosy*, Philadelphia: Lea & Febiger, 1988.

Wikipedia Encyclopedia, *wikipedia.org*.

Herbs, c. 60,000 BCE

Mathison, R. R., *The Eternal Search: The Story of Man and His Drugs*, New York: G.P. Putnam, 1958.

Reader's Digest Magic and Medicine of Plants, Pleasantville, NY: The Reader's Digest Association, 1986.

Alcohol, c. 10,000 BCE

Forney, R. B., Harger, R. N., "The Alcohols," in DiPalma, 1971.

Zernig, G., et al., eds., *Handbook of Alcoholism*. Boca Raton, FL: CRC Press, 2000.

Alchemy, c. 5000 BCE

Morris, R., *The Last Sorcerers: The Path from Alchemy to the Periodic Table*, Washington, DC: Joseph Henry Press, 2003.

Cannabis, c. 3000 BCE

Booth, M., *Cannabis: A History*, New York: Macmillan, 2005.

Tea, c. 2737 BCE

Bennett, B. A., Bealer, B. K., *The World of Caffeine: The Science and Culture of the World's Most Popular Drug*, New York: Routledge, 2001.

Opium, c. 2500 BCE

Gutstein, H. B., Huda, A., "Opioid Analgesics," in Brunton, Lazo, 2006.

Herz, A., ed., *Opioids I. Handbook of Experimental Pharmacology* 104/I and 104/II. Berlin: Springer-Verlag, 1993.

Smith and Ebers Papyri, c. 1550 BCE

Bryan, C. P., *tinyurl.com/24v2mox*.

Rauwolfia, c. 500 BCE

Patil, P. N., Gulati, O. D., Balaraman, R., *Topics in the History of Pharmacology*. Gujarat, India: B.S. Shah, 2009.

Hemlock, 399 BCE

Brickhouse, T. C., Smith, N. D., eds., *The Trial and Execution of Socrates*, New York: Oxford University Press, 2001.

Mandrake, c. 200 BCE

www.newworldencyclopedia.org/entry/Mandrake_(plant).

Osol, Farrar, 1960.

Theriac of Mithridates, c. 65 BCE
Mayor, A., *The Poison King: The Life and Legend of Mithradates*, Rome's Deadliest Enemy, Princeton, NJ: Princeton University Press, 2009.

Materia Medica, c. 60
nccam.nih.gov/health/homeopathy/abchomeopathy.com/matmed.htm.

Colchicine, c. 70
MayoClinic, *tinyurl.com/2ug88rq.*

Coffee, c. 800
Bennett, B. A., Bealer, B. K., *The World of Caffeine: The Science and Culture of the World's Most Popular Drug,* New York: Routledge, 2001.
Garattini, S., ed., *Caffeine, Coffee, and Health*, New York: Raven Press, 1993.

Arsenic, 1250
Whorton, J. C., *The Arsenic Century: How Victorian Britain Was Poisoned at Home, Work, and Play*, New York: Oxford University Press, 2010.

Witches' Flying Ointments, 1456
Murray, M. A., *The Witch-Cult in Western Europe*, Oxford: Clarendon Press, 1921.
Szasz, T. S., *Ceremonial Chemistry: The Ritual Persecution of Drugs, Addicts, and Pushers*, Syracuse, NY: Syracuse University Press, 2003.

Coca, 1532
Brecher, 1972.

Belladonna, 1542
Botanical.com, *tinyurl.com/2cg4pl.*
Osol, A., Farrar, 1960.

Antimonials, 1602
Osol, A., Farrar, 1960.

Patent Medicines, 1623
American Medical Association, *Nostrums and Quackery: Articles on the Nostrum Evil and Quackery*, Reprinted, with Additions and Modifications from *The Journal of the American Medical Association*, Chicago: American Medical Association Press, 1912.

Young, J. H., *The Toadstool Millionaires: A Social History of Patent Medicines in America Before Federal Regulation*, Princeton, NJ: Princeton University Press, 1961.

Cinchona Bark, 1639
Oaks Jr., S. C., Violaine, S. M., et al., eds., *Malaria: Obstacles and Opportunities*, Washington, DC: National Academies Press, 1991.
rain-tree.com/quinine.htm.

Ergot, 1670
Dale, H. H., *Annual Review of Pharmacology and Toxicology* **3**: 1; 1963.

Laudanum, 1676
Brecher, 1972.

Ferrous Sulfate, 1681
National Heart Lung and Blood Institute, *tinyurl.com/43sbl52.*

Ipecac, 1682
National Capital Poison Center, *poison.org/prepared/ipecac.asp.*

Hydrogen Cyanide, 1704
Goodman, Gilman, 1955.

Clinical Testing of Drugs, 1753
Bourgeois, F. T., Murthy, S., Mandl, K. D., *Annals of Internal Medicine* **153**: 158; 2010.
Oates, J. A., "The Science of Drug Therapy," in Brunton, Lazo, 2006.

Aconite, 1762
Osol, A., Farrar, 1960.

Tetrodotoxin, 1774
Medscape Reference, *tinyurl.com/36jvnzh reference.com/browse/Tetrodotoxin.*

Digitalis, 1775
Goodman, Gilman, 1955.
Sollmann, 1942.

Calomel, 1793
Swiderski, R. M., *Calomel in America: Mercurial Panacea, War, Song and Ghosts*, Boca Raton, FL: BrownWalker Press, 2009.

Smallpox Vaccine, 1796
Koplow, D. A., *Smallpox: The Fight to Eradicate a Global Scourge*, Berkeley: University of California Press, 2003.

Homeopathic Medicine, 1796
Barrett, S., *tinyurl.com/54sad.*
NaturalNews, *tinyurl.com/295dvvv.*
NCCAM Clearinghouse, *nccam.nih.gov/health/homeopathy/.*

Absinthe, 1797
Hulsman, M., et al., *International Journal of Epidemiology* **36**: 738; 2007.
Lachenmeier, D. W., Nathan-Maister, D., *Journal of Agriculture and Food Chemistry* **56**: 3073; 2008.

Alkaloids, 1806
Hesse, M., *Alkaloids: Nature's Curse or Blessing?* Zürich: Verlag Helvetica Chimica Acta, 2002.
Robinson, T., *Scientific American* **201**: 113; 1959.

Morphine, 1806
Gutstein, H. B., Huda, A., "Opioid Analgesics," in Brunton, Lazo, 2006.
Huxtable, R. J., Schwarz, S.K.W., *Molecular Interventions* **1**: 189; 2001.

Strychnine, 1818
Sollmann, 1942.

Caffeine, 1819
Bennett, B. A., Bealer, B. K., *The World of Caffeine: The Science and Culture of the World's Most Popular Drug*, New York: Routledge, 2001.
Fredholm, B. B., et al., *Pharmacological Reviews* **51**: 83; 1999.

Quinine, 1820
Centers for Disease Control and Prevention, *tinyurl.com/2797rs5.*
Oaks Jr., S. C., Violaine, S. M., et al., eds., *Malaria: Obstacles and Opportunities*, Washington, DC: National Academies Press, 1991.

Atropine, 1831
RxMed, *tinyurl.com/38anxlq drugs.com/ppa/atropine.html.*

Codeine, 1832

Gasche, Y., Youssef, D., Fathi, M., *New England Journal of Medicine* **351**: 2827, 2002.

Gutstein, H. B., Huda A, "Opioid Analgesics," in Brunton, Lazo 2006.

Medical Marijuana, 1839

Joy, J. E., Watson Jr., S. J., Benson Jr., J. A., eds., *Marijuana and Medicine: Assessing the Science Base*, Washington, D.C.: National Academy Press, 1999.

ProCon, *medicalmarijuana.procon.org*.

Nitrous Oxide, 1844

Orth, O. S., "General Anesthetics II: Gaseous Agents," in Drill, 1954.

Robinson, V., *Victory Over Pain: A History of Anesthesia*, New York: Henry Schuman, 1946.

Ether, 1846

Orth, O. S., "General Anesthetics I: Volatile Agents," in Drill, 1954.

Robinson, V., *Victory Over Pain: A History of Anesthesia*, New York: Henry Schuman, 1946.

Chloroform, 1847

Orth, O. S., "General Anesthetics I: Volatile Agents," in Drill, 1954.

Robinson, V., *Victory Over Pain: A History of Anesthesia*, New York: Henry Schuman, 1946.

Curare, 1850

McIntyre, A. R., *Curare: Its History, Nature, and Clinical Use*, Chicago: University of Chicago Press, 1947.

Bromides, 1857

Goodman, Gilman, 1955.

Phenol, 1867

McDonnell, G., Russell, A. D., *Clinical Microbiology Reviews* **12**: 147; 1999.

Chloral Hydrate, 1869

RxList. "Noctec," *rxlist.com/ noctec-drug.htm.*

Digitoxin, 1875

Chen, K. K., Kovaríková, A., *Journal of Pharmaceutical Sciences* **56**: 1535; 1967.

Koch-Weser, J., Schechter, P. J., *Life Sciences* **22**: 1361; 1978.

Physostigmine, 1875

Goodman, Gilman1955.

Rodin, F. H., *American Journal of Ophthalmology* **30**: 19; 1947.

Nitroglycerin, 1879

Elkayam, U., *Annals of Internal Medicine* **114**: 667; 1991.

Fant, K., *Alfred Nobel: A Biography*, New York: Arcade Publishing, 1993.

Parker, J. D., Parker, J. O., *New England Journal of Medicine* **338**: 520; 1998.

Scopolamine, 1881

Centers for Disease Control and Prevention, *tinyurl.com/38mb2zr.*

medicinenet.com/motion_sickness/ article.htm.

Paraldehyde, 1882

Drugs.com, *tinyurl.com/2v7ut2g.*

Cocaine, 1884

Brecher, 1972.

Kahn, E. J., *The Big Drink: The Story of Coca-Cola*, New York: Random House, 1960.

Petersen, R. C., Stillman, R. C., eds., *Cocaine: 1977*, (NIDA Research Monograph 13). Washington, DC: U.S. Department of Health and Human Services, 1977.

Theophylline, 1888

eMedTV, tinyurl.com/2d68mnv.

Mescaline, 1897

Brecher, 1972.

Heroin, 1898

Askwith, R., *opioids.com/heroin/ heroinhistory.html.*

Brecher, 1972.

Aspirin, 1899

Andermann, A.A.J., *tinyurl.com/3af5zr5.*

Jeffreys, D., *Aspirin: The Remarkable Story of a Wonder Drug*, New York: Bloomsbury, 2004.

Sneader, W., *British Medical Journal* **321** (7276): 1591; 2000.

Epinephrine/Adrenaline, 1901

Cannon, W. B., *The Way of an Investigator: A Scientist's Experience in Medical Research*, New York: W.W. Norton, 1945.

Goodman, Gilman, 1955.

Phenolphthalein, 1902

Drill, 1954.

Goodman, Gilman, 1955.

Barbital, 1903

López-Muñoz, F., Ucha-Udabe, R., Alamo, C., *Neuropsychiatric Disease and Treatment* **1**: 329; 2005.

Maynert, E. W., "Sedatives and Hypnotics II. Barbiturates," in Drill, 1971.

Atoxyl, 1905

Steverding, D., *parasitesandvectors.com/ content/2/1/29.*

Time Magazine, *tinyurl.com/36s744y.*

Novocain, 1905

Carpenter, R. L., and Mackey, D. C., "Local Anesthetics," in *Clinical Anesthesia*, Barash, P. G., Cullen, B. F., Stoelting, R. K., eds., Philadelphia: Lippincott, 1992.

Fortunato, P. M., *tinyurl.com/2e5ctrs.*

Drug Receptors, 1905

Pruell, C. R., Maehle, A. H., Halliwell, R. F., *A Short History of the Drug Receptor Concept*, New York: Palgrave Macmillan, 2009.

Pure Food and Drug Act, 1906

Young, J. H., *The Toadstool Millionaires: A Social History of Patent Medicines in America Before Federal Regulation*, Princeton, NJ: Princeton University Press, 1961.

U.S. Food and Drug Administration, 1906

U.S. Food and Drug Administration, *tinyurl.com/63pa6xk.*

Young, J. H., *The Toadstool Millionaires: A Social History of Patent Medicines in America Before Federal Regulation*, Princeton, NJ: Princeton University Press, 1961.

Oxytocin, 1909
Lee, H J., MacBeth, A. H., et al., *Progress in Neurobiology* 88: 127; 2009.

Salvarsan, 1910
Nobelprize.org, *tinyurl.com/37kgefa*.

Phenobarbital, 1912
Aviado, D. M., *Krantz and Carr's Pharmacological Principles of Medical Practice*, Baltimore: Williams & Wilkins, 1972.

Quinidine, 1912
Grace, A. A., Camm, A. J., *New England Journal of Medicine* 338: 35; 1998.

Thyroxine, 1914
Braverman, L. E., Utiger, R. D., eds., *Werner and Ingbar's The Thyroid*, New York: Lippincott Williams & Wilkins, 2005.
Norman, J., *tinyurl.com/4nctkau*

Heparin, 1916
Marcum, J. A., *jhmas.oxfordjournals.org/content/55/1/37*.

Neurotransmitters, 1920
Rubin, R. P., *Pharmacological Reviews* 59: 289; 2007.
Westfall, T. C., Westfall, D. P., "Neurotransmission: the Autonomic and Somatic Motor Nervous Systems," in Brunton, Lazo, 2006.

Merbaphen, 1920
Vogl, A., *Diuretic Therapy*, Baltimore: Williams & Wilkins, 1953.

Carbon Tetrachloride, 1921
Centers for Disease Control and Prevention, *tinyurl.com/3y537v3*.
Recknagel, R. O., *Pharmacological Reviews* 19: 145; 1967.

Insulin, 1921
LeRoith, D., Taylor, S. I., Oleksky, J. M., eds., *Diabetes Mellitus: A Fundamental and Clinical Text*, Philadelphia: Lippincott Williams & Wilkins, 2003.
Pickup, J. C., Williams, J., eds., *Textbook of Diabetes*, Oxford: Blackwell Publishing, 2003.

Hexylresorcinol, 1924
Osol, Farrar, 1960.

Ergotamine and Ergonovine, 1925
Goodman, Gilman, 1955.
Ruzicka, L., *jstor.org/pss/769674*.

Insulin Shock Therapy, 1927
American Experience, *tinyurl.com/2gyu3wy*.
Sabbatini, R.M.E., *tinyurl.com/2b37gsz*.

Thimerosal, 1927
Parker, S. K., et al., *Pediatrics* 114: 793; 2004.
Specter, M., *The New Yorker*, May 30, 2011, p. 80.

Penicillin, 1928
Mandell, G. L., Bennett, J. E., Dolin, R., eds., *Mandell, Douglas, and Bennett's Principles and Practice of Infectious Diseases*, Philadelphia: Churchill Livingstone, 2000.
Petri Jr., W. A., "Penicillins, Cephalosporins, and Other B-Lactam Antibiotics," in Brunton, Lazo, 2006.

Nembutal and Seconal, 1928
Lacey, M., *tinyurl.com/5fbyes*.

Estrone and Estrogen, 1929
Loose, D. S., Stancel, G. M., "Estrogens and Progestins," in Brunton, Lazo, 2006.
Watkins, E. S., *The Estrogen Elixir: A History of Hormone Replacement Therapy in America*, Baltimore: Johns Hopkins University Press, 2007.

Amphetamine, 1932
Brecher, 1972.
Hart, C. L., Ksir, C., *Drugs, Society and Human Behavior*, New York: McGraw-Hill, 2012.

Progesterone and Progestin, 1933
Djerassi, C., *This Man's Pill: Reflections on the 50th Birthday of the Pill*, New York: Oxford University Press, 2001.
MayoClinic, *tinyurl.com/2bza87t*.

Dinitrophenol, 1933
Sollmann, 1942.

Thiopental, 1934
Lasson, K., *tinyurl.com/6pwxal*.

Tubocurarine, 1935
McIntyre, A. R., "Curare and Related Compounds," in Drill, 1954.

Prontosil, 1935
Kiefer, D.M., *tinyurl.com/25qyxh2*.
Time Magazine, *tinyurl.com/25q4lsv*.

Testosterone, 1935
Bagatelle, C. J., Bremmer, W. J., *New England Journal of Medicine* 334: 707; 1996.

Neostigmine and Pyridostigmine, 1935
Golomb, B. A., *Proceedings of the National Academy of Sciences* 105: 4295; 2008.
MedlinePlus, *tinyurl.com/6aughxn*.

Tabun and Sarin, 1936
Centers for Disease Control and Prevention, *bt.cdc.gov/agent/sarin/basics/facts.asp*.
Romano, J. A., Lukey, B. J., Salem, H., eds., *Chemical Warfare Agents: Chemistry, Pharmacology, Toxicology, and Therapeutics*, Boca Raton, FL: CRC Press, 2008.

Sulfanilamide, 1936
Goodman, Gilman, 1955.
WW2 U.S. Medical Research Centre, *med-dept.com/sulfa.php#mil*.

Dapsone, 1937
MedlinePlus, *tinyurl.com/93bcd*.
World Health Organization, *who.int/lep/en/*.

Diethylstilbestrol, 1938
Giusti, R. M., Iwamoto, K., Hatch, E. E., *annals.org/content/122/10/778.full*.
National Cancer Institute, *cancer.gov/cancertopics/factsheet/Risk/DES*.

Dilantin, 1938
Rowland, L. P., *The Legacy of Tracy J. Putnam and H. Houston Merritt: Basic Neurology in the United States*, New York: Oxford University Press, 2009.

Federal Food, Drug, and Cosmetic Act, 1938
Dunn, J. H., *Federal Food, Drug, and Cosmetic Act*, Chicago: Clearinghouse Press, 1938.
Martin, B., *tinyurl.com/29a6wdd*.

DDT, 1939
Ecobichon, D. J., "Toxic Effects of Pesticides, " in *Casarett & Doull's Toxicology: The Basic Science of Poisons*, Klaassen, C.D., ed., New York: McGraw-Hill, 2001.
Lear, L., *Rachel Carson: Witness for Nature*, New York: Henry Hoyten, 1997.

Percorten, 1939
Dallek, R., *Atlantic Monthly*, December 2002, 49.

Warfarin, 1940
PubMed Health, *tinyurl.com/2vwxjrk*.
Wardrop, D., Keeling, D., *British Journal of Haematology* 141: 757; 2008.

Premarin, 1941
Watkins, E. S., *The Estrogen Elixir: A History of Hormone Replacement Therapy in America*, Baltimore: Johns Hopkins University Press, 2007.

Nitrogen Mustard, 1942
Hirsch, J., *Journal of the American Medical Association* 296: 1518; 2006.

LSD, 1943
Cooper, J. R., Bloom, F. E., Roth, R. H., *The Biochemical Basis of Neuropharmacology*, New York: Oxford University Press, 2003.
Hoffer, A., *Clinical Pharmacology & Therapeutics* 6: 183; 1965.
Khatchadourian, R., *The New Yorker*, December 17, 2012.

Streptomycin, 1944
Rom, W. N., Gray, S. M., eds., *Tuberculosis*, Boston: Little Brown, 1996.

Neo-Antergan, 1944
Dale, H. H., *Annual Review of Pharmacology and Toxicology* 3: 1; 1963.

Methamphetamine, 1944
National Institute on Drug Abuse, *tinyurl.com/3qp4t2d*.

Fluoride, 1945
American Public Health Association, *tinyurl.com/6yk4vvj*.
Jones, S., Burt, B. A., *Bulletin of the World Health Organization* 83(9): 670; 2005.

Benadryl, 1946
Rocha e Silva, M., ed., *Histamine and Anti-Histamines: Handbook of Experimental Pharmacology*, Vol. 18, Berlin: Springer-Verlag, 1966.
Rocha e Silva, M., ed., *Histamine II and Anti-Histaminics: Chemistry, Metabolism and Physiological and Pharmacological Actions: Handbook of Experimental Pharmacology*, Vol. 18, Part 2, Berlin: Springer-Verlag, 1978.

Radioiodine, 1946
Braverman, L. E., Utiger, R. D., eds., *Werner and Ingbar's The Thyroid*, New York: Lippincott Williams & Wilkins, 2005.
Saha, G. P., *Fundamentals of Nuclear Pharmacy*, New York: Springer-Verlag, 2004.

Methadone, 1947
O'Brien, C. P., Jaffe, J. H., eds., *Addictive States*, New York: Raven Press, 1992.

Drug Metabolism, 1947
Bachmann, C., Bickel, M. H., *Drug Metabolism Reviews* 16: 185; 1985-86.
Conti, A., Bickel, M .H., *Drug Metabolism Reviews* 6: 1; 1977.

Chloroquine, 1947
Centers for Disease Control and Prevention, *www.cdc.gov/malaria/traveldoctor.co.uk/malaria.htm*.

Amethopterin and Methotrexate, 1947
MedlinePlus, *tinyurl.com/44se6t*.

Tetracyclines, 1948
Merck, *merck.com/mmpe/sec14/ch170/ch170o.html*.
Tredwin, C. J., Scully, C., Bagan-

Sebastian, J. V., *Journal of Dental Research* 84: 596; 2005.

Xylocaine, 1948
Carpenter, R. L., and Mackey, D. C., "Local Anesthetics," in *Clinical Anesthesia*, Barash, P. G., Cullen, B. F., Stoelting, R. K., eds., Philadelphia: Lippincott, 1992.

Lithium, 1949
Cade, J. F., "The Story of Lithium," in *Discoveries in Biological Psychiatry*, Ayd, F. J., Blackwell, B., eds., Baltimore: Ayd Medical Communications, 1970.

Chloramphenicol, 1949
MedlinePlus, *tinyurl.com/3ewbqzu*.

Cortisone, 1949
Marks, H. M., *Bulletin of the History of Medicine* 66(3): 419; 1992.
MedlinePlus, *tinyurl.com/2as6ksb*

Succinylcholine, 1951
Kalow W., *Pharmacogenetics: Heredity and the Response to Drugs*, Philadelphia: WB Saunders, 1962.

Isoniazid, 1951
Kalow, W., *Pharmacogenetics: Heredity and the Response to Drugs*, Philadelphia: W.S. Saunders, 1962.
MedlinePlus, *tinyurl.com/3jxsgr9*.

Malathion, 1951
EXTOXNET, *tinyurl.com/o3p6ob*.

Phenergan, 1951
Popik, B., *tinyurl.com/23f7ydk*.
Supreme Court of the United States Blog, *tinyurl.com/3wk5ptw*.

Benemid, 1951
MedlinePlus, *tinyurl.com/6yyn47s*.

Chlorpromazine, 1952
Baldessarini, R. J., Tarazi, F. I., "Pharmacotherapy of Psychosis and Mania," in Brunton, Lazo, 2006.
Muñoz, L., Alamo, C., et al., *Annals of Clinical Psychiatry* 17: 113; 2005.
Rosenbloom, M., *The Journal of the American Medical Association* 287: 1860; 2002.

Reserpine, 1952
Domino, E. F., "Antipsychotics: Phenothiazines, Thioxanthines, Butyrophenones, and Rauwolfia Alkaloids," in DiPalma, 1971.
Osol, Farrar, 1960.

Iproniazid, 1952
Rees, L., Benaim, S., *tinyurl.com/4xz72z5*.

Erythromycin, 1952
MedlinePlus, *tinyurl.com/3kqax56*.

Diamox, 1952
Forward, S. A., Landowne, M., et al., *New England Journal of Medicine* **279**: 839; 1968.
traveldoctor.co.uk/altitude.htm.

Acetaminophen/Paracetamol, 1953
Thomas, S. H., *Pharmacology & Therapeutics* **60**: 91; 1993.
PubMed Health, *tinyurl.com/22lx2mr*.

Mercaptopurine, 1953
MIT, *web.mit.edu/invent/iow/elion2.html*.
Nobel Prize, *tinyurl.com/24fwor5*.

Nystatin, 1954
Hildick-Smith, G., "Chemotherapy of Fungal Infections," in DiPalma, 1971.

Polio Vaccine, 1954
Plotkin, S. A., Orenstein, W. A., Offit, P. A., eds., *Vaccines*, New York: Saunders Elsevier, 2008.

Meprobamate, 1955
Greenblatt, D. J., Shader, R. I., *American Journal of Psychiatry* **127**: 1297; 1971.
Ramchandani, D., López-Muñoz, F., Alamo, C., *Psychiatric Quarterly* **77**: 43; 2006.

Placebos, 1955
Beecher, H. K., *The Journal of the American Medical Association* **159**: 1602; 1955.
Moerman, D. E., *Meaning, Medicine and the "Placebo Effect,"* New York: Cambridge University Press, 2002.
Shapiro, A. K., Shapiro, E., *The Powerful Placebo: From Ancient Priest to Modern Physician*, Baltimore: Johns Hopkins University Press, 2000.

Ritalin, 1955
Fisher, B. C., ed., *Attention Deficit Disorder*, New York: Informa Healthcare USA, 2007.

Dianabol, 1956
Kochakian, C. D., *Anabolic Steroids in Sport and Exercise*, Champaign, IL: Human Kinetics, 2000.

Amphotericin B, 1956
MedlinePlus, *tinyurl.com/44gnnb5* .

Orinase, 1957
Hurley, D., *Diabetes Rising: How a Rare Disease Became a Modern Pandemic, and What To Do About It*, New York: Kaplan Publishing, 2010.
Schwartz T.B., Meinert C.L., *Perspectives in Biology and Medicine* **47(4)**: 564; 2004.

Thalidomide, 1957
Little, B. B., *Drugs and Pregnancy: A Handbook*, London: Hodder Arnold, 2006.
Rogers, J. M., Kavlock, R. J, "Developmental Toxicology," in *Casarett & Doull's Toxicology: The Basic Science of Poisons*, Klaassen, C.D., ed., New York: McGraw-Hill, 2001.

Tofranil and Elavil, 1957
Schatzberg, A. F., Nemeroff, C. B., eds., *The American Psychiatric Press Textbook of Psychopharmacology*, Washington, DC: American Psychiatric Press, 1998.

Grieseofulvin, 1958
MayoClinic, *tinyurl.com/3qg5uas*.

Glucophage, 1958
PubMed Health, *tinyurl.com/29wvoa9*.
UK Prospective Diabetes Study Group, *Lancet* **352 (9131)**: 854; 1998.

Diuril, 1958
Ernst, M. E., Moser, M., *New England Journal of Medicine*, **361**: 2153; 2009.
Greene, J. A., *Bulletin of the History of Medicine* **79**: 749; 2005.

Haldol, 1958
Ayd Jr., F. J., *www.ncbi.nlm.nih.gov/pubmed/1019142*.
Baldessarini, R. J., Tarazi, F. I., "Pharmacotherapy of Psychosis and Mania," in Brunton, Lazo, 2006.

Vinca Alkaloids, 1958
Duffin, J., *Pharmacy in History* **44 (2)**: 64; **(3)**: 105; 2002.

Dextromethorphan, 1958
MedlinePlus, *tinyurl.com/4fbsgmg*.

Flagyl, 1959
MedlinePlus, *tinyurl.com/67dxxvf*.

Librium, 1960
MedlinePlus, *tinyurl.com/3hqzeog*.
Woods, J. H., Katz, J. L., Winger, G., *Pharmacological Reviews* **44**: 151; 1992.

Enovid, 1960
MayoClinic, *tinyurl.com/ds9dq*.
Watkins, E. S., *On the Pill: A Social History of Oral Contraceptives, 1950–1970*, Baltimore: Johns Hopkins University Press, 1998.

Ampicillin, 1961
Petri, Jr., W. A., "Penicillins, Cephalosporins, and Other B-Lactam Antibiotics," in Brunton, Lazo, 2006.

Hexachlorophene, 1961
wiki.medpedia.com/Clinical:Phisohex_(hexachlorophene).

Monoamine Oxidase Inhibitors, 1961
MedlinePlus, *tinyurl.com/3mt3xtx*.
Sadock, B. J., Sadock, V. A., *Kaplan and Sadock's Synopsis of Psychiatry: Behavioral Sciences/Clinical Psychiatry*, North American Edition, Philadelphia: Lippincott Williams & Wilkins, 2007.

Kefauver-Harris Amendment, 1962
Time Magazine, tinyurl.com/2878688.
Henninger, D., *econlib.org/library/Enc1/DrugLag.html*.

Off-Label Drug Use, 1962
Radley, D. C., *Archives of Internal Medicine* 166: 1021; 2006.
Stafford, R. S., *New England Journal of Medicine* 358: 1427; 2008.

Valium, 1963
Woods, J. H., Katz, J. L., Winger, G., *Pharmacological Reviews* 44: 151; 1992.

Gentamicin, 1963
Begg, E. J., Barclay, M. L., *British Journal of Clinical Pharmacology* 39: 597; 1995.
Chambers, H. F., "Aminoglycosides," in Brunton, Lazo, 2006.

Propranolol, 1964
Consumer Reports, *tinyurl.com/4qlx4tw.*
Kroll, D. J., *tinyurl.com/yjqzzx9.*

Cephalothin, 1964
Hamilton-Miller, J.M.T., *International Journal of Antimicrobial Agents* 15: 179; 2000.
merck.com/mmpe/sec14/ch170/ch170c.html.
Petri Jr., W. A., "Penicillins, Cephalosporins, and Other B-Lactam Antibiotics," in Brunton, Lazo, 2006.

Lasix, 1966
Brater, D. C., *European Heart Journal* 13 (Suppl G): 10; 1992.
Klabunde, R. E., *tinyurl.com/dbv3yz.*

Zyloprim, 1966
MedlinePlus, *tinyurl.com/6hqjyoj.*
Rundles, R. W., *Archives of Internal Medicine* 145: 1492; 1985.

Rifampin, 1967
MedlinePlus, *tinyurl.com/3euprdy.*
Sensi, P., *Reviews of Infectious Diseases* 5 (Suppl. 3): S402; 1983.

Clomid, 1967
health.google.com/health/ref/Infertility.
MedlinePlus, *tinyurl.com/3dzke7b.*

Valproic Acid, 1967
drugs.com/cons/valproic-acid.html.

Phencyclidine, 1967
Petersen, R. C., Stillman, R. C., eds., *Phencycline (PCP) Abuse:*

An Appraisal, (21), Washington, DC: U.S. Department of Health and Human Services, 1978.

Levodopa, 1968
Factor, S. A., Weiner, W. J., eds., *Parkinson's Disease: Diagnosis and Clinical Management*, New York: Demos Medical Publishing, 2008.
National Institute of Neurological Disorders and Stroke, *tinyurl.com/q7dqe.*

Albuterol/Salbutamol, 1968
The American Academy of Allergy Asthma and Immunology, *tinyurl.com/yeosjvy.*
Mayo Clinic, *tinyurl.com/6jvobv.*

RhoGAM, 1968
Medscape, *tinyurl.com/6kkr76m.*
U.S. National Library of Medicine, *tinyurl.com/3uk2b6e.*

Fentanyl, 1968
U.S. Department of Justice, *tinyurl.com/4t3ay36.*

Butazolidin, 1968
Fox News, *tinyurl.com/62aakx.*

Praziquantel, 1972
MedlinePlus, *tinyurl.com/3rnjk8d.*
Merck Veterinary Manual, *tinyurl.com/3kmxrqf.*

Artemisinin, 1972
Dondorp, A. D., Nosten, F., et al., *The New England Journal of Medicine* 361: 455; 2009.

Opioids, 1973
Brownstein, M. J., *Proceeding of the National Academy of Sciences USA* 90: 5391; 1993.
Gutstein, H. B, Akil, H., "Opioid Analgesics" in Brunton, Lazo, 2006.
O'Brien, C. P., Jaffe, J. H., eds., *Addictive States*, New York: Raven Press, 1992.

Tamoxifen, 1973
Jordan, V. C., *Nature Reviews Drug Discovery* 2: 205; 2003.
MedlinePlus, *tinyurl.com/69xhmfc.*

Rohypnol, 1975
University of Maryland, *cesar.umd.edu/cesar/drugs/rohypnol.asp.*

Beclovent, 1976
Mayo Clinic, *tinyurl.com/4gaalf4.*
Rau, J. L., *Respiratory Care* 50: 1083; 2005.

Tagamet, 1976
Altman, L. K., *tinyurl.com/yk9vnqt.*
Black, J. W., Duncan, W. A. M., *Nature* 236: 385; 1972.

MDMA/Ecstasy, 1976
wikipedia.org/wiki/MDMA.

Lethal Injection, 1977
Zimmers, T. A., Sheldon, J., et al., *tinyurl.com/3p54rqs.*

Timoptic, 1978
American Academy of Ophthalmology, *tinyurl.com/4vtg69l.*

Captopril, 1981
MedlinePlus, *tinyurl.com/6jsa5pf.*
Consumer Reports, *tinyurl.com/6xyymug.*

Xanax, 1981
MedlinePlus, *tinyurl.com/6juoxw.*
Verster, J. C., Volkerts, E. R., *CNS Drug Reviews* 10: 45; 2004.

Acyclovir, 1982
Balfour, H. H., *The New England Journal of Medicine* 340: 1255; 1999.
Hayden, F. G., "Antiviral Agents (Nonretroviral)," in Brunton, Lazo, 2006.

Biologic Drugs, 1982
European Medicines Agency, Committee for Medicinal Products for Human Use, "Guideline on Similar Biological Medicinal Products," (2005-10-30).
Giezen, T. J., Mantel-Teeuwisse, A. K., et al., *Journal of the American Medical Association* 300: 1887; 2008.

Human Insulin, 1982
DiabetesHealth, *tinyurl.com/2b75ah6.*
How Products Are Made, *madehow.com/Volume-7/Insulin.html.*
pi.lilly.com/us/humulin-r-ppi.pdf.

Accutane, 1982
Goldsmith, L. A., Bolognia, J. L., et al., *Journal of the American Academy of Dermatology* **50**: 900; 2004.

Cyclosporine/Ciclosporin, 1983
Encyclopedia of Surgery, tinyurl. com/43olb3f.
PubMed Health, *tinyurl.com/3aoodjp.*

Propofol, 1983
Taraborrelli, J. R., *Michael Jackson: The Magic, the Madness, the Whole Story, 1958–2009*, New York: Hachette Book Group, 2009.

Growth Hormone, 1985
Rudman, D., Feller, A. G., et al., *New England Journal of Medicine* **323**: 1; 1990.
Vance, M. L., Mauras, N., *The New England Journal of Medicine* **341**: 1206; 1999.

Crack Cocaine, 1986
Baker, P., *tinyurl.com/2dcxsmt.*
Watson, S., *tinyurl.com/24y96hw.*

BuSpar, 1986
MedlinePlus, *tinyurl.com/pyoo3j.*

AZT/Retrovir, 1987
Flexner, C. "Antiretroviral Agents and Treatment of HIV Infection," in Brunton, Lazo, 2006.
Richman, D. D., *Nature* **410**: 995; 2001.

Cipro, 1987
Centers for Disease Control and Prevention, *bt.cdc.gov/bioterrorism/.*
Van der Linden, P. D., Sturkenboom, M. C., et al., *Archives of Internal Medicine* **163**: 1801; 2003.

Mevacor, 1987
Consumer Reports Best Buy Drugs, Evaluating Statin Drugs to Treat: High Cholesterol and Heart Disease, 2010.
Li, J. J., *Triumph of the Heart: The Story of Statins*, New York: Oxford University Press, 2009.

Prozac, 1987
Baldessarini, R. J. "Drug Therapy of Depression and Anxiety Disorders," in Brunton, Lazo, 2006.
Frazer, A., *Journal of Clinical Psychopharmacology*, **17**: 2S; 1997.

Ivermectin, 1987
Omura, S., *International Journal of Antimicrobial Agents* **31**: 91; 2008.

tPA, 1987
Rivera-Bou, W. L., *tinyurl.com/yznkvss.*

Rogaine, 1988
Hogue, M. D., "Hair Loss," in *Handbook of Nonprescription Drugs: An Interactive Approach to Self-Care*, Berardi, R. R., Ferreri, S. P., Hume, A. L., Kroon, L. A., Newton, G. D., eds., Washington, DC: American Pharmaceutical Association, 2006.
Pray, W. S., *Nonprescription Prescription Therapeutics*, Philadelphia: Lippincott Williams & Wilkins, 2006.

Mifepristone, 1988
Feminist Women's Health Center, *tinyurl.com/5kvst.*
Food and Drug Administration, *tinyurl.com/3onrmlu.*

Prilosec, 1989
Chong, E., Ensom, M. H., *Pharmacotherapy* **23**: 460; 2003.
www.consumerreports.org/health/resources. "Drugs to Treat Heartburn and Stomach Acid Reflux: The Proton Pump Inhibitors," 2010.

Clozapine, 1989
Alvir, J. M. J., Lieberman, J. A., et al., *New England Journal of Medicine* **329**: 162, 1993.
Baldessarini, R. J., Tarazi, F. I., "Pharmacotherapy of Psychosis and Mania," in Brunton, Lazo, 2006.

Epoetin, 1989
Borrione, P., Spaccamiglio, A., et al., *International SportMed Journal* **10**: 45; 2009.
Nelson, M. T., *tinyurl.com/yaox98d.*

Botox, 1989
Allergen, *allergen.com/assets/pdf/botox_ cosmetic_pi.pdf.*
Singer, N., *tinyurl.com/cs9gm2.*

Imitrex, 1991
Davidoff, R. A., *Migraine: Manisfestations, Pathogenesis, and Management*, New York: Oxford University Press, 2002.
Humphrey, P., Ferrari, M., Olesen, J., eds., *The Triptans: Novel Drugs for Migraine*, New York: Oxford University Press, 2001.

Nicotine Replacement Therapy, 1991
Centers for Disease Control and Prevention, *tinyurl.com/4p62x6l. tobacco.org/Documents/documents.html.*

Neupogen, 1991
tinyurl.com/3fhuwto.

Proscar and Propecia, 1992
Bihari, M., *tinyurl.com/386lgaf.*
National Kidney and Urologic Diseases Information Clearinghouse, *tinyurl. com/jl8nr.*

Ambien, 1992
Holm, K. J., Goa, K. L., *Drugs* **59**: 865, 2000.
MedlinePlus, *tinyurl.com/3wdbto6.*

Cognex and Aricept, 1993
Crystal, H., *tinyurl.com/38nwcwg.*
Shankle, W. R., Amen, D. G., *Preventing Alzheimer's: Ways to Help Prevent, Delay, Detect, and Even Halt Alzheimer's Disease and Other Forms of Memory Loss*, New York: Penguin Group, 2004.

Claritin, 1993
Holgate, S.T., Canonica, G. W., et al., *Clinical & Experimental Therapy* **33**: 1305; 2003.
MedlinePlus, *tinyurl.com/3pynhvz.*

Ephedra/Ephedrine, 1994
Drugs.com/ephedrine.html. mayoclinic.com/health/ephedra/NS_ patient-ephedra/.

Dietary Supplements, 1994

Institute of Medicine and National Research Council of the National Academies, *Dietary Supplements: Committee on the Framework for Evaluating the Safety of Dietary Supplements*, Washington, DC: The National Academies, 2005.

Office of Dietary Supplements, *ods.od.nih. gov/factsheets/list-all*.

U.S. Food and Drug Administration, *tinyurl.com/2dadvxr*

Fosamax, 1995

Mayo Clinic, tinyurl.com/ywtzqe.

OxyContin, 1996

PubMed Health, *tinyurl.com/3wyjj57*.

U.S. Drug Enforcement Administration, *tinyurl.com/2bln2fn*.

HAART, 1996

Biotechnology Encyclopedia, edinformatics.com/biotechnology/antiretroviral_drugs.htm

Current Programmes, 27802211.com/ice/program/program23.htm.

Zyprexa, 1996

Geddes, J., Freemantle, N., et al., *BMJ* **321**: 1371; 2000.

Goode, E., *biopsychiatry.com/misc/antipsychotic*.

Plavix, 1997

MedlinePlus, *tinyurl.com/5vsgawz*

Patrono, C., Coller, B., et al., *European Heart Journal* **25**: 166; 2004.

Direct-to-Consumer Ads, 1997

Donohue, J. M., Cevasco, M., Rosenthal, M .B., *New England Journal of Medicine* **357**:673; 2007.

Gerald, M. C., *Pharmacy in History* **52**: 3; 2010.

U.S. Food and Drug Administration, *fda. gov/downloads/RegulatoryInformation/Guidances/ucm125064*.

Synthroid, 1997

Braverman, L. E., Utiger, R. D., eds., *Werner and Ingbar's* The Thyroid, New York: Lippincott Williams & Wilkins, 2005.

Wertheimer, A. I., *Formulary* **40**: 258; 2005.

Evista, 1997

Delmas, P. D., Bjarnason, N. H., et al. *New England Journal of Medicine* **337**: 1641, 1997.

Mitlak, B. H., Cohen, F. J., *Hormone Research in Pediatrics* **48**: 155; 1997.

Flomax, 1997

Lepor, H, Roehrborn, C.G., eds., *Reviews in Urology* **7**: S1-S55 (Suppl. 4); 2005.

National Kidney and Urologic Diseases Information Clearinghouse, *tinyurl. com/56kt9*.

Celebrex and Vioxx, 1998

New York Times, tinyurl.com/4frab6b.

U.S. Food and Drug Administration, *tinyurl.com/68zw776*.

Viagra, 1998

Edwards, G., ed., *British Journal of Clinical Pharmacology*, **53S**: Suppl. 1; 2002.

Lue, T. F., *New England Journal of Medicine* **342**: 1802, 2000.

Herceptin, 1998

Bazell, R., *HER-2: The Making of Herceptin, a Revolutionary Treatment for Breast Cancer*, New York: Random House, 1998.

National Cancer Institute, *tinyurl. com/4xbj4rl*.

Enbrel, Remicade, and Humira, 1998

Matsumoto, A. K., Banthon, J., Bingham, C. O., *tinyurl.com/c9c66d*.

National Cancer Institute, *tinyurl. com/4xbj4rl*.

Plan B, 1999

Mayo Clinic, *tinyurl.com/42w8233*.

Stewart F., et al., "Emergency Contraception," in *Contraceptive Technology*, Hatcher R. A., Trussell, J., Nelson, A. L., et al., eds., New York: Ardent Media, 2007.

Gleevec/Glivec, 2001

Pray, L. A., *tinyurl.com/49vp9z4*.

Iressa and Erbitux, 2003

Cummings, J., Ward, T. H., et al., *British Journal of Clinical Pharmacology* **153**: 646; 2008.

National Cancer Institute, *tinyurl. com/5b3eo*.

17P/Progesterone Injections and Gel, 2003

Meis, P. J., Kiebanoff, M., et al., *New England Journal of Medicine* **348**: 2379; 2003.

UNC Center for Maternal and Infant Health, *mombaby.org/index. php?c=2&s=58*.

Resveratrol, 2003

New York Times, tinyurl.com/4w7euqr.

Weintraub, A., *tinyurl.com/n74fx4*.

Avastin, 2004

National Cancer Institute, *tinyurl. com/3pgkbud*.

Pollack, A., *tinyurl.com/3n5h6kn*.

Gardasil, 2006

Centers for Disease Control and Prevention, *tinyurl.com/6khpnev*.

Chantix/Champix, 2006

PubMed Health, *tinyurl.com/5whef4q*.

Singh, S, Loke, Y. K., et al., *tinyurl. com/3khecc3*.

Lucentis, 2006

European Medicines Agency, *tinyurl. com/4dsej8e*.

Haddrill, M., *tinyurl.com/ygdfm7z*.

Avandia, 2010

Harris, G., *tinyurl.com/2ga672j*.

Hurley, D., *Diabetes Rising: How a Rare Disease Became a Modern Pandemic, and What To Do About It*, New York: Kaplan Publishing, 2010.

Provenge, 2010

U.S. Food and Drug Administration, *tinyurl.com/2bwfh8b*.

Gilenya, 2010

Multiple Sclerosis Resource Centre, *tinyurl.com/655uawg*.

Prescription Drug Abuse, 2010

Galanter, M., Kleber, H. D., *The American Psychiatric Publishing Textbook of Substance Abuse Treatment*, Arlington, VA: American Psychiatric Publishing, 2008.

MedlinePlus, *tinyurl.com/dcf73h*.

Weight-Loss Drugs, 2010

Centers for Disease Control and Prevention, *tinyurl.com/q2tzej*.

Hobson, K., *tinyurl.com/35pvna6*.

Pradaxa, 2010

European Drug Encyclopedia, *tinyurl.com/8rrtmf9*.

U.S. Food and Drug Administration, *tinyurl.com/6n6uta2*.

Viread, 2011

Abdool Karin, Q., Abdool Karin, S. S., et al., *Science* **329** (5996): 1168; 2010.

Current Opinion in HIV and AIDS **5** (5), September 1, 2010. (HIV vaccine research).

Victrelis and Incivek, 2011

Bacon, B. R., Gordon, S. C., et al., *New England Journal of Medicine* **364**: 1207; 2011.

Poordad, F., McCone Jr., J., et al., *New England Journal of Medicine* **364**: 1195; 2011.

Benlysta, 2011

U.S. Food and Drug Administration, *tinyurl.com/6d6znse*.

Broad-Spectrum Sunscreens, 2012

U.S. Food and Drug Administration, *tinyurl.com/45xxz8r*.

Shaath, N., ed., *Sunscreens: Regulation and Commercial Development*, Boca Raton, FL: Taylor & Francis, 2005.

Kalydeco, 2012

tinyurl.com/7gfu26x.

Kearney, C., *tinyurl.com/d3bvptp*.

Anti-Alzheimer's Drugs, 2014

Rafii, M. S., Aisen, P. S., *biomedcentral.com/1741-7015/7/7*.

Shankle, W. R., Amen, D. G., *Preventing Alzheimer's: Ways to Help Prevent, Delay, Detect, and Even Halt Alzheimer's Disease and Other Forms of Memory Loss*, New York: Penguin Group, 2004.

Female Viagra, 2015

Martin, D., *tinyurl.com/9vvawae*. *tinyurl.com/3xvn5ly*.

Smart Drugs, 2018

Gazzaniga, M. S., "Smarter on Drugs," *Scientific American Mind*, September 21, 2005.

Talbot, M, "Brain Gain," *The New Yorker*, April 27, 2009.

Antiaging Drugs, 2020

Kahn, A. J., *Gerontology: Biological Sciences* **60A** (2): 142; 2005.

Gene Therapy, 2020

Mayo Clinic, *tinyurl.com/7uowybl*.

National Cancer Institute, *tinyurl.com/mhko24*.

National Library of Medicine, *tinyurl.com/7yfxmnm*.

Index

Photo Credits